Crash Course 1000 SBAs for Finals and the MLA

Medicine and Surgery

First edition author

Neel Sharma

Second edition author

Philip Xiu

3rd Edition

CRASH COURSE

SERIES EDITOR

Philip Xiu

MA (Cantab), MB BChir, MRCP, MRCGP, MScClinEd, FHEA, MAcadMEd, RCPathME

Honorary Senior Lecturer

Leeds University School of Medicine

PCN Educational Lead

Medical Examiner

Leeds Teaching Hospital Trust

Leeds, UK

Crash Course 1000 SBAs for Finals and the MLA

Medicine and Surgery

Pratheeshan Sabeshan

BSc (Hons), Final Year Medical Student

Imperial College London

London, UK

Hester Lacey

MBBS, MA, MAcadMEd

University Hospitals Sussex NHS Foundation Trust

Brighton, UK

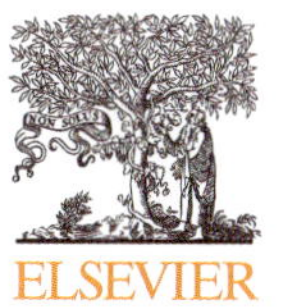

Elsevier

Publisher's note: Elsevier takes a neutral position with respect to territorial disputes or jurisdictional claims in its published content, including in maps and institutional affiliations.

First edition 1998

Second edition 2019

Third edition 2025

ISBN: 978-0-4432-8321-5

Content Strategist: Trinity Hutton
Content Development Specialist: Ayan Dhar
Project Manager: Ayan Dhar
Design: Miles Hitchen
Marketing Manager: Deborah Watkins

Printed in India by Thomson Press (Ltd)
Last digit is the print number: 9 8 7 6 5 4 3 2 1

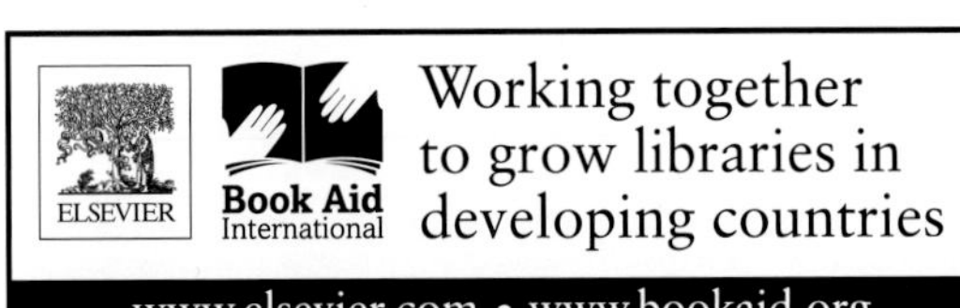

Series editor's Foreword

With great honour and pride, we present the latest edition of the *Crash Course* series. This series has traversed a journey of nearly a quarter-century, stemming from the vision of Dr. Dan Horton-Szar, and his legacy continues to walk with us on this pathway of knowledge.

The series has been popular with students worldwide, selling over **1 million copies** and being translated into more than **8 languages**, reinforcing our commitment to global learning.

We remain extremely grateful for your unwavering trust. The series has once again been refreshed and fully upgraded in accordance with the rapidly changing medical guidelines, ensuring the content is comprehensive, accurate and fully up-to-date.

This latest series continues our tradition of integrating clinical practice with basic medical sciences, tailored meticulously for today's medical undergraduate curriculum. A central highlight of this instalment is our emphasis on high-yield exam content designed specifically for the UKMLA curriculum.

The addition of the **Rapid UKMLA Index** at the beginning of the book enhances this offering, serving as a valuable aid to students to track their exam preparation efficiently. We have also revised all self-assessment questions to align with the single best answer format in line with the latest UKMLA examination style. We have also added ***High-Yield Association Tables***. These are essential tools designed to aid students in recognizing clinical patterns and acing vignette-style exam questions. By condensing complex medical scenarios into digestible, manageable insights, these tables ensure efficient learning. They connect symptoms, diagnosis, and treatment, bolstering understanding and confidence in tackling the rigorous UKMLA exams. This comprehensive approach makes these tables an indispensable asset in your exam preparations.

Utilizing student feedback, we have strived to maintain the core principles of this series: delivering precise and readable text that brings together depth and clarity. The authors are experienced junior doctors who successfully navigated these exams recently, ensuring practical and tested guidance. A team of expert faculty advisors from across the United Kingdom ensures the content's accuracy, making it resilient and reliable.

As we turn a new chapter with the latest edition, we honour the past, cherish the present, and embrace the promise of the future. We wish you every success in your journey of learning and growth and hope that this series adds value to your life, both as students and as future medical professionals.

Philip Xiu

Preface

Authors

Welcome to **Crash Course 1000 SBAs for Finals and the MLA, Medicine and Surgery**. With comprehensive coverage and UKMLA curriculum mapping, this self-assessment edition provides a complete overview of medical and surgical content for medical finals. This edition assesses understanding and application of knowledge through 1000 high-yield SBA questions structured in the style of UKMLA AKT exams, offering a representative question sample of core condition diagnosis, investigations, management and complications to aid exam preparation.

This volume was developed in response to student feedback, with adaptation of self-assessment material to maintain the clarity, coverage and conciseness that make the *Crash Course* series an essential revision companion. In this edition, question **difficulty** and **relevancy** are signposted to ensure study sessions can be tailored to meet individual educational goals. All content is related to **updated clinical guidelines** to ensure relevancy and reliability of learning.

We hope this volume will be a valuable resource and will support you to achieve your full potential in medical exams.

Pratheeshan Sabeshan and Hester Lacey

Author's acknowledgements

With thanks to Washington, Mum and Tom, for their support and encouragement, and Phil and the team at Elsevier for their guidance and expertise.

Hester Lacey

Series editor's acknowledgement

We would like to express our sincere gratitude to those who have provided their support and expertise in preparing this sixth edition of the *Crash Course* series. Our junior doctor contributors' participation in crafting the manuscript has been indispensable. Their first-hand experience and current medical knowledge have infused realism and practicality into our content.

Our faculty editors deserve a special note of thanks. They have extensively validated the correctness of the information, ensuring that the content is not just accurate but also contemporaneous, credible, and aligns with the latest medical standards.

We extend our heartfelt thanks to our publisher, Elsevier. Their staff have demonstrated an unwavering commitment to quality, maintaining the high standards set since the first edition. Their insights have routinely enriched the content and process alike.

Our Commissioning Editor, Jeremy Bowes, deserves a special mention for his consistent support and guiding hand throughout the development process. His directions and advice have bettered this edition and spurred us on our quest for excellence.

We are greatly indebted to Alex Mortimer for her wisdom, practical insights and valuable guidance. A big thank you to our Content Strategists, Trinity Hutton and Cloe Holland-Borosh, who need special acknowledgement for meticulously outlining the direction and scope of the content. They've managed to mix details with a strategic plan, keeping our readers in mind.

Lastly, much gratitude is owed to our Content Product Managers, Taranpreet Kaur, Ayan Dhar, Shivani Pal and Tapajyoti Chaudhuri, who have juggled the numerous day-to-day tasks with utmost dedication and perseverance. Despite the ever-approaching deadlines, they have shown remarkable patience and steadfast determination, ensuring that each step of the book's development was accomplished seamlessly.

In conclusion, we sincerely thank each of these wonderful people for their outstanding contributions and support, without which this work wouldn't have been achieved. Their passion, commitment and collaborative effort have helped us bring this edition together.

Philip Xiu

Rapid UKMLA Index

The UKMLA Curriculum Conditions Priority levels have been based on the below:

Level 1: Conditions that a newly qualified doctor should have a good knowledge of and be able to recognise and manage.
Level 2: Conditions requiring knowledge for recognising and confirming diagnosis and planning first–line management in straightforward cases.
Level 3: Conditions where recognition of clinical presentation and describing principles of management are important.

Table UKMLA Conditions and Where to Find Them

Priority	Topic	Chapter	Question ID (Chp-Q number)
3	Achalasia	Chapter 2: Gastroenterology Chapter 11: Gastrointestinal surgery	2–37, 2–46 10–40
1	Acid–base abnormality	Chapter 9: Trauma and surgical emergencies Chapter 10: Perioperative care Chapter 11: Gastrointestinal surgery Chapter 14: Urology	9–11 10–5 11–43 14–43
1	Acid–base balance and disorders	Chapter 9: Trauma and surgical emergencies Chapter 10: Perioperative care Chapter 11: Gastrointestinal surgery Chapter 14: Urology	9–11 10–5 11–43 14–43
3	Acoustic neuroma	Chapter 5: Neurology	5–70
2	Acromegaly	Chapter 7: Endocrine and diabetes	7–23, 7–38, 7–46
1	Acute bronchitis	Chapter 3: Respiratory	3–21
1	Acute cholangitis	Chapter 2: Gastroenterology Chapter 11: Gastrointestinal surgery	2–24, 2–32 2–32
1	Acute circulatory failure/ shock	Chapter 9: Trauma and surgical emergencies	9–10,9–11
1	Acute coronary syndromes	Chapter 1: Cardiology Chapter 9: Trauma and surgical emergencies Chapter 10: Perioperative care Chapter 12: Cardiothoracics and vascular	1–1,1–2,1–7, 1–14,1–17,1–27,1–34, 1–38, 1–53, 1–55, 1–62, 1–73, 1–75 9–2,38 10–2 12–16
1	Acute kidney injury	Chapter 4: Renal Chapter 9: Trauma and surgical emergencies Chapter 10: Perioperative care	4–2, 4–3, 4–5, 4–7, 4–8, 4–9, 4–10, 4–11, 4–12, 4–13 9–11 10–10
1	Acute pancreatitis	Chapter 2: Gastroenterology Chapter 11: Gastrointestinal surgery	2–1, 2–12 11–4, 11–8, 11–48, 11–50, 11–70
2	Acute Respiratory Distress Syndrome	Chapter 3: Respiratory	3–49
2	Addison's disease	Chapter 7: Endocrine and diabetes	7–17, 7–19, 7–22
2	Alcoholic hepatitis	Chapter 2: Gastroenterology	2–51

continued

Priority	Topic	Chapter	Question ID (Chp-Q number)
1	Allergic disorder	Chapter 3: Respiratory Chapter 10: Perioperative care	3–27, 3–53 10–6
3	Alpha–1 antitrypsin deficiency	Chapter 3: Respiratory	3–55
3	Amyloidosis	Chapter 4: Renal	4–36
1	Anaemia	Chapter 8: Haematology Chapter 9: Trauma and surgical emergencies Chapter 10: Perioperative care Chapter 11: Gastrointestinal surgery	8–3, 8–19 9–14 10–20 11–19, 11–32, 11–64
3	Anal carcinoma	Chapter 11: Gastrointestinal surgery	11–76
2	Anal fissure	Chapter 11: Gastrointestinal surgery	11–75,11–80
1	Aneurysms, ischaemic limb and occlusions	Chapter 12: Cardiothoracics and vascular	12–11, 12–26
2	Ankylosing spondylitis	Chapter 6: Rheumatology Chapter 13: Orthopaedics	6–16, 6–22, 6–27 13–51
1	Aortic aneurysm	Chapter 12: Cardiothoracics and vascular	12–5, 12–10, 12–20, 12–13
3	Aortic dissection	Chapter 1: Cardiology Chapter 12: Cardiothoracics and vascular	1–26, 1–29, 1–39, 1–47, 1–51 12–6,12–15
2	Aortic valve disease	Chapter 1: Cardiology Chapter 12: Cardiothoracics and vascular	1–40, 1–71 12–22
1	Appendicitis	Chapter 2: Gastroenterology Chapter 11: Gastrointestinal surgery	2–3, 2–8 11–11,11–24,11–7
1	Arrhythmias	Chapter 1: Cardiology Chapter 12: Cardiothoracics and vascular	1–10, 1–22, 1–24, 1–25, 1–28, 1–33, 1–35, 1–37, 1–44, 1–46, 1–59, 1–77 12–11
2	Arterial thrombosis	Chapter 1: Cardiology Chapter 11: Gastrointestinal surgery Chapter 12: Cardiothoracics and vascular	1–76 11–76 12–12
1	Arterial ulcers	Chapter 12: Cardiothoracics and vascular	12–18
3	Asbestos–related lung disease	Chapter 3: Respiratory	3–31, 3–36, 3–52, 3–60
2	Ascites	Chapter 11: Gastrointestinal surgery	11–58,11–74
1	Asthma	Chapter 3: Respiratory	3–3, 3–10, 3–13
2	Asthma COPD overlap syndrome	Chapter 3: Respiratory	3–59
2	Barret's oesophagus	Chapter 11: Gastrointestinal surgery	11–21
3	Behcet's disease	Chapter 6: Rheumatology	6–37
2	Bell's palsy	Chapter 5: Neurology	5–27
2	Benign Paroxysmal Positional Vertigo	Chapter 5: Neurology	5–71
1	Benign prostatic hyperplasia	Chapter 14: Urology	14–31, 14–5, 14–10, 14–20, 14–49
2	Bladder cancer	Chapter 14: Urology	14–9, 14–12, 14–14
2	Boeerhaave's syndrome	Chapter 2: Gastroenterology	2–71, 2–74
3	Bone tumours	Chapter 6: Rheumatology	6–39, 6–44
3	Brain abscess	Chapter 5: Neurology	5–65, 5–72

Priority	Topic	Chapter	Question ID (Chp-Q number)
2	Brain metastases	Chapter 5: Neurology Chapter 15: Breast surgery	5–67 15–1
2	Breast abscess/ mastitis	Chapter 15: Breast surgery	15–2, 15–21, 15–16, 15–24, 15–3, 15–8
1	Breast cancer	Chapter 15: Breast surgery	15–17, 15–30, 15–5, 15–7, 15–9, 15–26, 15–17, 15–18, 15–20, 15–30, 15–4, 15–6, 15–10, 15–23, 15–19
1	Breast cysts	Chapter 15: Breast surgery	15–14, 15–15
1	Breathlessness	Chapter 9: Trauma and surgical emergencies Chapter 10: Perioperative care Chapter 12: Cardiothoracics and vascular	9–7,9–8, 9–15, 9–20 10–8, 10–11, 1–14 12–6,12–15, 12–16, 12–29, 12–7, 12–4
3	Bronchiectasis	Chapter 3: Respiratory	3–1, 3–8, 3–11, 3–18
1	Bronchiolitis	Chapter 3: Respiratory	3–51
3	Bursitis	Chapter 13: Orthopaedics	13–56
1	Cardiac arrest	Chapter 1: Cardiology Chapter 9: Trauma and surgical emergencies Chapter 10: Perioperative care Chapter 12: Cardiothoracics and vascular	1–11, 1–19, 1–21, 1–23 9–10 10–2 12–16
1	Cardiac failure	Chapter 1: Cardiology Chapter 10: Perioperative care	1–3, 1–5, 1–12, 1–16 10–2
2	Cardiac tamponade	Chapter 1: Cardiology Chapter 12: Cardiothoracics and vascular	1–9 12–16
3	Cardiomyopathies	Chapter 1: Cardiology	1–31, 1–43, 1–52, 1–67, 1–72
1	Cellulitis	Chapter 13: Orthopaedics	13–1, 13–9
3	Cerebellar disorders	Chapter 5: Neurology	5–50
1	Chest pain	Chapter 9: Trauma and surgical emergencies Chapter 10: Perioperative care Chapter 12: Cardiothoracics and vascular	9–8 10–10 12–16, 12–29, 12–6,12–15, 12–19, 12–7, 12–4
1	Cholecystitis	Chapter 2: Gastroenterology Chapter 11: Gastrointestinal surgery	2–2, 2–4 11–22, 1–45
3	Chronic fatigue syndrome	Chapter 6: Rheumatology	6–43
1	Chronic kidney disease	Chapter 4: Renal Chapter 14: Urology	4–1, 4–4, 4–6 14–43
1	Chronic obstructive pulmonary disease	Chapter 3: Respiratory	3–4, 3–9, 3–17, 3–54
1	Chronic pancreatitis	Chapter 2: Gastroenterology Chapter 11: Gastrointestinal surgery	2–45 11–48, 1–50
2	Cirrhosis	Chapter 2: Gastroenterology	2–25, 2–57, 2–62
2	Cluster Headache	Chapter 5: Neurology	5–4, 5–19
2	Coeliac disease	Chapter 2: Gastroenterology	2–14, 2–23
1	Colorectal polyps	Chapter 11: Gastrointestinal surgery	11–28
1	Colorectal tumours	Chapter 11: Gastrointestinal surgery	11–25,11–32,11–46
1	Compartment syndrome	Chapter 9: Trauma and surgical emergencies Chapter 13: Orthopaedics	9–6 13–17, 13–3, 13–8, 13–53, 13–60

continued

Priority	Topic	Chapter	Question ID (Chp-Q number)
3	Congenital Adrenal Hyperplasia	Chapter 7: Endocrine and diabetes	7–49
1	Constipation	Chapter 2: Gastroenterology Chapter 11: Gastrointestinal surgery	2–49 11–4
2	Cough	Chapter 9: Trauma and surgical emergencies Chapter 10: Perioperative care Chapter 12: Cardiothoracics and vascular	9–7,9–8, 9–15, 9–20 10–11 12–60
1	Covid–19	Chapter 3: Respiratory	3–7
2	Cranial nerve palsies	Chapter 5: Neurology	5–32, 5–43, 5–61
1	Crystal arthropathy	Chapter 6: Rheumatology	6–6, 6–10, 6–12
3	Cushing's syndrome	Chapter 7: Endocrine and diabetes	7–7, 7–11, 7–14, 7–16, 7–21
2	Cyanosis	Chapter 10: Perioperative care Chapter 12: Cardiothoracics and vascular	10–11 12–7, 12–4, 12–19, 12–29
2	Cystic fibrosis	Chapter 3: Respiratory	3–26, 3–33
1	Decreased/loss of consciousness	Chapter 9: Trauma and surgical emergencies Chapter 10: Perioperative care Chapter 12: Cardiothoracics and vascular	9–2, 9–3, 9–4, 9–5 10–15 12–16
1	Deep vein thrombosis	Chapter 12: Cardiothoracics and vascular	12–3
1	Dehydration	Chapter 9: Trauma and surgical emergencies Chapter 10: Perioperative care Chapter 11: Gastrointestinal surgery	9–11 10–10 11–59
1	Delirium	Chapter 10: Perioperative care	10–18
1	Dementias	Chapter 5: Neurology	5–11, 5–13, 5–22, 5–25
1	Deteriorating patient	Chapter 9: Trauma and surgical emergencies Chapter 10: Perioperative care	9–10 10–4, 10–2
2	Diabetes in pregnancy (gestational and pre)	Chapter 7: Endocrine and diabetes	7–43, 7–47
3	Diabetes insipidus	Chapter 7: Endocrine and diabetes	7–26, 7–32
1	Diabetes mellitus type 1 and 2	Chapter 7: Endocrine and diabetes	7–2, 7–4, 7–12, 7–18, 7–20, 7–65, 7–69
1	Diabetic ketoacidosis	Chapter 7: Endocrine and diabetes	7–3, 7–8, 7–10
1	Diabetic nephropathy	Chapter 4: Renal	4–29
2	Diabetic neuropathy	Chapter 7: Endocrine and diabetes	7–40, 7–60
2	Diabetic retinopathy	Chapter 7: Endocrine and diabetes	7–36, 7–44
1	Diarrhoea	Chapter 11: Gastrointestinal surgery	11–32, 11–33, 11–39, 11–41, 11–43, 11–47, 11–52,11–69
2	Difficulty with breast feeding	Chapter 15: Breast surgery	15–24, 15–25, 15–21, 15–2, 15–8, 15–3
1	Disease prevention/screening	Chapter 10: Perioperative care Chapter 12: Cardiothoracics and vascular Chapter 14: Urology Chapter 15: Breast surgery	10–13 12–13 14–41 15–7
1	Disseminated intravascular coagulation	Chapter 8: Haematology	8–30
1	Diverticular disease	Chapter 2: Gastroenterology Chapter 11: Gastrointestinal surgery	2–16 11–4,11–20,11–37,11–41,11–61

Priority	Topic	Chapter	Question ID (Chp-Q number)
1	Encephalitis	Chapter 5: Neurology	5–45
3	Epididymitis and orchitis	Chapter 14: Urology	14–18, 14–11, 14–7, 14–54
1	Epilepsy	Chapter 5: Neurology	5–2, 5–14, 5–23, 5–26
1	Epistaxis	Chapter 8: Haematology	8–16
3	Essential or secondary hypertension	Chapter 1: Cardiology Chapter 12: Cardiothoracics and vascular	1–8, 1–13, 1–20, 1–36, 1–45, 1–70 12–2, 12–5, 12–6, 12–11, 12–13, 12–14, 12–15, 12–17, 12–20, 12–21, 12–22
2	Essential tremor	Chapter 5: Neurology	5–44, 5–51
1	Extradural haemorrhage	Chapter 5: Neurology Chapter 9: Trauma and surgical emergencies	5–20 9–3
3	Factor V Leiden	Chapter 8: Haematology	8–18
1	Fever	Chapter 10: Perioperative care Chapter 11: Gastrointestinal surgery Chapter 14: Urology Chapter 15: Breast surgery	10–8, 10–7 11–59 14–4, 14–15, 14–50, 14–51, 14–54, 14–58 15–16
3	Fibromyalgia	Chapter 6: Rheumatology	6–34, 6–42
3	Fibrotic lung disease	Chapter 3: Respiratory	3–58
3	Food intolerance	Chapter 11: Gastrointestinal surgery	11–1,11–2, 11–14, 11–38
1	Frailty Urinary incontinence	Chapter 14: Urology	14–29, 14–32, 14–53, 14–57
1	Gallstones and biliary colic	Chapter 2: Gastroenterology Chapter 11: Gastrointestinal surgery	2–6 11–56
1	Gangrene	Chapter 12: Cardiothoracics and vascular	12–9
2	Gastric cancer	Chapter 11: Gastrointestinal surgery	11–30, 11–62, 11–78
2	Gastric cancer	Chapter 2: Gastroenterology	2–31, 2–36, 2–76
2	Gastrointestinal perforation	Chapter 2: Gastroenterology Chapter 11: Gastrointestinal surgery	2–33 11–59
2 1	Gastro–oesophageal reflux disease	Chapter 2: Gastroenterology Chapter 11: Gastrointestinal surgery	2–7, 2–20 11–6, 11–21, 11–29
3	Gilbert's syndrome	Chapter 2: Gastroenterology	2–59
2	Glomerulonephritis	Chapter 4: Renal	4–19, 4–21, 4–23, 4–25, 4–31, 4–33, 4–39, 4–41
3	Glucose–6–phosphatase deficiency	Chapter 8: Haematology	8–38, 8–42
3	Granulomatosis with Polyangiitis	Chapter 3: Respiratory	3–64
2	Gynaecomastia	Chapter 7: Endocrine and diabetes	7–35, 7–54
1	Haematuria	Chapter 9: Trauma and surgical emergencies Chapter 14: Urology	9–11 14–52
2	Haemochromatosis	Chapter 2: Gastroenterology	2–39, 2–42, 2–52
2	Haemoglobinopathies	Chapter 8: Haematology	8–17, 8–20, 8–22
3	Haemolytic Uraemic Syndrome	Chapter 8: Haematology	8–26, 8–28
3	Haemophilia	Chapter 8: Haematology	8–5, 8–8, 8–10

continued

Priority	Topic	Chapter	Question ID (Chp-Q number)
2	Haemorrhoids	Chapter 11: Gastrointestinal surgery	11–65, 11–67
2	Hepatitis	Chapter 2: Gastroenterology	2–28, 2–41, 2–43, 2–51, 2–60
2	Hepatocellular carcinoma	Chapter 2: Gastroenterology	2–47
3	Hepatorenal syndrome	Chapter 4: Renal	4–40
1	Hernias	Chapter 11: Gastrointestinal surgery	11–16, 11–26, 11–31, 11–57, 11–72
2	Hiatus hernia	Chapter 11: Gastrointestinal surgery	11–72
3	Hirschsprung's disease	Chapter 2: Gastroenterology	2–79
2	Huntington's disease	Chapter 5: Neurology	5–34
3	Hydrocephalus	Chapter 5: Neurology	5–68, 5–82
2	Hypercalcaemia of malignancy	Chapter 7: Endocrine and diabetes	7–27, 7–52
2	Hyperlipidaemia	Chapter 1: Cardiology	1–65
3	Hyperosmolar hyperglycaemic state	Chapter 7: Endocrine and diabetes	7–45
2	Hyperparathyroidism	Chapter 7: Endocrine and diabetes	7–24, 7–30, 7–35, 7–59
1	Hypertension	Chapter 12: Cardiothoracics and vascular	12–2, 12–5, 12–6, 12–11, 12–13, 12–14, 12–15, 12–17, 12–20, 12–21, 12–22
3	Hyperthermia and hypothermia	Chapter 9: Trauma and surgical emergencies Chapter 14: Urology	9–19 14–49
1	Hyperventilation (panic attack)	Chapter 3: Respiratory	3–16
1	Hypoglycaemia	Chapter 7: Endocrine and diabetes	7–5
2	Hypogonadism	Chapter 7: Endocrine and diabetes	7–29, 7–67
2	Hypokalaemia	Chapter 7: Endocrine and diabetes	7–61
2	Hypoparathyroidism	Chapter 7: Endocrine and diabetes	7–39
3	Hypopituitarism	Chapter 7: Endocrine and diabetes	7–29, 7–67
2	Hyposplenism/splenectomy	Chapter 8: Haematology	8–15
1	Hypothermia	Chapter 7: Endocrine and diabetes	7–13
1	Hypothyroidism	Chapter 7: Endocrine and diabetes	7–28, 7–51
2	Idiopathic arthritis	Chapter 6: Rheumatology	6–13
3	Idiopathic Intracranial Hypertension	Chapter 5: Neurology	5–33
3	Idiopathic pulmonary fibrosis	Chapter 3: Respiratory	3–43
2	Ileus	Chapter 2: Gastroenterology Chapter 11: Gastrointestinal surgery	2–66, 2–72 11–13, 11–79, 11–23
2	Infant feeding problems	Chapter 15: Breast surgery	15–25, 15–21, 15–2, 15–24, 15–8, 15–3
2	Infections and infestations of the gastro–intestinal tract	Chapter 2: Gastroenterology	2–27, 2–30, 2–78
1	Infectious colitis	Chapter 2: Gastroenterology Chapter 11: Gastrointestinal surgery	2–54, 2–58 11–52
1	Infectious diarrhoea	Chapter 11: Gastrointestinal surgery	11–52
1	Infectious mononucleosis	Chapter 2: Gastroenterology	2–26

Priority	Topic	Chapter	Question ID (Chp-Q number)
2	Infective endocarditis	Chapter 1: Cardiology	1–41, 1–48, 1–50, 1–56, 1–58, 1–78
2	Inflammatory bowel disease	Chapter 2: Gastroenterology Chapter 11: Gastrointestinal surgery	2–5, 2–18, 2–19, 2–22 11–55, 11–43
2	Influenza	Chapter 3: Respiratory	3–6
2	Inhaled foreign body	Chapter 3: Respiratory	3–37
3	Intestinal ischaemia	Chapter 11: Gastrointestinal surgery	11–47, 11–73, 11–39, 11–69
2	Intestinal obstruction	Chapter 2: Gastroenterology Chapter 11: Gastrointestinal surgery	2–40 2–50
2	Intestinal obstruction and ileus	Chapter 11: Gastrointestinal surgery	11–13, 11–79, 11–23
2	Intracranial tumours and space occupying lesions	Chapter 5: Neurology	5–73, 5–74, 5–81
2	Irritable bowel syndrome	Chapter 2: Gastroenterology Chapter 11: Gastrointestinal surgery	2–21 11–33
1	Ischaemic heart disease	Chapter 11: Gastrointestinal surgery Chapter 12: Cardiothoracics and vascular	11–68 12–1, 12–26
1	Jaundice	Chapter 11: Gastrointestinal surgery	11–3, 11–10, 11–12, 11–53, 11–56, 11–74, 11–17, 11–36, 11–55, 11–60
3	Kartagener Syndrome	Chapter 3: Respiratory	3–62
2	Leukaemia	Chapter 8: Haematology	8–2, 8–4, 8–6, 8–11, 8–14
2	Limp	Chapter 13: Orthopaedics	13–56
3	Limp Lower limb soft tissue injury	Chapter 13: Orthopaedics	13–34, 13–37, 13–55, 13–56
2	Liver abscess	Chapter 2: Gastroenterology	2–77
2	Liver failure	Chapter 2: Gastroenterology Chapter 11: Gastrointestinal surgery	2–9, 2–11, 2–13, 2–15 11–74
2	Loss of libido	Chapter 14: Urology	14–47
2	Lower limb fractures	Chapter 13: Orthopaedics	13–41, 13–44, 13–20, 13–40, 13–07, 13–18, 13–29, 13–35, 13–47
3	Lower limb soft tissue injury	Chapter 13: Orthopaedics	13–34, 13–37, 13–55, 13–56, 13–30, 13–25, 13–34, 13–37, 13–55, 13–56, 13–32, 13–33, 13–58
3	Lung abscess	Chapter 3: Respiratory	3–30
2	Lung cancer	Chapter 3: Respiratory Chapter 12: Cardiothoracics and vascular	3–39, 3–56 12–29
3	Lupus	Chapter 6: Rheumatology	6–32
3	Lymphoedema	Chapter 12: Cardiothoracics and vascular	12–18
2	Lymphoma	Chapter 8: Haematology	8–1, 8–12, 8–13, 8–31
2	Malabsorption	Chapter 2: Gastroenterology Chapter 11: Gastrointestinal surgery	2–68 11–53, 11–48, 11–50
2	Malnutrition	Chapter 2: Gastroenterology Chapter 10: Perioperative care Chapter 11: Gastrointestinal surgery	2–17 10–18 11–64
3	Melanosis coli	Chapter 2: Gastroenterology	2–64

continued

Priority	Topic	Chapter	Question ID (Chp-Q number)
2	Ménière's disease	Chapter 5: Neurology	5–47
1	Meningitis	Chapter 5: Neurology	5–38, 5–42
3	Mesenteric adenitis	Chapter 2: Gastroenterology	2–10
1	Mesenteric ischaemia	Chapter 11: Gastrointestinal surgery	11–39, 11–47
2	Metastatic disease	Chapter 3: Respiratory Chapter 11: Gastrointestinal surgery Chapter 14: Urology Chapter 15: Breast surgery	3–48 11–34 14–56 15–1
1	Migraine	Chapter 5: Neurology	5–5, 5–24
2	Mitral valve disease	Chapter 1: Cardiology Chapter 12: Cardiothoracics and vascular	1–54, 1–60, 1–64, 1–68, 1–69 12–60
3	Motor neurone disease	Chapter 5: Neurology	5–30, 5–46
2	Multi–organ dysfunction syndrome	Chapter 9: Trauma and surgical emergencies Chapter 10: Perioperative care	9–19 10–2
2	Multiple myeloma	Chapter 8: Haematology	8–24, 8–33
2	Multiple sclerosis	Chapter 5: Neurology	5–40, 5–57, 5–60, 5–62
3	Muscular dystrophies	Chapter 5: Neurology	5–76
3	Musculoskeletal deformities	Chapter 13: Orthopaedics	13–51
3	Myasthenia gravis	Chapter 5: Neurology	5–36, 5–54
3	Myeloproliferative disorders	Chapter 8: Haematology	8–36, 8–43, 8–45
1	Myocardial infarction	Chapter 10: Perioperative care Chapter 12: Cardiothoracics and vascular	10–2 12–16
3	Myocarditis	Chapter 1: Cardiology	1–61, 1–66
2	NAFLD	Chapter 2: Gastroenterology	2–48
3	Narcolepsy	Chapter 5: Neurology	5–75
3	Necrotising fasciitis	Chapter 13: Orthopaedics	13–16, 13–15, 13–9
2	Nephrotic syndrome	Chapter 4: Renal	4–15, 4–17, 4–28, 4–30, 4–34, 4–37
3	Neuroendocrine Tumours	Chapter 7: Endocrine and diabetes	7–62, 7–64. 7–68
3	Neuroleptic outlet syndrome	Chapter 5: Neurology	5–80
1	Neutropenic sepsis	Chapter 8: Haematology	8–34, 8–40, 8–44
1	Obesity	Chapter 7: Endocrine and diabetes	7–6, 7–9
2	Obstructive sleep apnoea	Chapter 3: Respiratory	3–32, 3–41
3	Occupational lung disease	Chapter 3: Respiratory	3–50, 3–57
2	Oesophageal cancer	Chapter 2: Gastroenterology Chapter 11: Gastrointestinal surgery	2–44 11–49, 11–54
2	Oesophageal disorders	Chapter 2: Gastroenterology	2–50, 2–55, 2–61, 2–75
1	Osteoarthritis	Chapter 6: Rheumatology Chapter 13: Orthopaedics	6–1, 6–3, 6–5 13–22, 13–4, 13–14, 13–24
3	Osteomalacia	Chapter 6: Rheumatology	6–7
1	Osteomyelitis	Chapter 13: Orthopaedics	13–28, 13–5
1	Osteoporosis	Chapter 6: Rheumatology Chapter 13: Orthopaedics	6–4, 6–8, 6–11 13–38, 13–23, 13–57

Priority	Topic	Chapter	Question ID (Chp-Q number)
3	Paget's disease of the bone	Chapter 6: Rheumatology	6–35
1	Pallor	Chapter 9: Trauma and surgical emergencies Chapter 10: Perioperative care Chapter 11: Gastrointestinal surgery Chapter 12: Cardiothoracics and vascular	9–14 10–20 11–19, 11–32 12–6,12–15
2	Pancreatic cancer	Chapter 2: Gastroenterology Chapter 11: Gastrointestinal surgery	2–38, 2–42 11–36, 11–60, 11–53
3	Pancytopenia	Chapter 8: Haematology	8–21
2	Parkinson's disease	Chapter 5: Neurology	5–29, 5–37, 5–59, 5–64
2	Pathological fracture	Chapter 13: Orthopaedics	13–54
1	Patient on anti–coagulant therapy	Chapter 10: Perioperative care	10–3
1	Patient on anti–platelet therapy	Chapter 10: Perioperative care	10–3
2	Peptic ulcer disease and gastritis	Chapter 2: Gastroenterology Chapter 11: Gastrointestinal surgery	2–29, 2–33 11–1,11–2, 11–14, 11–38
2	Perianal abscesses and fistulae	Chapter 11: Gastrointestinal surgery	11–51, 11–71
3	Pericardial disease	Chapter 1: Cardiology Chapter 12: Cardiothoracics and vascular	1–4, 1–6, 1–63 12–19
2	Peripheral nerve injuries/palsies	Chapter 5: Neurology Chapter 13: Orthopaedics	5–28, 5–39, 5–48, 5–63 13–26, 13–45
1	Peripheral oedema and ankle swelling	Chapter 13: Orthopaedics	13–17, 13–3, 13–8, 13–53, 13–60
3	Peripheral polyneuropathy including Guillain Barré syndrome	Chapter 5: Neurology	5–31, 5–35, 5–49, 5–52, 5–55, 5–77
2	Peripheral vascular disease	Chapter 12: Cardiothoracics and vascular	12–1, 12–17, 12–9, 12–10
3	Peritoneal Dialysis	Chapter 4: Renal	4–38
2	Peritonitis	Chapter 2: Gastroenterology Chapter 11: Gastrointestinal surgery	2–53, 2–56 11–58
3	Phaeochromocytoma	Chapter 7: Endocrine and diabetes	7–31, 7–33, 7–58
2	Pituitary tumours	Chapter 7: Endocrine and diabetes	7–34, 7–48
2	Pleural Effusion	Chapter 3: Respiratory	3–45
1	Pneumonia	Chapter 3: Respiratory Chapter 10: Perioperative care	3–23, 3–28, 3–38, 3–42, 3–63 10–11
1	Pneumothorax	Chapter 3: Respiratory Chapter 9: Trauma and surgical emergencies Chapter 12: Cardiothoracics and vascular	3–2, 3–12, 3–19 9–15 12–7
3	Polycystic kidney disease	Chapter 4: Renal	4–14, 4–16, 4–27
3	Polycythaemia	Chapter 8: Haematology	8–25, 8–32
1	Polymyalgia rheumatica	Chapter 6: Rheumatology	6–18, 6–25
3	Polymyositis and dermatomyositis	Chapter 6: Rheumatology	6–38, 6–40, 6–41
2	Portal hypertension	Chapter 11: Gastrointestinal surgery	11–3
2	Primary hyperaldosteronism	Chapter 7: Endocrine and diabetes	7–25, 7–41
1	Prostate cancer	Chapter 14: Urology	14–16, 14–38, 14–13, 14–41

continued

Priority	Topic	Chapter	Question ID (Chp-Q number)
2	Psoriasis	Chapter 6: Rheumatology	6–21, 6–31
2	Pulmonary embolism	Chapter 1: Cardiology	1–15,1–30,1–32,1–49,1–57
1		Chapter 10: Perioperative care	10–14
2		Chapter 12: Cardiothoracics and vascular	12–4
3	Pulmonary hypertension	Chapter 3: Respiratory	3–61
3	Radiculopathies	Chapter 13: Orthopaedics	13–26, 13–45
2	Raised intracranial pressure	Chapter 5: Neurology Chapter 9: Trauma and surgical emergencies	5–12 9–3,9–6
3	Raynaud's syndrome	Chapter 12: Cardiothoracics and vascular	12–25
2	Reactive arthritis	Chapter 6: Rheumatology	6–19, 6–29
3	Refeeding syndrome	Chapter 10: Perioperative care	10–18
3	Renal artery stenosis	Chapter 4: Renal	4–20, 4–22, 4–24
2	Renal cancer	Chapter 4: Renal	4–18
1	Respiratory distress syndrome	Chapter 11: Gastrointestinal surgery	11–70
1	Respiratory failure	Chapter 3: Respiratory Chapter 9: Trauma and surgical emergencies	3–20 9–1
2	Rheumatoid arthritis	Chapter 6: Rheumatology Chapter 13: Orthopaedics	6–2, 6–9, 6–14 13–4 13–6, 13–32, 13–48, 13–49, 13–58
2	Sarcoidosis	Chapter 3: Respiratory	3–25, 3–29, 3–44, 3–47
3	Scleroderma	Chapter 6: Rheumatology	6–36, 6–45
2	Scrotal/testicular pain and/or lump/swelling	Chapter 14: Urology	14–59, 14–35, 14–26, 14–40, 14–60
1	Sepsis	Chapter 10: Perioperative care	10–12
1	Septic arthritis	Chapter 6: Rheumatology Chapter 13: Orthopaedics	6–26, 6–30, 6–33 13–6, 13–12, 13–2
1	Shock	Chapter 9: Trauma and surgical emergencies Chapter 10: Perioperative care Chapter 12: Cardiothoracics and vascular	9–10,9–11 10–8,10–12 12–6,12–15, 12–16
3	SIADH	Chapter 4: Renal Chapter 7: Endocrine and diabetes	4–32 7–50
2	Sickle cell disease	Chapter 8: Haematology	8–7, 8–9
2	Sigmoid volvulus	Chapter 11: Gastrointestinal surgery	11–9, 11–18
3	Sinus thrombosis	Chapter 5: Neurology	5–83
2	Sjogren's Syndrome	Chapter 6: Rheumatology	6–20, 6–24, 6–28
1	Spinal cord compression	Chapter 13: Orthopaedics	13–19, 13–13
2	Stridor	Chapter 10: Perioperative care	10–6
1	Stroke	Chapter 5: Neurology Chapter 12: Cardiothoracics and vascular	5–3, 5–7, 5–10, 5–16, 5–18, 5–66, 5–69 12–21
1	Subarachnoid haemorrhage	Chapter 5: Neurology Chapter 9: Trauma and surgical emergencies	5–15, 5–17, 5–21 9–4
1	Subdural haemorrhage	Chapter 5: Neurology Chapter 9: Trauma and surgical emergencies	5–6 9–2
3	Superior vena cava thrombosis/ obstruction	Chapter 12: Cardiothoracics and vascular	12–30

Priority	Topic	Chapter	Question ID (Chp-Q number)
1	Surgical site infection	Chapter 10: Perioperative care	10–7
3	Syringomyelia	Chapter 5: Neurology	5–78
3	Systemic lupus erythematosus	Chapter 6: Rheumatology	6–15, 6–17, 6–23
3	Systemic Sclerosis	Chapter 6: Rheumatology	6–36, 6–45
2	Temporal arteritis	Chapter 5: Neurology	5–53
1	Tension headache	Chapter 5: Neurology	5–1
2	Testicular cancer	Chapter 14: Urology	14–33, 14–46, 14–1, 14–19, 14–56
1	Testicular torsion	Chapter 14: Urology	14–8, 14–21, 14–6
3	Thoracic outlet syndrome	Chapter 5: Neurology	5–79
3	Thrombocytopenia	Chapter 8: Haematology	8–23
3	Thrombotic thrombocytopenic purpura	Chapter 8: Haematology	8–41
3	Thyroid cancer	Chapter 7: Endocrine and diabetes	7–53, 7–55
1	Thyroid eye disease	Chapter 7: Endocrine and diabetes	7–15, 7–56, 7–66
1	Thyroid nodules	Chapter 7: Endocrine and diabetes	7–1, 7–42, 7–63, 7–68
1	Thyrotoxicosis	Chapter 7: Endocrine and diabetes	7–15, 7–37
1	Transfusion reactions	Chapter 8: Haematology Chapter 10: Perioperative care	8–35, 8–37 10–17
1	Transient ischaemic attacks	Chapter 5: Neurology	5–8, 5–9
2	Trauma	Chapter 9: Trauma and surgical emergencies Chapter 13: Orthopaedics	9–17,9–18,9–20 13–41, 13–44, 13–20, 13–40, 13–07, 13–18, 13–29, 13–35, 13–47, 13–54
3	Trigeminal neuralgia	Chapter 5: Neurology	5–56
2	Tuberculosis	Chapter 3: Respiratory	3–22, 3–24, 3–35, 3–46
2	Undescended testes	Chapter 14: Urology	14–21
2	Upper limb fractures	Chapter 13: Orthopaedics	13–54
3	Upper limb soft tissue injury	Chapter 13: Orthopaedics	13–46, 13–50, 13–52, 13–31, 13–36, 13–43, 13–59
2	Upper respiratory tract infection	Chapter 3: Respiratory	3–52
3	Urethral stricture	Chapter 14: Urology	14–55
1	Urinary incontinence	Chapter 14: Urology	14–29, 14–32, 14–53, 14–57
1	Urinary symptoms	Chapter 14: Urology	14–29, 14–32
1	Urinary tract calculi	Chapter 14: Urology	14–42
1	Urinary tract infection	Chapter 14: Urology	14–4, 14–43, 114–2, 14–15, 14–52, 14–51
3	Urticaria	Chapter 10: Perioperative care	10–6
2	Varicose veins	Chapter 12: Cardiothoracics and vascular	12–12, 12–24
1	Vasovagal syncope	Chapter 1: Cardiology	1–42
1	Venous ulcers	Chapter 12: Cardiothoracics and vascular	12–18
2	Vitamin B, C and D deficiency	Chapter 2: Gastroenterology	2–63
2	Vitamin B12 and/or folate deficiency	Chapter 2: Gastroenterology Chapter 10: Perioperative care Chapter 11: Gastrointestinal surgery	2–34 10–18 11–64

continued

Priority	Topic	Chapter	Question ID (Chp-Q number)
2	Volvulus	Chapter 11: Gastrointestinal surgery	11–9, 11–18
1	Vomiting	Chapter 10: Perioperative care Chapter 11: Gastrointestinal surgery	10–4 11–7, 11–8, 11–23, 11–11, 11–59, 11–5, 11–13, 11–42
3	Von Willebrand Disease	Chapter 8: Haematology	8–27, 8–29
3	Waldenstrom's macroglobulinaemia	Chapter 8: Haematology	8–39
2	Wernicke's encephalopathy	Chapter 5: Neurology	5–58
3	Whipple's disease	Chapter 2: Gastroenterology	2–65, 2–80

Contents

Normal values

HAEMATOLOGY

Haemoglobin	
Male	135–177 g/L
Female	115–165 g/L
Mean corpuscular haemoglobin (MCH)	27–32 pg
Mean corpuscular haemoglobin concentration (MCHC)	32–36 g/dL
Mean corpuscular volume (MCV)	80–96 fL
Packed cell volume (PCV)	
Male	0.40–0.54 L/L
Female	0.37–0.47 L/L
White blood count (WBC)	4–11 × 10^9/L
Basophil granulocytes	<0.01–0.1 × 10^9/L
Eosinophil granulocytes	0.04–0.4 × 10^9/L
Lymphocytes	1.5–4.0 × 10^9/L
Monocytes	0.2–0.8 × 10^9/L
Neutrophil granulocytes	2.0–7.5 × 10^9/L
Platelet count	150–400 × 10^9/L
Serum B_{12}	160–925 ng/L (150–675 pmol/L)
Serum folate	2.9–18 μg/L (3.6–63 nmol/L)
Red cell folate	149–640 μg/L
Red cell mass	
Male	25–35 mL/kg
Female	20–30 mL/kg
Reticulocyte count	0.5–2.5% of red cells (50–100 × 10^9/L)
Erythrocyte sedimentation rate (ESR)	<20 mm in 1 hour

COAGULATION

Bleeding time (Ivy method)	3–9 min
Activated partial thromboplastin time (APTT)	23–31s
Prothrombin time	12–16s
International Normalized Ratio (INR)	1.0–1.3
D-dimer	<500 ng/mL

LIPIDS AND LIPOPROTEINS

Cholesterol	3.5–6.5 mmol/L (ideal <5.2 mmol/L)
HDL cholesterol	
Male	0.8–1.8 mmol/L
Female	1.0–2.3 mmol/L
LDL cholesterol	<4.0 mmol/L
Triglycerides	
$[H^+]$	35–45 nmol/L
pH	7.35–7.45

BIOCHEMISTRY (SERUM/PLASMA)

Alanine aminotransferase (ALT)	5–40 U/L
Albumin	35–50 g/L
Alkaline phosphatase	39–117 U/L
Amylase	25–125 U/L
Aspartate aminotransferase (AST)	12–40 U/L
Bicarbonate	22–30 mmol/L
Bilirubin	<17 μmol/L (0.3–1.5 mg/dL)
Calcium	2.20–2.67 mmol/L (8.5–10.5 mg/dL)
Chloride	98–106 mmol/L
C-reactive protein	<10 mg/L
Creatinine	79–118 μmol /L (0.6–1.5 mg/dL)
Creatine kinase (CPK)	
Female	24–170 U/L
Male	24–195 U/L
CK–MB fraction	<25 U/L (<60% of total activity)
Ferritin	
Female	6–100 μg/L
Male	20–260 μg/L
Postmenopausal	12–230 μg/L
α-Fetoprotein	<10 kU/L
Glucose (fasting)	4.5–5.6 mmol/L (70–110 mg/dL)
γ–Glutamyl transpeptidase (γ–GT)	
Male	11–58 U/L
Female	7–32 U/L
Glycosylated (glycated) haemoglobin (HbA_{1c})	3.7–5.1%
Iron	13–32 μmol /L (50–150 μg/dL)
Iron–binding capacity (total) (TIBC)	42–80 μmol /L (250–410 μg/dL)
Magnesium	0.7–1.1 mmol/L

Osmolality	275–295 mOsm/kg
Phosphate	0.8–1.5 mmol/L
Potassium	3.5–5.0 mmol/L
Prostate-specific antigen (PSA)	≤4.0 μg/L
Protein (total)	62–77 g/L
Sodium	135–146 mmol/L
Urate	0.18–0.42 mmol/L (3.0–7.0 mg/dL)
Urea	2.5–6.7 mmol/L (8–25 mg/dL)

BLOOD GASES (ARTERIAL)

P_aCO_2	4.8–6.1 kPa (36–46 mmHg)
P_aO_2	10–13.3 kPa (75–100mmHg)
Male	0.70–2.1 mmol/L
Female	0.50–1.70 mmol/L
Bicarbonate	22–26 mmol/L

Abbreviations

AAA	Abdominal aortic aneurysm
ABG	Arterial blood gas
ABPI	Ankle brachial pressure index
ACL	Anterior cruciate ligament
ACS	Acute chest syndrome
AD	Alzheimer disease
ADHD	Attention-deficit/hyperactivity disorder
ADPKD	Autosomal dominant polycystic kidney disease
AF	Atrial fibrillation
AIDS	Acquired immune deficiency syndrome
AKI	Acute kidney injury
ALI	Acute limb ischaemia
ALL	Acute lymphoblastic leukaemia
ALS	Advanced life support
ALT	Alanine aminotransferase
AMI	Acute mesenteric ischaemia
AMTS	Abbreviated Mental Test Score
APTT	Activated partial thromboplastin time
ASA	American Society of Anaesthesiologists
ASO	Antistreptolysin O
ATN	Acute tubular necrosis
AVPU	Alert, voice, pain, unconscious
AXR	Abdominal X-ray
BD	bis die; twice a day
BED	Binge eating disorder
BLS	Basic life support
BMI	Body mass index
BNF	British National Formulary
BNP	Brain natriuretic peptide
BP	Blood Pressure
BPD	Borderline personality disorder
BPH	Benign prostatic hyperplasia
BPPV	Benign paroxysmal positional vertigo
bpm	Beats per minute (for pulse only)
C1-6, T1-12, L1-6	Spinal cord/column levels
Ca^{2+}	Calcium
CAD	Coronary artery disease
CAH	Congenital adrenal hyperplasia
CAHMS	Child and Adolescent Mental Health Service
CAP	Community-acquired pneumonia
CBG	Capillary blood glucose
CBT	Cognitive behavioural therapy
CES	Cauda equina syndrome
CF	Cystic fibrosis
CFS	Clinical Frailty Score
CK	Creatine kinase
CKD	Chronic kidney disease
CLI	Critical limb ischaemia
CMN	Congenital melanocytic nevus
CO_2	Carbon dioxide
COCP	Combined oral contraceptive pill
COPD	Chronic obstructive pulmonary disease
CPAP	Continuous positive airway pressure
CPR	Cardiopulmonary resuscitation
Creat	Creatinine
CRP	C-reactive protein
CRT	Capillary refill time
CSF	Cerebrospinal fluid
CT	Computerized tomography
CT AP	CT abdomen and pelvis
CT KUB	CT kidneys, ureters and bladder
CT TAP	CT thorax, abdomen, pelvis
CTA	CT angiography
CTG	Cardiotocograph
CTPA	Computed tomography pulmonary angiogram
CVP	Central venous pressure
CXR	Chest X-ray
DDH	Developmental dysplasia of the hip
DIC	Disseminated intravascular coagulation
DIP	Distal interphalangeal
DKA	Diabetic ketoacidosis
DMARD	Disease-modifying antirheumatic drug
DMD	Duchenne muscular dystrophy
DRE	Digital rectal examination
DVT	Deep vein thrombosis

EAC	External auditory canal
ECG	Electrocardiogram
ECT	Electroconvulsive therapy
EBV	Epstein–Barr virus
ED	Emergency department
EEG	Electroencephalograph
EMDR	Eye movement desensitization and reprocessing therapy
eGFR	Glomerular filtration rate
ERCP	Endoscopic retrograde cholangiopancreatography
ERP	Exposure and response prevention
ESR	Erythrocyte sedimentation rate
ESWL	Extracorporeal shock wave lithotripsy
EUPD	Emotionally unstable personality disorder
EUS	Endoscopic ultrasound
FAST	Focussed assessment with sonography for trauma
FBC	Full blood count
FEV	Forced expiratory volume
FFP	Fresh-frozen plasma
FOOSH	Fall onto an outstretched hand
FSGS	Focal segmental glomerulosclerosis
FSH	Follicle stimulating hormone
FVC	Forced vital capacity
FVIII	Factor VIII
GAS	Group A beta-haemolytic streptococcal
GBS	Guillain–Barré syndrome
GCS	Glasgow Coma Scale
GORD	Gastroesophageal reflux disease
GTN	Glyceryl trinitrate
GUM	Genitourinary medicine
HBA1c	Glycated haemoglobin
HCG (or hCG)	Human chorionic gonadotropin
HIV	Human immunodeficiency virus
HPV	Human papillomavirus
HRCT	High-resolution computed tomography
HSV	Herpes simplex virus
HUS	Haemolytic uraemic syndrome
IBD	Inflammatory bowel disease
IBS	Irritable bowel syndrome
ICP	Intracranial pressure
ICU	Intensive care unit
IDA	Iron deficiency anaemia
IHD	Ischaemic heart disease
IM	Intramuscular
IO	Intraosseous
ITP	Immune thrombocytopaenia
IUGR	Intrauterine growth restriction
IV	Intravenous
IVDU	Intravenous drug use
IVF	In vitro fertilization
JIA	Juvenile idiopathic arthritis
JVP	Jugular venous pressure
K	Potassium
LBO	Large bowel obstruction
LDH	Lactate dehydrogenase
LFT	Liver function tests
LH	Luteinizing Hormone
LLQ	Left lower quadrant
LUQ	Left upper quadrant
LUTS	Lower urinary tract symptoms
MAU	Medical admissions unit
MCA	Middle cerebral artery
MCD	Minimal change disease
MCL	Medial collateral ligament
MCP	Metacarpophalangeal joints
MCV	Mean cell volume
MDI	Multiple daily injection
mmHg	Millimetres of mercury (for blood pressure only)
MMSE	Mini-mental state exam
MRI	Magnetic resonance imaging
MSU	Mid-stream urine
Na	Sodium
NAAT	Nucleic acid amplification test
NEC	Necrotizing enterocolitis
NEWS	National Early Warning System
NG	Nasogastric
NHS	National Health Service
NICE	The National Institute for Health and Clinical Excellence
NICU	Neonatal intensive care unit
NOF	Neck of femur
NPV	Negative predictive value
NRDS	Neonatal respiratory distress syndrome
NSAIDs	Nonsteroidal antiinflammatory drugs
NSTEMI	Non–ST-elevation myocardial infarction

OE	Otitis externa
OM	Otitis media
OME	Otitis media with effusion
ORIF	Open reduction and internal fixation
OSA	Obstructive sleep apnoea
P	Pulse
PAD	Peripheral arterial disease
PCR	Polymerase chain reaction
PDA	Patent ductus arteriosus
PE	Pulmonary embolism
PEFR	Peak expiratory flow rate
PIP	Proximal interphalangeal
PKU	Phenylketonuria
Plt	Platelet count
PPHN	Persistent pulmonary hypertension of the newborn
PPV	Positive predictive value
PPV	Positive pressure ventilation
PR	Per rectum
PRN	Pro re nata; as needed
PSA	Prostatic specific antigen
PSGN	Poststreptococcal glomerulonephritis
PT	Prothrombin time
PTH	Parathyroid hormone
PTSD	Posttraumatic stress disorder
PUD	Peptic ulcer disease
QDS	Quarter in die; four times a day
O_2	Oxygen
OGD	Oesophagogastroduodenoscopy
OR	Odds ratio
OSA	Obstructive sleep apnoea
RAAS	Renin-angiotensin-aldosterone system
RAPD	Relative afferent pupillary defect
RBC	Red blood cell count
RLQ	Right lower quadrant
ROP	Retinopathy of prematurity
RR	Respiratory rate
RSV	Respiratory syncytial virus
RUQ	Right upper quadrant
SAH	Subarachnoid haemorrhage
SBO	Small bowel obstruction
SBP	Spontaneous bacterial peritonitis
SIADH	Syndrome of inappropriate antidiuretic hormone
SJS	Stevens–Johnson syndrome
SLE	Systemic lupus erythematosus
SNHL	Sensorineural hearing loss
SNRI	Serotonin and norepinephrine reuptake inhibitors
SP	Spontaneous pneumothorax
SpO_2	Oxygen saturation (in %)
SSRI	Selective serotonin reuptake inhibitor
STEMI	ST-elevation myocardial infarction
STI	Sexually transmitted infection
SVC	Superior vena cava
T2DM	Type 2 diabetes mellitus
T4	Thyroxine
TAVR	Transcatheter aortic valve replacement
TB	Tuberculosis
TBSA	Total body surface area
TCA	Tricyclic antidepressant
TDS	ter die sumendus; three times a day
TFT	Thyroid function tests
TIA	Transient ischaemic attack
TM	Tympanic membrane
TOF	Tetralogy of Fallot
TSH	Thyroid stimulating hormone
TSS	Toxic shock syndrome
TURP	Transurethral resection of the prostate
U&E	Urea and electrolytes
UGIB	Upper gastrointestinal bleed
UPSI	Unprotected sexual intercourse
Ur	Urea
URTI	Upper respiratory tract infection
US	Ultrasound
UTI	Urinary tract infection
VDRL	Venereal disease research laboratory
VEGF	Vascular endothelial growth factor
VP	Ventriculoperitoneal
VSD	Ventricular septal defect
VTE	Venous thromboembolism
WBC	White blood cell count
Y-BOCS	Yale-Brown-Obsessive-Compulsive Scale

How to use the book and ace the UKMLA exams

This edition can be used by clinical students at any stage, from initial clinical placements to finals preparation. The book is split into **eight medical** chapters and **seven surgical** chapters, organized by specialty, difficulty and relevancy, with icons to indicate the relevancy, difficulty and question type, allowing for targeted, adaptable revision depending on individual goals.

a). Curriculum coverage: Essential -> Important -> Supplementary

 Essential

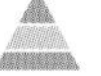 Important

 Supplementary

b). Difficulty: Easy -> Moderate -> Hard

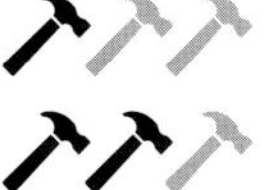 Easy

 Moderate

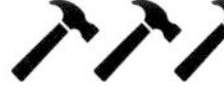 Hard

c). Question type: Remember, Understand, Apply

 Apply

ANATOMY OF A SINGLE BEST ANSWER QUESTION

Single best answer questions have a stem, presenting the problem. Five options are offered, all of which are plausible, with one which is clearly correct. Options are homogeneous (i.e., all the options should be diagnoses, investigations or mechanisms).

1. **Stem:** A stem presenting the problem.
2. **Lead-in:** A lead-in asking the question.
3. **Answer options:** 5 answer options for each question.

Example:
Stem: A 52-year-old woman has 6 hours of acute abdominal pain and vomiting, after episodes of right upper quadrant pain after meals lasting several hours for 3 months. She has hypercholesterolemia, managed with atorvastatin. Her temperature is 38.2°C, pulse 120 bpm and BP 98/73 mmHg. She is overweight, with dry mucous membranes and epigastric tenderness.

Lead-in rubric: Which is the most likely diagnosis?
Answer options:

A. Appendicitis
B. Cholangitis
C. Cholecystitis
D. Pancreatitis
E. Peptic ulcer disease

Answer: D. Pancreatitis

RELEVANCY LEVELS

The **Crash Course Curriculum Relevancy Levels** are carefully curated, based on an intensive mapping of medical school curriculums and frequency in examination scenarios.

This approach enhances exam preparation and ensures every study session is productive, with a focused and effective way to navigate the breadth of the medical school curriculum.

- **Essential:** Core topics of knowledge essential to pass exams. Should be covered early in revision to cement understanding of basic principles.
- **Important:** Significant topics covered by most medical curricula. Form the majority of questions in exams, and should be covered after you have a solid grasp of the basics.
- **Supplementary:** Additional knowledge beyond that expected – used to differentiate students aiming to just pass finals and the highest achievers.

SECOND-ORDER-LEVEL QUESTIONS (APPLY)

Apply-based questions are more clinically complex and require the application of knowledge and understanding, often known as second-order questions. An **Apply** question might require you to infer a diagnosis from a clinical stem and then answer a question such as, **'Which test is most likely to help confirm the diagnosis?'**. In contrast, an **Understand**-type question requires only one step, for example, **'Which is the most likely diagnosis?'**

The UKMLA AKT exam heavily favours the more challenging **Apply**-type questions. Over **56%** of the questions in this volume are **Apply**-based questions to represent the UKMLA accurately.

QUESTION DIFFICULTY

The difficulty of each question (Easy, Moderate, Hard) is based on the likely percentage of correct answers from a representative student cohort.

- **Easy:** 80% or higher
- **Moderate:** 50%–80%
- **Hard:** 50% or less

Difficulty is spread across the **15 topic chapters:**

Total	Easy	Moderate	Hard	
Essential	85	126	36	**247**
Important	69	244	53	**366**
Supplementary	31	124	37	**192**
	185	**494**	**126**	**805**

This volume and the companion Volume 2 cover **every topic in the UKMLA index**. Question mapping ensures you can determine complete curriculum coverage and identify strengths and areas for improvement. Each chapter has a UKMLA topic mapping index, highlighting the question type and number test for a given topic:

- Aetiology/risk factors/pathophysiology
- Investigations
- Diagnosis
- Management
- Prognosis/complications

HOW TO MAKE THE BEST USE OF THIS BOOK

The table below represents question difficulty and relevancy tagging in the Cardiology chapter as an example.

Cardiology	Easy	Moderate	Hard
Essential	10	14	4
Important	8	31	9
Supplementary	4	15	5

We recommend you attempt the **Essential questions** in each chapter prior to a clinical rotation or when you are trying to understand the basics.

Once you are 100% confident with the Essential questions, **Important questions** should be attempted. Taking time to fully understand the explanations will allow you to answer these types of questions confidently in your exams.

The **Supplementary questions** should be left to the end and may be done as "additional revision" for those looking to excel in exams. These questions should be attempted at least once even if you are only looking to pass. There are a lot of easy marks available in the Supplementary questions, so being able to answer some of these will be valuable.

DIAGNOSTIC MOCKS AND UKMLA MOCK

Two **Diagnostic Mocks** for **medicine** and **surgery totalling 100 questions** are included, reflective of the topic splits in the UKMLA exam. These mini-mocks enhance your diagnostic skills by understanding key features of the most common topics, to aid in spot diagnosis and increase speed and accuracy in second-order questions.

A comprehensive **100-question UKMLA-style mock** is included at the end, with a diverse and representative mix of question relevancy and difficulty, offering a realistic representation of the UKMLA exam.

The diagnostic mocks may be used early in revision to gain insight into areas of weakness and strength, and the UKMLA-specific mock close to the final exam date to provide a realistic expectation of your performance and highlight areas for prioritization.

Section 1
MEDICINE QUESTIONS

Cardiology

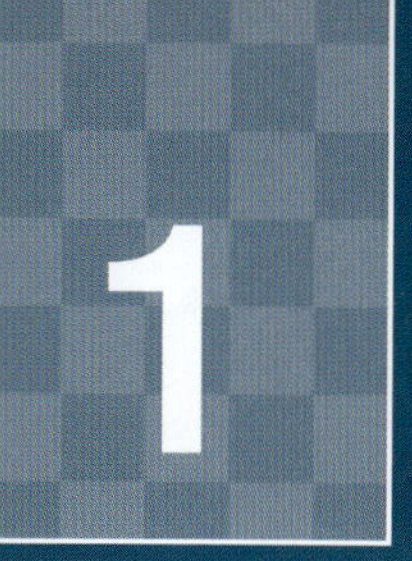

1. A 51-year-old man has sudden, severe chest pain radiating to his left jaw. He has hyperlipidaemia, managed with atorvastatin. He is pale and clammy to the touch.

Investigations:
Troponin: Elevated
ECG: ST elevation in leads I, V5 and V6

Which is the most likely diagnosis?
A. Anterior STEMI
B. Anterolateral STEMI
C. Inferior STEMI
D. Lateral STEMI
E. Posterior STEMI

2. A 54-year-old woman has sudden crushing chest pain radiating to the left jaw. Her father had a coronary artery bypass graft two months ago.

Investigations:
Troponin: elevated
ECG: ST elevation in leads II, III and aVF.

Which is the most likely coronary artery affected?
A. Left anterior descending artery
B. Left circumflex artery
C. Left main stem
D. Posterior ascending artery
E. Right coronary artery

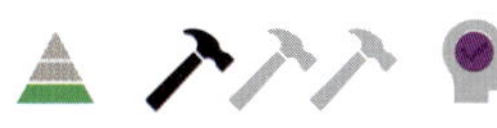

3. A 62-year-old man has shortness of breath and fatigue. He has hypertension, managed with amlodipine. He has pitting oedema bilaterally up to the knees, and bibasal crepitations on chest auscultation and an S3 heart sound are heard.

Which is the most suitable diagnostic investigation?
A. Aortic US
B. Chest X-ray
C. Coronary angiography
D. Echocardiogram
E. Electrocardiogram

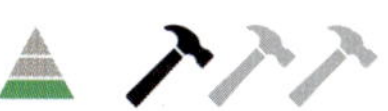

4. A 21-year-old woman has chest pain worse on inspiration. She has recovered from an upper respiratory tract infection two weeks ago. A friction rub is heard in systole and diastole.

Investigations:
ECG: widespread concave ST elevation.

Which is the most likely diagnosis?
A. Acute pericarditis
B. Constrictive pericarditis
C. Pulmonary embolism
D. ST-elevated myocardial infarction
E. Unstable angina

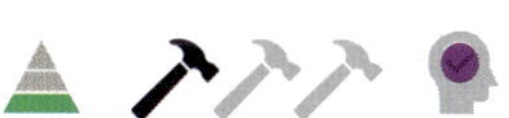

5. A 67-year-old woman has reduced exercise tolerance and shortness of breath whilst lying down. She had an ST-elevated myocardial infarction three years ago. She has a raised JVP and a displaced apex beat.

Investigations:
Echocardiogram: ejection fraction of 0.38.

Which is the most appropriate management?
A. Amlodipine
B. Bisoprolol
C. Furosemide
D. Losartan
E. Ramipril

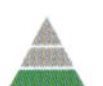  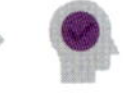

6. A 32-year-old woman has a non-productive cough and pleuritic chest pain. She had Coxsackie B virus 1 month ago, which resolved. Her temperature is 38.7°C.

Investigations:
ECG: concave ST elevation and PR depression in most leads.

Which is the most appropriate management?
   A. Implantable cardioverter-defibrillator
   B. NSAID + colchicine
   C. Pericardiectomy
   D. Pericardiocentesis
   E. Percutaneous coronary intervention

7. A 53-year-old man has sudden central chest pain at rest. He has hyperlipidaemia, managed with atorvastatin.

Investigations:
ECG: ST depression in the lateral leads.

Which is the most likely diagnosis?
   A. Non-ST-elevated myocardial infarction
   B. Prinzmetal angina
   C. Stable angina
   D. ST-elevated myocardial infarction
   E. Unstable angina

 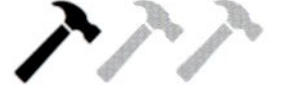 

8. A 62-year-old woman has had occasional headaches and fatigue for 3 months. She has type 2 diabetes mellitus, managed with metformin. Her BP is 167/84 mmHg.

Which is the most appropriate management?
   A. Amlodipine
   B. Furosemide
   C. Losartan
   D. Phenoxybenzamine
   E. Ramipril

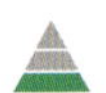 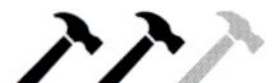 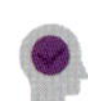

9. A 38-year-old woman has shortness of breath after a cycling accident. Her BP is 88/55 mmHg. She has left chest bruising, dampened heart sounds and a raised JVP.

Investigations:
ECG: electrical alternans.

Which is the most appropriate management?
   A. Implantable cardioverter-defibrillator
   B. Open heart surgery
   C. Pericardiocentesis
   D. Surgical aortic valve replacement
   E. Transcatheter aortic valve replacement

  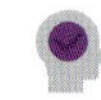

10. A 60-year-old woman has a racing heartbeat for three hours and lightheadedness. She has type 2 diabetes mellitus, managed with metformin and empagliflozin. Her pulse is 162 bpm, and BP is 88/55 mmHg.

Investigations:
ECG: Figure 1.1 (see Chapter 37).

Which is the most appropriate management?
   A. Immediate DC cardioversion
   B. Implantable cardioverter-defibrillator
   C. IV adenosine
   D. IV atropine
   E. Radiofrequency ablation of the accessory pathway

 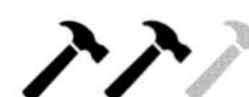

11. A 55-year-old man has sudden central chest pain. He is pale and clammy to touch and becomes unresponsive during cardiovascular examination.

Investigations:
ECG: irregular deflections of varying amplitude, with no discernable p waves and QRS complexes.

Which is the most likely diagnosis?
   A. Atrial fibrillation
   B. Torsades des pointes
   C. Ventricular fibrillation
   D. Ventricular tachycardia
   E. Wolff-Parkinson-White syndrome

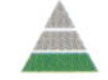 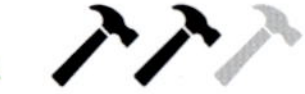 

12. A 78-year-old man has shortness of breath, often waking him up at night. He has heart failure, managed with bisoprolol and ramipril. He has pitting oedema bilaterally to the shins, and a S3 heart sound.

Investigations:
Echocardiogram: left ventricular ejection fraction of 36%.

Which is the most appropriate management?
A. Candersartan
B. Digoxin
C. Diltiazem
D. Dobutamine
E. Spironolactone

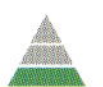 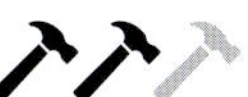 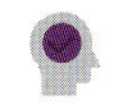

13. A 64-year-old woman has her annual medication check-up. She is asymptomatic but has struggled to control her BP with amlodipine, with an average reading of 152/96 mmHg for the past week. She has gout, managed with allopurinol. Her clinic BP is 159/101 mmHg.

Which is the most appropriate management?
A. Candersartan
B. Doxazosin
C. Indapamide
D. Spironolactone
E. Verapamil

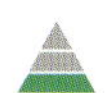  

14. A 72-year-old man has had shortness of breath for three hours. He has hyperlipidaemia, managed with atorvastatin.

Investigations:
ECG: W-shaped wave in lead V1, an M-shaped wave in lead V6, and ST elevation in leads V1-V4.

Which is the most appropriate management?
A. Aspirin and Fondaparinux
B. Immediate DC cardioversion
C. IV adenosine
D. No management required
E. Percutaneous Coronary Intervention

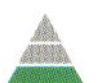  

15. A 79-year-old man has sudden pleuritic chest pain. He had an elective left knee replacement 3 weeks ago. He has left-sided crepitations on chest auscultation.

Which is the most suitable investigation?
A. Chest X-ray
B. CT pulmonary angiogram
C. ECG
D. Proximal leg vein US
E. V/Q scan

16. A 65-year-old woman has difficulty breathing gradually worsening for 2 weeks. She has hyperlipidaemia, managed with atorvastatin. Her pulse is 108 bpm. She has a raised JVP, hepatomegaly and bibasal crepitations on chest auscultation.

Which of the following may be seen on CXR?
A. Consolidation
B. Kerley B lines
C. Lobar collapse
D. Lower lobe diversion
E. Widened mediastinum

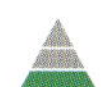  

17. A 62-year-old man has chest discomfort on exertion for 6 months, relieved by rest. He has stable angina managed with glyceryl trinitrate spray and bisoprolol.

Which is the most appropriate management?
A. Amlodipine
B. Isosorbide mononitrate
C. Ivabradine
D. Nicorandil
E. Ranolazine

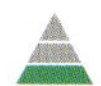 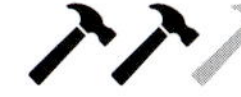

18. A 58-year-old woman has had a dry cough for 3 weeks. She was diagnosed with heart failure four months ago.

Which medication is most likely to be related to her presentation?
A. Amlodipine
B. Bisoprolol
C. Furosemide
D. Losartan
E. Ramipril

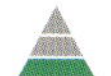  

19. A 75-year-old woman recovering in the respiratory ward from community-acquired pneumonia suddenly became unresponsive. No one states to have been monitoring or witnessing her becoming unresponsive.

Investigations:
ECG: irregular deflections with varying amplitudes and a lack of p waves and QRS complexes

Which is the most appropriate management?
A. One shock followed by one minute of CPR
B. One shock followed by two minutes of CPR
C. Three shocks followed by three minutes of CPR
D. Two shocks followed by three minutes of CPR
E. Two shocks followed by two minutes of CPR

 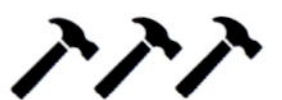 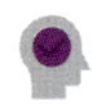

20. A 42-year-old woman was diagnosed with congestive heart failure 3 years ago. She is now unable to carry out any physical activity without discomfort and has extreme shortness of breath at rest. She has bilateral swelling of her legs up to her knees.

Based on this woman's presentation, which New York Heart Association class is she in?
A. NYHA Class I
B. NYHA Class II
C. NYHA Class III
D. NYHA Class IV
E. NYHA Class V

21. A 62-year-old woman is transferred to the coronary care unit after an anterior ST-elevated myocardial infarction. However, she became unresponsive 10 minutes after being transferred to the Coronary Care Unit (CCU).

Investigations:
ECG: irregular deflections with varying amplitudes and a lack of p waves and QRS complexes
He is shocked by a defibrillator three consecutive times. However, the ECG trace is still the same as it was before.

Which is the most appropriate management?
A. Amiodarone 1 mg and adrenaline 300 mg
B. Amiodarone 150 mg and adrenaline 1 mg
C. Amiodarone 300 mg and adrenaline 2 mg
D. Amiodarone 300 mg and adrenaline 1 mg
E. Atropine 300 mg and adrenaline 1 mg

22. A 74-year-old woman has her annual check-up. She has an ischaemic stroke, managed with aspirin and clopidogrel.

Investigations:
ECG: PR interval of 240 ms

Which is the most likely diagnosis?
A. Complete heart block
B. First-degree heart block
C. Left bundle branch block
D. Mobitz I heart block
E. Right bundle branch block

 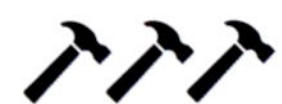 

23. A 21-year-old man is brought in via ambulance after a serious car accident. He was conscious in the ambulance, but when examined in the emergency department, he was unresponsive and pulseless.

Investigations:
ECG: regular broad complex tachycardia.
Based on the ECG, advanced life support (ALS) is started; however, intravenous access cannot be gained for medication.

Which is the most appropriate route to administer the medications for ALS?
A. Central line
B. Endotracheal line
C. Intramuscular route
D. Intraosseous line
E. Rectal route

 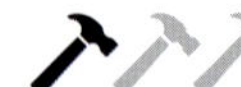 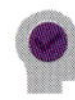

24. A 34-year-old man has had intermittent sensations of a racing heartbeat for 2 months. He uses cocaine recreationally every two weeks on average.

Investigations:
ECG: narrow complex tachycardia with absent P waves.

Which is the most appropriate management?
A. Adenosine
B. Amlodipine
C. Carotid sinus massage
D. DC Cardioversion
E. Verapamil

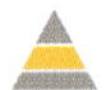 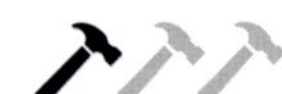

25. A 73-year-old woman has had shortness of breath and a racing heartbeat for 3 hours. She has hyperlipidaemia, managed with atorvastatin.

Investigations
ECG: narrow complex tachycardia with rapid, undulating waves in leads II, III and aVF.

Which is the most likely diagnosis?

A. Atrial fibrillation
B. Atrial flutter
C. Supraventricular tachycardia
D. Torsades de pointes
E. Wolff-Parkinson-White syndrome

 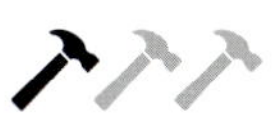 

26. A 46-year-old man has sudden chest pain and shortness of breath. He has hypertension, managed with ramipril and uses cocaine recreationally monthly. He has weak brachial pulses bilaterally and on chest auscultation, an early diastolic murmur is heard.

Which of the following signs are you likely to see on the X-ray of this man?

A. Consolidation
B. Kerley B lines
C. Lobar collapse
D. Lower lobe diversion
E. Widened mediastinum

27. A 56-year-old man has chest pain that radiates to the left shoulder that started 1 hour ago. He has stable angina, managed with glyceryl trinitrate spray and bisoprolol.

Investigations:
Troponin: elevated
ECG: ST depression and tall R waves in leads V1-V3.

Which is the most likely diagnosis?

A. Anterior ST-elevated myocardial infarction (STEMI)
B. Anterolateral non-ST-elevated myocardial infarction (NSTEMI)
C. Inferior NSTEMI
D. Inferior STEMI
E. Posterior STEMI

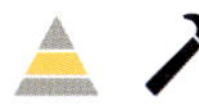

28. A 29-year-old woman has a racing heartbeat occurring intermittently for 6 months. She has thyrotoxicosis, managed with propranolol and carbimazole.

Investigations:
ECG: Figure 1.2 (see Chapter 37).

Which is the most likely diagnosis?

A. Atrial fibrillation
B. Superventricular tachycardia
C. Torsades de pointes
D. Ventricular fibrillation
E. Wolff-Parkinson-White syndrome

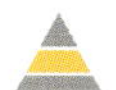 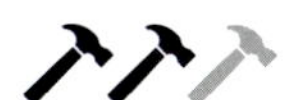

29. A 37-year-old man has sudden chest pain. He has Marfan syndrome. He has weak brachial pulses bilaterally.

Investigations:
CT angiogram: false lumen in the ascending aorta.

Which is the most likely diagnosis?

A. Abdominal Aortic Aneurysm
B. Aortic dissection
C. Carotid artery dissection
D. ST-elevated myocardial infarction
E. Unstable angina

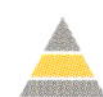 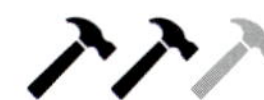 

30. A 64-year-old man has had pleuritic chest pain for 2 days. He has testicular cancer diagnosed 4 months ago. He has just returned from holiday in South Africa three days ago. His pulse is 108 bpm and respiratory rate 23 breaths per minute.

What is the % probability of a PE if zero of the PERC criteria are fulfilled?

A. <2%
B. <4%
C. <6%
D. <8%
E. <10%

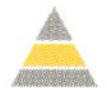 

31. A 22-year-old man presents after collapsing during a rugby match. He has since regained consciousness and he has a jerky carotid pulse, and an ejection systolic murmur is heard.

Investigations:
ECG: signs of left ventricular hypertrophy with T wave inversion in leads V1-V5 and deep Q waves in leads III and aVF.

Which is the most likely inheritance pattern?
A. Autosomal dominant
B. Autosomal recessive
C. Mitochondrial
D. X-linked dominant
E. X-linked recessive

  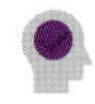

32. An 82-year-old woman has sudden pleuritic chest pain after an elective right total hip replacement 2 weeks ago. Her temperature is 38.6°C, pulse is 120 bpm and BP is 84/56 mmHg.

Which is the most appropriate management?
A. IV alteplase
B. Rivaroxaban for six months
C. Rivaroxaban for three months
D. Warfarin for six months
E. Warfarin for three months

 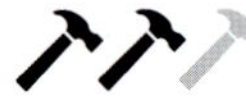 

33. A 37-year-old woman has had shortness of breath for 48 hours. She had *a mycoplasma pneumoniae* infection two weeks ago, managed with erythromycin. She has dizziness.

Investigations:
ECG: ventricular tachycardia with a prolonged QT interval.

Which is the most appropriate management?
A. Immediate DC cardioversion
B. IV adenosine
C. IV atropine
D. IV magnesium sulphate
E. Temporary pacemaker

34. A 41-year-old man has chest pain radiating to his left shoulder, which started around 45 minutes ago. He has hyperlipidaemia, managed with atorvastatin.

Investigations:
Troponin: elevated
ECG shows T wave inversion in the leads I, aVL, and V3-V6.

Which is the most likely diagnosis?
A. Anterior non-ST-elevated myocardial infarction (NSTEMI)
B. Anterolateral NSTEMI
C. Inferior NSTEMI
D. Inferior ST-elevated myocardial infarction (STEMI)
E. Lateral STEMI

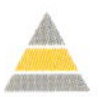 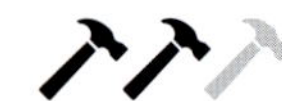 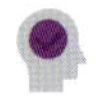

35. A 42-year-old woman has a racing heartbeat for four hours. She has rheumatoid arthritis, managed with methotrexate. Her pulse is 114 bpm and BP of 85/56 mmHg.

Investigations:
ECG: irregularly irregular rhythm.

Which is the most appropriate management?
A. Adenosine
B. Cardioversion after three weeks of anticoagulation
C. Immediate flecainide
D. Immediate synchronised DC cardioversion
E. Verapamil

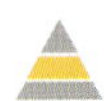 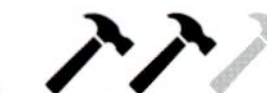 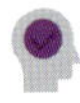

36. A 41-year-old man has muscle weakness and vomiting for 24 hours. He has hypertension, managed with ramipril.

Investigations:
Serum sodium = 139 mmol/L (137–144)
Serum potassium = 6.4 mmol/L (3.5–4.9)
ECG: tall tented T waves and broad QRS complexes.

Which is the most appropriate next step in the management?
A. Calcium resonium
B. Haemodialysis
C. Insulin/dextrose infusion
D. IV calcium gluconate
E. Nebulised salbutamol

 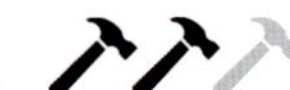 

37. A 21-year-old man has a racing heartbeat that is noticeable after going on his morning walk. His older brother suddenly died at the age of 23 due to cardiac issues.

Investigations:
ECG: short PR intervals, delta waves and widened QRS complexes.

Which is the most appropriate management?
A. Implantable cardioverter-defibrillator
B. Immediate DC cardioversion
C. IV adenosine
D. IV atropine
E. Radiofrequency ablation of the accessory pathway

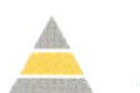 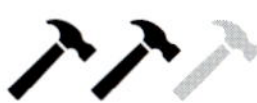

38. A 70-year-old woman has sudden central, crushing chest pain radiating to the left shoulder. She has hypercholesterolaemia, managed with atorvastatin.

After 12 hours of the PCI, she is pale and clammy to touch and her pulse is 48 bpm.

Investigations now:
ECG: complete P: QRS dissociation

Which coronary artery is most likely affected?
A. Left anterior descending artery
B. Left circumflex artery
C. Left main stem
D. Posterior ascending artery
E. Right coronary artery

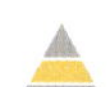 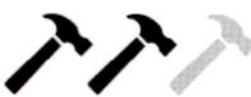 

39. A 50-year-old man has sudden chest pain that radiates to the back. He has Ehlers-Danlos syndrome. His pulse is 114 bpm and BP is 82/54 mmHg. He has absent femoral pulses bilaterally and an early diastolic murmur.

Which is the most suitable investigation?
A. Chest X-ray
B. CT angiography chest/abdomen/pelvis
C. Transoesophageal echocardiogram
D. Transthoracic echocardiogram
E. US Doppler of the lower limb

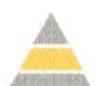 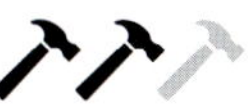 

40. A 78-year-old woman has chest pain that is worse on inspiration and feeling dizzy for a week. She has type 2 diabetes mellitus, managed with metformin and chronic kidney disease. She has a loud ejection systolic murmur with a soft S2 heart sound.

Which is the most appropriate definitive management?
A. Implantable cardioverter-defibrillator
B. Percutaneous mitral balloon valvotomy
C. Pericardiocentesis
D. Surgical aortic valve replacement
E. Transcatheter aortic valve replacement

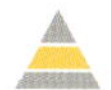 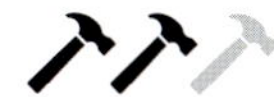

41. A 40-year-old woman has shortness of breath. She has multiple petechial lesions on her palms and soles, and a pansystolic murmur at the left sternal border is heard.

Investigations:
Echocardiogram: vegetation on the valvular leaflet.

Which is the most likely cause of the murmur heard on chest auscultation?
A. Aortic regurgitation
B. Aortic stenosis
C. Mitral regurgitation
D. Mitral stenosis
E. Tricuspid regurgitation

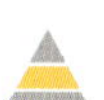 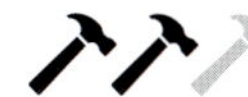 

42. A 17-year-old boy presents in an ambulance after collapsing in football training. He has since regained consciousness, and he remembered feeling dizzy before collapsing.

Which is the most suitable initial investigation?
A. Chest X-ray
B. Echocardiogram
C. Electrocardiogram
D. Electroencephalography
E. Tilt-table test

 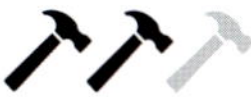

43. A 24-year-old man has chest pain and shortness of breath. His younger sister died suddenly from cardiac problems. He has prominent a waves in his JVP.

Investigations:
Echocardiogram: marked left ventricular hypertrophy and systolic anterior motion of the mitral valve.

Which is the most likely diagnosis?
A. Arrhythmogenic right ventricular cardiomyopathy
B. Dilated cardiomyopathy
C. Hypertrophic obstructive cardiomyopathy
D. Restrictive cardiomyopathy
E. Takotsubo cardiomyopathy

44. A 64-year-old woman has palpitations. She had myocarditis three months ago.

Investigations:
ECG: M-shaped wave in lead V1 and a W-shaped wave in lead V6.

Which is the most likely diagnosis?
A. First-degree heart block
B. Left bundle branch block
C. Mobitz-II heart block
D. Right bundle branch block
E. Trifascicular block

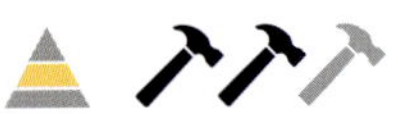

45. A 65-year-old man has visual disturbances. He has hypertension managed poorly with amlodipine. Visual field examination reveals an enlarged blindspot.

Investigations:
Fundoscopy: blurring of the optic margins with venous engorgement.

Which is the most likely cause of his presentation?
A. Stage I hypertensive retinopathy
B. Stage II hypertensive retinopathy
C. Stage III hypertensive retinopathy
D. Stage IV hypertensive retinopathy
E. Stage V hypertensive retinopathy

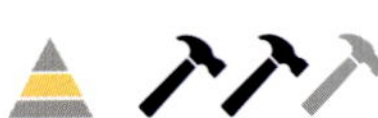

46. A 56-year-old man has dizziness causing a fall and a racing heartbeat. He has never had this issue in the past. He had community-acquired pneumonia a month ago, managed with erythromycin.

Investigations:
ECG: QT interval of 520ms and signs of ventricular tachycardia.

Which is the most likely diagnosis?
A. Atrial fibrillation
B. Atrial flutter
C. Supraventricular tachycardia
D. Torsades de pointes
E. Wolff-Parkinson-White syndrome

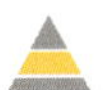 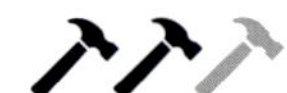 

47. A 72-year-old man has had chest pain for four hours. He has hypertension, managed with amlodipine. His pulse is 108 bpm and BP 182/121 mmHg. He has weak femoral pulses bilaterally.

Investigations:
CT angiogram: false lumen in the descending aorta.

Which is the most appropriate management?
A. Implantable cardioverter-defibrillator
B. IV labetalol
C. Open heart surgery
D. Percutaneous mitral balloon valvotomy
E. Surgical aortic valve replacement

 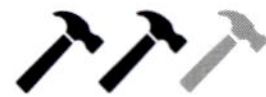

48. A 51-year-old man has shortness of breath and fever. He has splinter haemorrhages on the nails, Osler nodes in the hands bilaterally and he has a pansystolic murmur loudest on expiration.

Investigations:
Transthoracic echocardiogram: vegetation on the mitral valve.

Based on the likely diagnosis, which might be seen on fundoscopy?
A. Neovascularisation
B. Papilloedema
C. Reduced red reflex
D. Retinal detachment
E. Roth spots

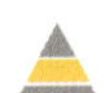 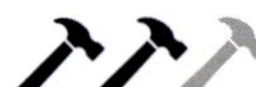 

49. A 70-year-old woman has sudden pleuritic chest pain and blood in her sputum. She had an elective left hip replacement around 3 weeks ago. Her pulse is 120 bpm. He has bibasilar crepitations on chest auscultation and leg swelling bilaterally, with dilated, swollen, tender lower leg veins.

Which is the most appropriate management?
A. IV alteplase
B. Rivaroxaban for six months
C. Rivaroxaban for three months
D. Warfarin for six months
E. Warfarin for three months

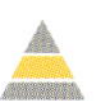 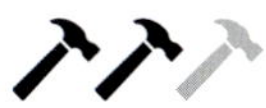

50. A 74-year-old woman has had shortness of breath and chest pain for 3 weeks. She had a mitral valve replacement six weeks ago. She has a pansystolic murmur heard best on expiration and Janeway lesions bilaterally.

Investigations:
Transoesophageal echocardiogram: vegetation on the mitral valve.

Which is the most appropriate tool to use to diagnose?
A. ABCD2 score
B. CHA2DS2-VASc score
C. Modified Duke criteria
D. NYHA classification
E. Wells score

51. A 74-year-old woman has sudden tearing chest pain and shortness of breath. She has hypertension, managed with amlodipine. She has weak brachial pulses bilaterally and an early diastolic murmur best heard on expiration is present.

Investigations:
Transthoracic echocardiogram: false lumen in the ascending aorta.

Which is the likely murmur heard on auscultation?
A. Aortic regurgitation
B. Aortic stenosis
C. Mitral regurgitation
D. Mitral stenosis
E. Pulmonary regurgitation

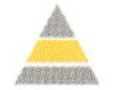 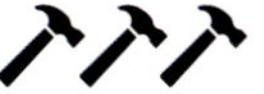 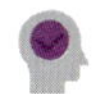

52. A 21-year-old man has had a racing heartbeat for a week.

Investigations:
ECG: T wave inversion in leads V1-3, and a terminal notch is seen in the QRS complex.
MRI chest: enlarged, hypokinetic right ventricle with a thin free wall.

Which is the most appropriate management?
A. Implantable cardioverter-defibrillator
B. Open heart surgery
C. Pericardiocentesis
D. Surgical aortic valve replacement
E. Transcatheter aortic valve replacement

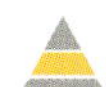 

53. A 57-year-old man has had shortness of breath for a week. He had a lateral STEMI 1 week ago which was managed with percutaneous coronary intervention. His pulse is 114 bpm and BP is 82/57 mmHg. His JVP is elevated and dampened heart sounds and crepitations are heard on chest auscultation.

Investigations:
ECG: electrical alternans.

Which is the most likely diagnosis?
A. Dressler syndrome
B. Left ventricular aneurysm
C. Left ventricular free wall rupture
D. Ventricular Septal Defect
E. Viral pericarditis

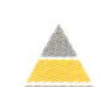 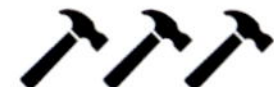 

54. A 54-year-old woman has blood in her sputum and shortness of breath. She had rheumatic fever 3 weeks ago, managed with oral penicillin V. She has blueish-red discolouration of her cheeks and a mid-late diastolic murmur is best heard on expiration.

Investigations:
ECG: right axis deviation, a tall R wave in lead V1, and a prominent biphasic P wave in lead V1.

Which is the most appropriate management?
A. Percutaneous mitral balloon valvotomy
B. Regular monitoring with echocardiograms
C. Surgical aortic valve replacement
D. Transcatheter aortic valve replacement
E. Warfarin

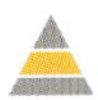 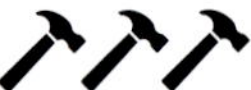

55. A 56-year-old man has central pleuritic chest pain, which is worse when lying down. He had an anterior ST-elevated myocardial infarction four weeks ago managed by percutaneous coronary intervention. His temperature is 38.4°C and pulse is 102 bpm.

Investigations:
ECG: concave ST elevation in leads I-III, VF and V3-V6.

Which is the most likely diagnosis?
- A. Dressler syndrome
- B. Left ventricular aneurysm
- C. Left ventricular free wall rupture
- D. Ventricular Septal Defect
- E. Viral pericarditis

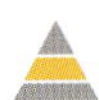  

56. A 28-year-old woman has had chest pain and shortness of breath for 2 weeks. She has had prior heart valve replacement surgery. Her temperature is 38.4°C.
She has splinter haemorrhages and a pansystolic murmur best heard on expiration.

Which is the most suitable investigation?
- A. Chest MRI
- B. CT chest/abdomen/pelvis
- C. PET Scan
- D. Transesophageal echocardiography
- E. Transthoracic echocardiography

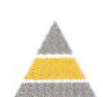  

57. A 68-year-old woman has sudden chest pain worse on inspiration and shortness of breath. Her pulse is 102 bpm. She has crepitations in the base of her left lung and leg swelling bilaterally, with dilated, swollen, tender lower leg veins.

Which is the most suitable investigation?
- A. Chest X-ray
- B. CT pulmonary angiogram
- C. D-dimer
- D. Proximal leg vein US
- E. V/Q scan

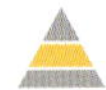  

58. A 53-year-old man has had a fever, chills, and fatigue for 1 week. He also has a new onset of shortness of breath and chest pain. He admits to recreational IV drug use. He has a grade 2/6 systolic murmur at the left sternal border.

Investigations:
Blood cultures: Streptococcus viridans
Transthoracic echocardiogram: vegetation on the anterior mitral valve leaflet.

Which of the following would be an indication for surgery?
- A. Low complement levels
- B. Presence of Roth spots on fundoscopy
- C. Prosthetic valve
- D. Severe valvular incompetence
- E. Streptococcus viridans infection

 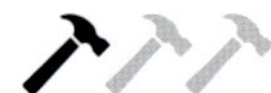

59. A 24-year-old man has had a racing heartbeat and lightheadedness for 1 week. His pulse is 126 bpm.

Investigations:
ECG: QT interval of 520ms.

Which of the following electrolyte abnormalities can cause the ECG findings seen?
- A. Hypercalcaemia
- B. Hypermagnesemia
- C. Hyperphosphataemia
- D. Hypokalaemia
- E. Hyponatraemia

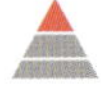 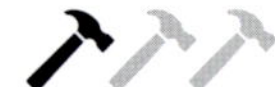

60. A 47-year-old woman has had shortness of breath and blood in her sputum for three weeks. She has a mid-late diastolic murmur with a loud S1.

Which is the most likely cause?
- A. Bicuspid aortic valve
- B. Ehlers-Danlos syndrome
- C. Marfan syndrome
- D. Rheumatic fever
- E. Valve calcification

 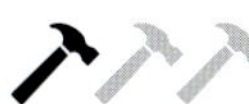 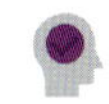

61. A 23-year-old man has chest pain, shortness of breath, and fatigue for a week. He had an upper respiratory tract infection three weeks ago that has since resolved. He has bilateral crepitations and muffled heart sounds on chest auscultation.

Investigations:
C-reactive protein (CRP): 38 mg/L (<10)

Which of the following is a likely complication?
A. Aortic dissection
B. Arrhythmogenic right ventricular cardiomyopathy
C. Dilated cardiomyopathy
D. Dressler syndrome
E. Restrictive cardiomyopathy

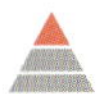 

62. A 24-year-old woman presents after collapsing whilst walking to work in the morning. She has regained consciousness fully. Her younger brother suddenly collapsed due to an abnormal heartbeat.

Investigations:
ECG: partial right bundle branch block and convex ST elevation of 3 mm in leads V1-V2 followed by a negative T wave.

Which is the most likely diagnosis?
A. Anterior ST-elevated myocardial infarction (STEMI)
B. Brugada syndrome
C. Inferior STEMI
D. Wellen syndrome
E. Wolff-Parkinson-White Syndrome

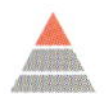  

63. A 48-year-old man has gradually worsening shortness of breath and swelling in his legs bilaterally for 2 months. He has hyperlipidaemia, managed with atorvastatin. He has a paradoxical rise in JVP during inspiration and a loud S3 heart sound is heard.

Investigations:
CXR: pericardial calcifications.

Which is the most appropriate management?
A. Implantable cardioverter-defibrillator
B. NSAID + colchicine
C. Open heart surgery
D. Pericardiectomy
E. Pericardiocentesis

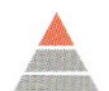 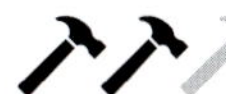

64. A 46-year-old woman has had worsening breathlessness and blood in her sputum for 6 weeks. She has a ventricular septal defect diagnosed in her childhood. She is cyanotic, has clubbing of her fingers bilaterally and has a fixed, widely split-second heart sound.

Investigations:
CXR: gross dilatation of the main, left and right pulmonary arteries.

Which is the most likely diagnosis?
A. Atrial myxoma
B. Coarctation of the aorta
C. Eisenmenger syndrome
D. Hypertrophic obstructive cardiomyopathy
E. Tetralogy of Fallot

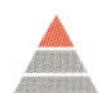 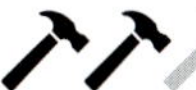

65. An 85-year-old woman has severe pain at rest in both her feet. She has unstable angina, managed with cardiac catheterisation last week. Her toes are cold and purple, but the major arterial pulses in her lower limbs are still present.

Investigations:
Renal biopsy: intravascular cholesterol clefts.

Which is the most likely cause?
A. Allergic reaction to the heparin
B. Cholesterol embolism
C. Haemorrhage from recent anticoagulation
D. Heparin-induced thrombocytopenia
E. Sepsis

 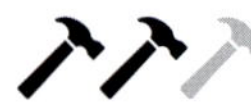

66. A 31-year-old man has had shortness of breath for 4 days. He had a viral illness from which he recovered a week ago. His temperature is 38.1°C and pulse is 114 bpm. He has bibasilar crepitations on chest auscultation.

Investigations:
CXR: bilateral pulmonary infiltrates and cardiomegaly.

Which is the most likely diagnosis?
  A. Dilated cardiomyopathy
  B. Infective endocarditis
  C. Myocarditis
  D. Pericarditis
  E. Rheumatic heart disease

67. A 52-year-old man has exertional shortness of breath that gradually gets worse for 2 months. He has shortness of breath when lying down and pitting ankle oedema.

Investigations:
Echocardiogram: dilation of all four chambers and thinning of both ventricular walls.

Which is the most likely cause?
  A. Alcoholism
  B. Amyloidosis
  C. Obesity
  D. Smoking
  E. Stress

 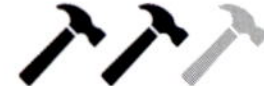

68. A 56-year-old woman has shortness of breath and unintentional weight loss of 4kg over 3 months. She has clubbing of the fingers bilaterally, and a mid-diastolic murmur is heard.

Investigations:
Echocardiogram: pedunculated heterogeneous mass attached to the fossa ovalis.

Which is the most likely diagnosis?
  A. Aortic dissection
  B. Arrhythmogenic right ventricular cardiomyopathy
  C. Atrial myxoma
  D. Hypertrophic obstructive cardiomyopathy
  E. Infective endocarditis

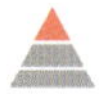 

69. A 21-year-old man has chest pain and exertional shortness of breath. Around six months ago, he had an upwards lens dislocation. He has a high-arched palate and pectus excavatum, and a mid-to-late systolic murmur is heard.

Which is the most likely diagnosis?
  A. Aortic stenosis
  B. Coarctation of the aorta
  C. Ebstein anomaly
  D. Mitral valve prolapse
  E. Ventricular septal defect

 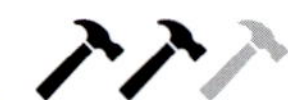 

70. A 27-year-old woman has blurred vision and swelling of her limbs. She is currently 30 weeks pregnant. Her BP is 167/98 mmHg. She has pitting oedema in her limbs.

Which is the most appropriate management?
  A. Indapamide
  B. Labetalol
  C. Losartan
  D. Nifedipine
  E. Rampiril

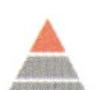 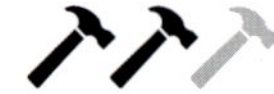

71. A 13-year-old boy has had severe headaches and chest pain for five days. He has a radio-femoral delay and has a mid-systolic murmur best heard over the back.

Investigations:
CXR: irregular notching of the inferior margins of the posterior ribs.

Which is the most likely diagnosis?
  A. Aortic stenosis
  B. Coarctation of the aorta
  C. Ebstein abnormality
  D. Mitral valve prolapse
  E. Ventricular septal defect

72. A 54-year-old woman has severe chest pain and shortness of for 1 month. She has type 2 diabetes mellitus, managed with metformin and sitagliptin.

Investigations:
Echocardiogram: severe hypokinesis of the mid and apical segment of the left ventricle.

Which is the most likely diagnosis?
A. Arrhythmogenic right ventricular cardiomyopathy
B. Dilated cardiomyopathy
C. Hypertrophic obstructive cardiomyopathy
D. Restrictive cardiomyopathy
E. Takotsubo cardiomyopathy

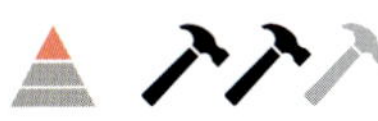

73. A 65-year-old woman has had shortness of breath for 2 weeks. Two weeks ago, she had an inferolateral STEMI, which was treated with percutaneous coronary intervention. She has pitting oedema in the legs bilaterally and has an S3 heart sound.

Investigations:
ECG: ST elevation in the inferolateral leads.

Which is the most likely diagnosis?
A. Dressler syndrome
B. Left ventricular aneurysm
C. Left ventricular free wall rupture
D. Ventricular Septal Defect
E. Viral pericarditis

74. A 4-month-old boy has a routine check-up. His parents say that he has been feeding well and that they have noticed nothing untoward with his progress. He has a harsh pansystolic murmur best heard at the lower left sternal border.

Investigations:
Echocardiogram: left-to-right shunt.

Which is the most likely diagnosis?
A. Atrial septal defect
B. Coarctation of the aorta
C. Tetralogy of Fallot
D. Transposition of the great arteries
E. Ventricular Septal Defect

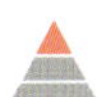 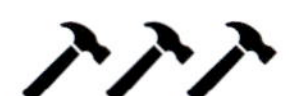 

75. A 28-year-old man has palpitations and dizziness, worsened by exertion for 3 weeks. His sister passed away from cardiac arrest, aged 27.

Investigations:
ECG: T wave inversion in leads V1-3 and a terminal notch in the QRS complex
Echocardiogram: enlarged, hypokinetic right ventricle with a thin free wall.

Which gene is most likely to be mutated in this man?
A. DES
B. MYBPC3
C. MYH7
D. PKP2
E. TTN

76. A 32-year-old woman has sudden chest pain worse on inspiration. She has systemic lupus erythematosus and has had two miscarriages in the past four years. When asked, she reports no recent travel or hospitalisations.

Investigations:
Activated partial thromboplastin time (aPTT): 47 seconds (30-40)
D-dimer: 1.8 mg/L (<0.5)

Which of the following antibodies would be elevated?
A. Anti-beta2 glycoprotein I antibody
B. Anti-CCP antibody
C. Anti-Mi-2 antibody
D. Anti-smooth muscle antibody
E. TSH receptor antibodies

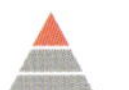 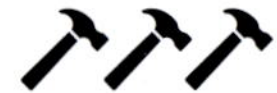

77. A 41-year-old man presents after collapsing on the bus. He has since regained consciousness. His ECG shows saddleback ST elevation in leads V1-V3 and then he is given a challenge of a medication.

Investigations:
ECG: Convex ST elevation >2 mm in leads V1-V3 followed by a negative T wave

Which medication is given to the patient before his second ECG?

A. Adenosine
B. Ajmaline
C. Amiodarone
D. Heparin
E. Verapamil

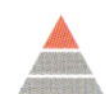 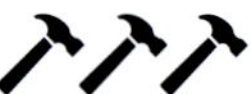

78. A 42-year-old man has fever and myalgia for 1 week. He has bilateral lower leg swelling and bibasilar crackles on chest auscultation.

Investigations:
Blood cultures: Streptococcus gallolyticus growth

Which is the most appropriate management?

A. Amoxicillin and clarithromycin
B. Benzylpenicillin and colonoscopy
C. Benzylpenicillin and Mitral Valve Replacement
D. Ceftriaxone and vancomycin
E. Dobutamine and furosemide

Gastroenterology

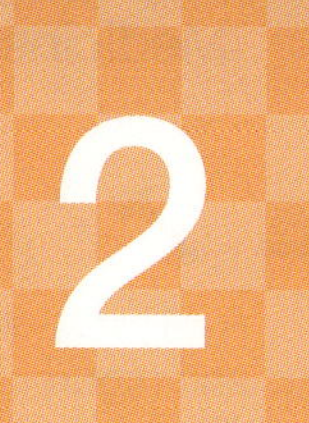

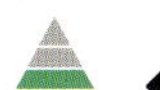 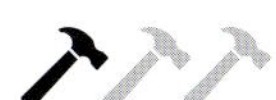

1. A 43-year-old woman has severe epigastric pain radiating to the back for 2 hours. She is diaphoretic, with epigastric tenderness and guarding.

Investigations:
Serum amylase: 1300 U/L (60-180).

Which is the most likely diagnosis?
   A. Acute cholecystitis
   B. Acute pancreatitis
   C. Aortic dissection
   D. Ascending cholangitis
   E. Myocardial infarction

 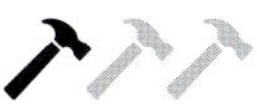

2. A 54-year-old man has sudden right upper quadrant pain radiating to his right shoulder. He has tenderness and guarding in the right upper quadrant.

Which is the most likely diagnosis?
   A. Acute cholecystitis
   B. Acute pancreatitis
   C. Ascending cholangitis
   D. Liver abscess
   E. Splenic infarct

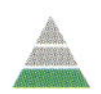 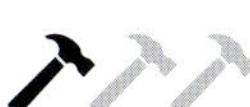

3. A 24-year-old woman has a generalized, dull ache in the lower abdomen, with nonbloody vomiting and loss of appetite for 3 hours. Her temperature is 38.4°C. She has rebound tenderness and guarding in the lower abdomen.

Investigations:
Neutrophils: 9.2×10^9/L (1.5–7.0)

Which is the most likely diagnosis?
   A. Acute appendicitis
   B. Acute cholecystitis
   C. Ectopic pregnancy
   D. Mesenteric adenitis
   E. Ovarian torsion

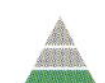  

4. A 41-year-old man has severe, intermittent right upper quadrant pain radiating to his right shoulder for 4 hours. He has tenderness and guarding in the right upper quadrant.

Investigations:
Abdominal US: stones in the gall bladder.

Which is the most appropriate definitive management?
   A. Diclofenac
   B. IV antibiotics
   C. Laparoscopic cholecystectomy
   D. Mesalazine
   E. Ursodeoxycholic acid

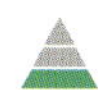 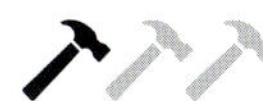

5. A 32-year-old man has had diarrhoea 5 times a day and rectal bleeding for 3 weeks. His mother had inflammatory bowel disease. He has severe abdominal pain in the left lower quadrant.

Which is the most likely diagnosis?
   A. Coeliac disease
   B. Crohn disease
   C. Gastric cancer
   D. Giardiasis
   E. Ulcerative colitis

 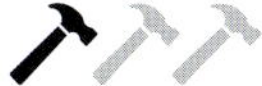

6. A 43-year-old woman has severe right upper quadrant pain radiating to her right shoulder that started after a fatty meal 2 hours ago. She has tenderness in her right upper quadrant but does not have an inspiratory arrest on palpation of the right hypochondrium.

Which is the most likely diagnosis?
   A. Acute appendicitis
   B. Acute cholecystitis
   C. Acute pancreatitis
   D. Ascending cholangitis
   E. Biliary colic

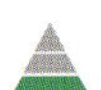 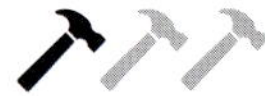

7. A 34-year-old man has recurrent central chest pain and regurgitation of food after meals, leaving an unpleasant taste. His symptoms are relieved by antacids. He has smoked 20 cigarettes a day for 20 years.

Which is the most likely diagnosis?

A. Gastric cancer
B. Gastro-oesophageal reflux disease (GORD)
C. Helicobacter pylori infection
D. Hiatus hernia
E. Peptic ulcer disease

 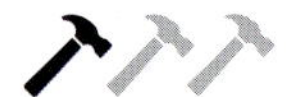

8. A 27-year-old woman has had lower abdominal pain for 1 day. Her temperature is 38.0°C. She has tenderness and guarding one-third of the distance from the anterior superior iliac spine to the umbilicus, and palpation of the left lower quadrant elicits pain in the right lower quadrant.

What would be the first change seen in the bloods of this woman?

A. Elevated C-reactive Protein (CRP)
B. Elevated Erythrocyte Sedimentation Rate (ESR)
C. Elevated neutrophils
D. Elevated serum amylase
E. Elevated temperature

9. A 21-year-old woman, who is 30 weeks pregnant, has severe abdominal pain for one day. She has yellowing of the sclera and right upper quadrant pain.

Investigations:
Alanine transaminase (ALT): 524 U/L (5–35)
Aspartate transaminase (AST): 300 U/L (1–31)

Which is the most likely diagnosis?

A. Acute fatty liver of pregnancy
B. Budd-Chiari syndrome
C. HELLP syndrome
D. Obstetric cholestasis
E. Primary biliary cirrhosis

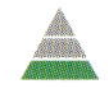 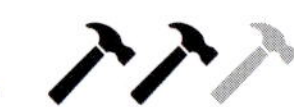

10. A 9-year-old boy has right iliac fossa pain for 2 days. He had an upper respiratory tract infection 1 week ago. His abdomen is soft, with mild tenderness in the right lower quadrant.

Which is the most likely diagnosis?

A. Acute appendicitis
B. Acute cholecystitis
C. Acute pancreatitis
D. Infectious mononucleosis
E. Mesenteric adenitis

 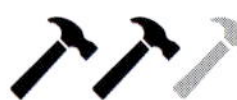 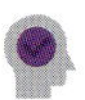

11. A 24-year-old man was found unconscious with three empty packets of paracetamol. He has depression, managed with fluoxetine. He has yellowing of his skin and sclera.

Investigations:
Prothrombin time: 28 seconds (11.5–15.5)

Which is the most appropriate management?

A. Acetylcysteine
B. Activated charcoal
C. Intravenous fluids and supportive care
D. Haemodialysis
E. Vitamin K administration

 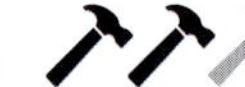 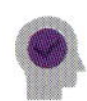

12. A 46-year-old woman has severe epigastric pain radiating through her back. She has discolouration of the flank regions and epigastric tenderness.

Investigations:
Abdominal US: stones in the bile duct

Which is the most appropriate management?

A. Creon
B. Endoscopic drainage
C. Endoscopic retrograde cholangiopancreatography (ERCP)
D. Laparoscopic cholecystectomy
E. Metronidazole

 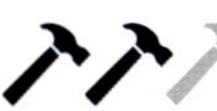 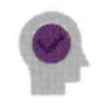

13. A 22-year-old woman has confusion and asterixis for 3 hours. She had a paracetamol overdose 3 days ago, managed with acetylcysteine. She had yellow sclera and right upper quadrant pain on presentation.

Which is the most appropriate investigation?
  A. Liver US
  B. Prothrombin time
  C. Serum alanine transaminase (ALT)
  D. Serum aspartate aminotransferase (AST)
  E. Serum gamma glutamyl transferase (GGT)

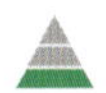 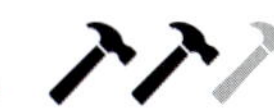 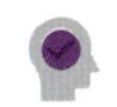

14. A 37-year-old woman has had stomach cramps and pale diarrhoea for three months. She has type 1 diabetes mellitus, managed with a basal-bolus insulin regime. She has abdominal bloating.

Investigations:
Duodenal biopsy: intraepithelial lymphocytes

Which is the most appropriate management?
  A. Gluten-free diet
  B. Mesalazine
  C. Metoclopramide
  D. Metronidazole
  E. Prednisolone

 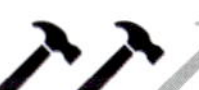

15. A 26-year-old man is confused after ingesting three full packets of paracetamol. He has yellowing of his sclera and is not oriented to time, person, or place.

Investigations:
Prothrombin time: 18.2 seconds (11.5–15.5).

What are the most likely liver function tests for this man?
  A. Alanine transaminase (ALT) high, Alkaline phosphatase (ALP) high
  B. ALT high, ALP normal
  C. ALT high, ALP low
  D. ALT high, Aspartate aminotransferase (AST) low
  E. ALT high, Gamma glutamyl transferase (GGT) high

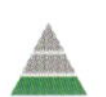 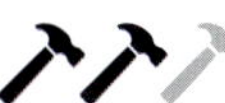

16. A 63-year-old man has sudden left lower quadrant pain and alternating constipation and diarrhoea. He has tenderness and guarding in the left lower quadrant and has reduced bowel sounds.

Investigations:
White cell count: 14.2 x 10^9/L (3.0–10.0).

Which is the most likely diagnosis?
  A. Anal cancer
  B. Acute diverticulitis
  C. Crohn disease
  D. Sigmoid colon tumour
  E. Ulcerative Colitis

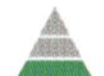 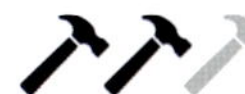 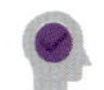

17. A 71-year-old woman has had unintentional weight loss and muscle weakness for 5 months. She also has a poor appetite and has decreased food intake. She has a BMI of 17 kg/m^2 and has muscular wasting and generalized weakness throughout the body.

Which is the most appropriate prognostic tool?
  A. Alvarado Score
  B. Child-Pugh Score
  C. Glasgow-Blatchford Score
  D. Maddrey Discriminant function
  E. Malnutrition Universal Screening Tool

 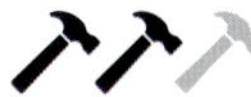 

18. A 31-year-old man has bloody diarrhoea, an urgency to defecate and left lower quadrant pain for 6 months. He has bilaterally tender red nodules on his shins and tenderness in the left lower quadrant.

Which is the most appropriate diagnostic investigation?
  A. Abdominal X-ray
  B. Colonoscopy and biopsy
  C. CT abdomen
  D. Jejunal biopsy
  E. US abdomen

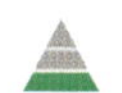 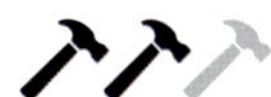 

19. A 43-year-old man has had non-bloody diarrhoea and weight loss for 6 months. He has tenderness in his right lower quadrant and perianal skin tags.

Investigations:
Colonic biopsy: noncaseating granuloma and serosal inflammation.

Which is the most appropriate management?

A. Gluten-free diet
B. Mesalazine
C. Metronidazole
D. Paracetamol
E. Prednisolone

 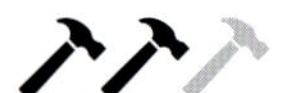 

20. A 47-year-old man has recurrent retrosternal discomfort and difficulty swallowing solids for 5 months. His symptoms are exacerbated by meals and when lying down. He has tried losing weight and avoiding spicy food, which have not solved his symptoms.

Which is the most appropriate management?

A. Amoxicillin, clarithromycin and metronidazole
B. Omeprazole
C. Metoclopramide
D. Pneumatic dilatation via oesophagogastroduodenoscopy (OGD)
E. Ranitidine

 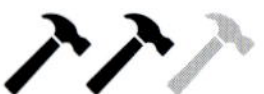 

21. A 34-year-old woman has had recurrent abdominal pain and changes in her bowel habits for 6 months. Her bowel movements alternate between diarrhoea constipation, and abdominal bloating. She is primarily concerned about her episodes of diarrhoea and how it affects her daily activities.

Which is the most appropriate management?

A. Amitriptyline
B. Isphagula husk
C. Lactulose
D. Loperamide
E. Senna

22. A 47-year-old man has had fatigue and itching for a month. He has yellowing of his sclera and the liver is palpated 4 cm below the costal margin.

Investigations:
Endoscopic retrograde cholangiopancreatography (ERCP): multiple biliary strictures

Which is the most likely diagnosis?

A. Autoimmune hepatitis
B. Cholangiocarcinoma
C. Crohn disease
D. Primary biliary cirrhosis
E. Primary sclerosing cholangitis

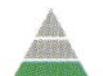 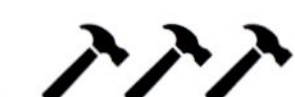

23. A 28-year-old man has had fatigue and diarrhoea for 4 months. He has Hashimoto thyroiditis, managed with levothyroxine. He has pruritic, vesicular skin lesions on his elbows and knees.

Investigations:
Serum IgA: 0.6 g/L (0.8–3.0)
IgA tissue transglutaminase: 13.9U/mL (<15).

What is the skin lesion that he has?

A. Dermatitis herpetiformis
B. Eczema
C. Pemphigus vulgaris
D. Psoriasis
E. Pyoderma gangrenosum

 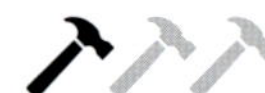

24. A 61-year-old woman has right upper quadrant pain and a mild fever for 5 hours. Her temperature is 38.7°C. She has yellowing of her sclera and tenderness and rigidity in the right upper quadrant.

Investigations:
AXR: stones in the bile duct.

Which is the most likely diagnosis?

A. Acute cholecystitis
B. Acute pyelonephritis
C. Ascending cholangitis
D. Gallstone ileus
E. Liver abscess

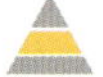 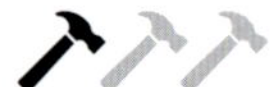

25. A 44-year-old woman has had right upper quadrant pain and abdominal swelling for 1 month. She has yellowing of her sclera, leukonychia, visible blood vessels on the abdomen and shifting dullness.

Investigations:
Alanine transaminase (ALT): 43 U/L (5-35)
Aspartate transaminase (AST): 146 U/L (1-31)

Which is the most likely diagnosis?
A. Acute liver failure
B. Haemochromatosis
C. Hepatocellular carcinoma
D. Liver cirrhosis
E. Wilson disease

26. An 18-year-old man has a sore throat and left upper quadrant pain for 1 week. His temperature is 38.3°C. He has lymphadenopathy in the cervical and axillary regions.

Which is the most likely diagnosis?
A. Diverticulitis
B. Duodenal ulcer
C. Gastritis
D. Infectious mononucleosis
E. Mesenteric adenitis

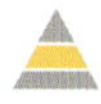 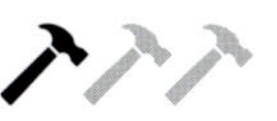 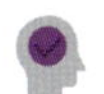

27. A 32-year-old woman has generalized abdominal pain, watery diarrhoea, and persistent vomiting for 24 hours. She denies any recent travel or exposure to sick contacts. She is lethargic and has diffuse tenderness and hyperactive bowel sounds but no guarding or rebound tenderness.

Which is the most appropriate management?
A. Bed rest and oral rehydration solution
B. Call an ambulance and admitted to the hospital
C. IV fluids + IV antibiotics
D. Oral antibiotics
E. Refer to a gastroenterologist for further investigation

 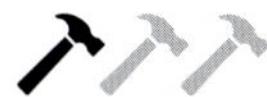

28. A 45-year-old man has had fatigue, nausea, and abdominal discomfort for 3 weeks. He has a history of IV drug use and unprotected sexual activity with multiple partners. He has yellowing of his skin and an enlarged, tender liver.

Investigations:
Complement levels: low C4

Which is the most likely diagnosis?
A. Hepatitis A
B. Hepatitis B
C. Hepatitis C
D. Hepatitis D
E. Hepatitis E

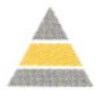 

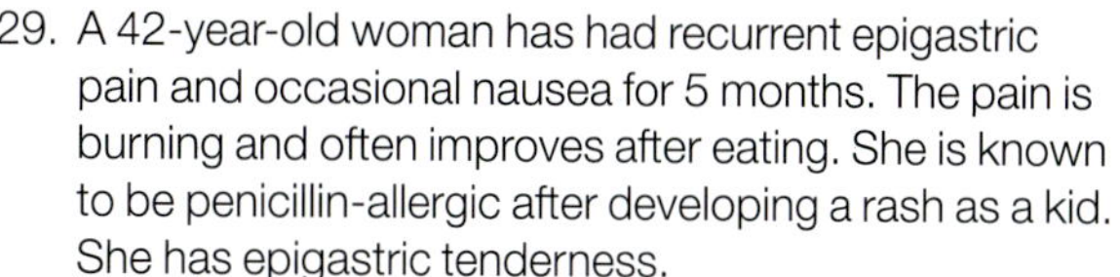

29. A 42-year-old woman has had recurrent epigastric pain and occasional nausea for 5 months. The pain is burning and often improves after eating. She is known to be penicillin-allergic after developing a rash as a kid. She has epigastric tenderness.

Investigations:
Urea breath test: positive

Which is the most appropriate management?
A. Omeprazole
B. Omeprazole, amoxicillin + clarithromycin
C. Omeprazole + bismuth
D. Omeprazole, clarithromycin + metronidazole
E. Omeprazole + levofloxacin

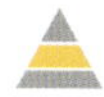 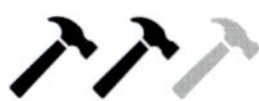

30. A 28-year-old woman has had a dull, frontal headache and diarrhoea for 5 days. She recently returned from a trip to South Asia where she had street food. Her temperature is 38.9°C. She has blanching erythematous maculopapular lesions on her chest and diffuse abdominal tenderness.

Which is the most likely diagnosis?
A. Brucellosis
B. Dengue fever
C. Infectious mononucleosis
D. Norovirus
E. Typhoid fever

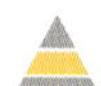 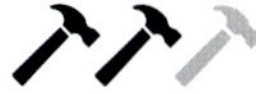

31. A 32-year-old woman has persistent epigastric pain and unintentional weight loss of 9 kg for four months. She is pale and has epigastric tenderness.

Investigations:
OGD: Large, ulcerated mass in the pyloric antrum.

Which is the most likely diagnosis?
A. Acute pancreatitis
B. Duodenal ulcer
C. Gastric cancer
D. Gastric ulcer
E. Pancreatic cancer

 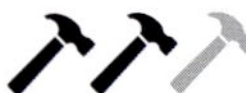

32. A 47-year-old man has had intermittent right upper quadrant pain for 24 hours. He has biliary colic but has never had pain as severe as this. His temperature is 38.2°C. He has yellowing of his sclera and right upper quadrant tenderness.

Which is the most likely cause?
   A. *Campylobacter jejuni*
   B. *Clostridium difficile*
   C. *Enterobacter cloacae*
   D. *Enterococcus faecalis*
   E. *Escherichia coli*

 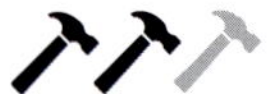 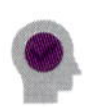

33. A 47-year-old woman has sudden severe epigastric pain that has progressively worsened. She has recurrent peptic ulcers, but her pain is typically mild. Her pulse is 120 bpm, and BP is 87/58 mmHg. She has guarding and rebound tenderness of the epigastric region.

Which is the most appropriate initial investigation?
   A. Chest x-ray
   B. CT abdomen
   C. Gastric biopsy
   D. Oesophagogastroduodenoscopy (OGD)
   E. US abdomen

 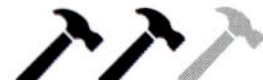

34. A 54-year-old woman has fatigue and numbness in her hands and feet for 2 months. She has type 1 diabetes mellitus, managed with a basal-bolus insulin regime.

Investigations:
Blood Film: Macrocytic hypochromic cells

Which is the most likely diagnosis?
   A. Anaemia of chronic disease
   B. Vitamin B1 deficiency
   C. Vitamin B3 deficiency
   D. Vitamin B6 deficiency
   E. Vitamin B12 deficiency

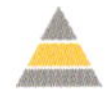 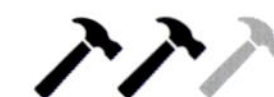 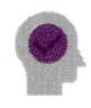

35. A 19-year-old man has had difficulty writing and slurred speech for 4 months. He is aggressive, with a resting tremor bilaterally.

Investigations:
Alanine transaminase (ALT): 49 U/L (5–35)
Aspartate transaminase (AST): 53 U/L (1–31)

Which is the most appropriate investigation?
   A. Liver US
   B. Prothrombin time
   C. Serum caeruloplasmin
   D. Transferrin saturation
   E. Transient elastography

 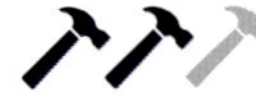 

36. A 64-year-old man has persistent epigastric pain and unintentional weight loss of 5 kg for 2 months. He has mild epigastric tenderness and a palpable left supraclavicular lymph node.

Investigations:
OGD: large, ulcerated mass in the pyloric antrum.

Which is the most appropriate management?
   A. Chemotherapy
   B. Omeprazole
   C. Radiofrequency ablation
   D. Subtotal gastrectomy
   E. Sleeve gastrectomy

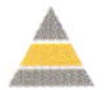 

37. A 38-year-old woman has difficulty swallowing both solids and liquids and a foul taste in her mouth after eating meals for 5 months.

Investigations:
Barium Swallow: grossly expanded distal oesophagus with tapering at the gastroesophageal junction

Which is the most likely diagnosis?
   A. Achalasia
   B. Boerhaave syndrome
   C. Hiatus hernia
   D. Oesophageal cancer
   E. Pharyngeal pouch

 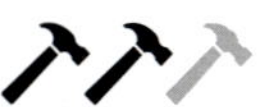 

38. A 50-year-old man has back pain and unintentional weight loss of 5 kg for 2 months. He has smoked 10 cigarettes a day for 20 years. He has a yellow tinge to his sclera and a palpable gall bladder.

Which is the most appropriate diagnostic investigation?
A. CA 19-9
B. CT pancreas
C. Liver US
D. Oesophagogastroduodenoscopy
E. Serum lipase

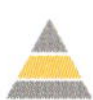 

39. A 45-year-old woman has had generalized joint pain and right upper quadrant pain for two months and gradual darkening of her skin. She has hepatomegaly.

Which is the most likely diagnosis?
A. Acute liver failure
B. Haemochromatosis
C. Hepatocellular carcinoma
D. Liver cirrhosis
E. Wilson disease

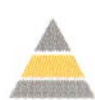 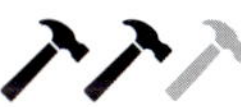 

40. A 24-year-old woman has severe abdominal pain, inability to pass stool or flatus and bilious vomiting for 1 day. She had acute appendicitis a year ago, managed with a laparoscopic appendectomy. She has abdominal distension and high-pitched bowel sounds.

Which is the most appropriate diagnostic investigation?
A. Beta-hCG
B. Chest X-ray
C. CT abdomen
D. Serum lactate
E. US abdomen

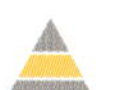  

41. A 43-year-old homeless man has muscle and joint pains and mild abdominal discomfort for 1 week. He has a history of intravenous drug use for two years and drinks 15 units of alcohol per week. He has yellowing of his sclera and mild hepatomegaly.

Investigations:
HBsAg: positive
Anti-Hbs: negative
IgM anti-Hbc: positive

Which is the most likely diagnosis?
A. Acute hepatitis B infection
B. Alcoholic liver disease
C. Chronic hepatitis B infection
D. Hepatitis C infection
E. Previous hepatitis B vaccination

 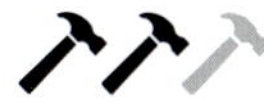 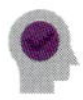

42. A 73-year-old man has oily, foul-smelling stools that are difficult to flush away and unintentional weight loss of 7 kg for three months. He has yellowing of his sclera and has a palpable gall bladder.

Investigations:
CT Pancreas: pancreatic malignancy at the head of the pancreas; staged as T2N0M0.

Which is the most appropriate management?
A. Chemoradiotherapy
B. Creon
C. Endoscopic stent insertion
D. Immunotherapy
E. Surgical resection

 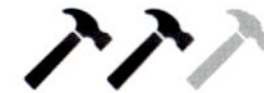 

43. A 41-year-old woman has had irregular menstrual periods and fatigue for 4 months. She has type 1 diabetes mellitus, managed with a basal-bolus insulin regime. She has visible blood vessels on the abdomen and hepatomegaly.

Investigations:
Antinuclear antibodies (ANA): positive
Anti-smooth muscle antibodies (SMA): positive

Which blood test is most likely to be positive?
A. Antiliver/kidney microsomal type 1 (anti-LKM1) antibodies
B. Antimitochondrial (AMA) antibodies
C. Antineutrophil cytoplasmic (cANCA) antibodies
D. Antismooth muscle (SMA) antibodies
E. Perinuclear antineutrophil cytoplasmic (pANCA) antibodies

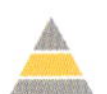 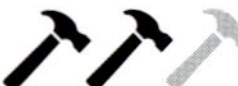 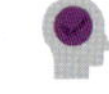

44. A 69-year-old woman has difficulty swallowing solids and liquids, progressively worsening for 4 months. She has lost 6 kg of weight unintentionally and had blood in her vomit. She has mild cervical lymphadenopathy.

Investigations:
Upper GI endoscopy with biopsy: T1N0M0 lesion in the lower third of the oesophagus.

Which is the most appropriate management?
A. Endoscopic diverticulectomy
B. Ivor-Lewis oesophagectomy
C. Omeprazole
D. Pneumatic dilation
E. Thoracotomy and stent placement

 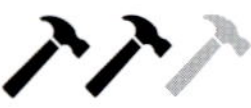 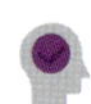

45. A 38-year-old woman has had constant, dull epigastric pain radiating to the back for 2 years. She drinks around 30 units of alcohol per week. She is malnourished and has a palpable, tender mass in the epigastrium.

Investigations:
AXR: calcifications throughout the pancreas.

Which is the most appropriate management?
A. Coeliac plexus block
B. Creon
C. Endoscopic decompression
D. Distal pancreatectomy
E. Laparoscopic Cholecystectomy

46. A 44-year-old man has painful swallowing solids and liquids, progressively worsening for 6 months.

Investigations:
Barium swallow: dilated distal oesophagus with tapering at the gastroesophageal junction

Which is the most appropriate first-line management?
A. Chemotherapy
B. Heller cardiomyotomy
C. Omeprazole
D. Pneumatic dilatation
E. Thoracotomy and stent placement

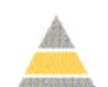 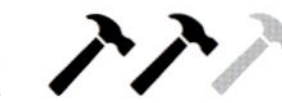 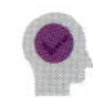

47. A 53-year-old woman has right upper quadrant pain and unintentional weight loss of 8 kg for 4 months. She has a chronic hepatitis B infection. She has yellowing of her sclera and hepatomegaly.

Investigations:
Serum alpha-fetoprotein (AFP): elevated

Which is the most appropriate diagnostic investigation?
A. Liver biopsy
B. Liver CT
C. Liver US
D. Prothrombin time
E. Transient elastography

 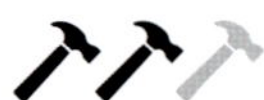

48. A 45-year-old man has fatigue and right upper quadrant discomfort for 2 months. He has type 2 diabetes mellitus, managed with metformin and empagliflozin. His liver is palpable 5 cm below the costal margin.

Investigations:
Liver US: diffuse hyperechoic echotexture

Which is the most appropriate diagnostic investigation?
A. CT abdomen
B. Enhanced liver fibrosis blood test
C. Prothrombin time
D. Serum amylase
E. Transient elastography

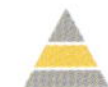 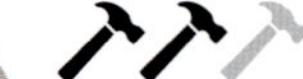 

49. An 82-year-old woman has abdominal bloating and cannot pass stool for 2 weeks. She has infrequent bowel movements with the stool consistency being hard. She had an elective left hemiarthroplasty 3 weeks ago and has been managing her pain with oxycodone. She has generalized abdominal discomfort.

Which is the most appropriate management?
A. Bisacodyl and docusate suppository
B. Ispaghula husk and senna
C. Ispaghula husk and macrogol
D. Macrogol and senna
E. Sodium phosphate enema and senna

 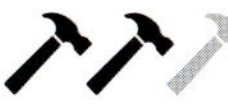

50. A 57-year-old man has had frequent heartburn and a sour taste in his mouth after meals for 8 months. He has been trying to manage this with over-the-counter antacids, which has not provided symptomatic relief. His BMI is 32 kg/m^2.

Investigations:
OGD: columnar epithelium in the oesophagus with irregular mucosal pits

Which is the correct time period for endoscopic surveillance in the first year?
A. Every 1 month
B. Every 2 months
C. Every 3 months
D. Every 6 months
E. Every 12 months

51. A 52-year-old woman has had right upper quadrant pain for 3 months. She has 40 units of alcohol per week. She has abdominal tenderness around the right upper quadrant.

Investigations:
Alanine transaminase (ALT): 42 U/L (5–35)
Aspartate transaminase (AST): 138 U/L (1–31)
Gamma-glutamyl transferase (GGT): 76 U/L (4–35)

Which is the most appropriate management?
A. Cholestyramine
B. Desferrioxamine
C. Penicillamine
D. Prednisolone
E. Ursodeoxycholic acid

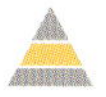 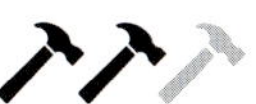 

52. A 37-year-old man has had pain in his hands and erectile dysfunction for 2 months. Both his parents had liver issues when he was younger. He has skin hyperpigmentation and the liver is palpable 4 cm below the costal margin.

Investigations:
Liver MRI: abnormally low liver signal

Which is the most appropriate management?
A. Hepatic vein angioplasty
B. Octreotide
C. Surgical resection
D. Ursodeoxycholic acid
E. Venesection

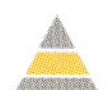  

53. A 68-year-old woman has severe right upper quadrant pain and abdominal swelling. She has cirrhosis secondary to chronic alcohol misuse. Her temperature is 38.7°C. She has shifting dullness.

Which is the most appropriate diagnostic investigation?
A. Abdominal US
B. CT abdomen
C. Liver function tests
D. Paracentesis
E. Serum lipase

 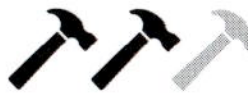 

54. A 62-year-old woman has non-bloody diarrhoea and generalized abdominal pain. She had a urinary tract infection 2 weeks ago, managed with ciprofloxacin. Her BP is 84/57 mmHg.

Investigations:
Stool sample: clostridium difficile toxin positive.

Which is the most appropriate management?
A. IV vancomycin + oral metronidazole
B. Oral fidaxomicin
C. Oral metronidazole
D. Oral vancomycin
E. Oral vancomycin + IV metronidazole

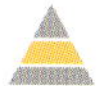 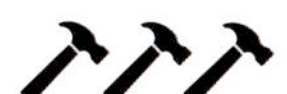 

55. A 34-year-old man has had painful swallowing and the sensation of food getting stuck in his chest for 5 months, especially when eating dry foods. He has allergic rhinitis, managed with nasal fluticasone. He has constant chest discomfort, even at rest, that he attributes to the narrowing of his windpipe.

Investigations:
OGD: white mucosal plaques with oesophageal stenosis

Which is the most appropriate definitive management?
A. Endoscopic dilation
B. Heller cardiomyotomy
C. Oesophageal stent
D. Omeprazole
E. Oral budesonide

 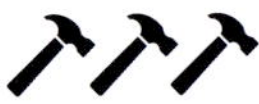 

56. A 65-year-old has had abdominal swelling and right upper quadrant pain for 4 days. He has advanced cirrhosis. He has shifting dullness.

Investigations:
Ascitic tap: protein concentration of 14 g/L; no organisms.

Which is the most appropriate prophylaxis?
A. IV cefotaxime
B. IV ciprofloxacin
C. No prophylaxis needed
D. Oral azithromycin
E. Oral ciprofloxacin

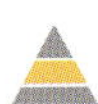  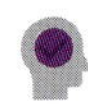

57. A 54-year-old woman has had right upper quadrant pain and abdominal swelling for 6 weeks. She has been drinking 45 units of alcohol per week. She has a fine tremor bilaterally in her hands, shifting dullness, and her breath smells sweet.

Which is the most appropriate diagnostic investigation?
A. Abdominal US
B. Enhanced liver fibrosis blood test
C. Liver biopsy
D. Paracentesis
E. Transient elastography

58. An 84-year-old woman had nonbloody diarrhoea and colicky abdominal pain for 5 days, after an elective right hemiarthroplasty a week ago. She had amoxicillin-associated diarrhoea 6 weeks ago, managed with vancomycin, She has generalised abdominal tenderness.

Which is the most appropriate management?
A. IV metronidazole
B. IV vancomycin
C. Oral fidaxomicin
D. Oral metronidazole
E. Oral vancomycin

59. A 24-year-old man has recurrent episodes of jaundice, that he notices after playing football every Sunday. He has no family history of liver disease.

Investigations:
Serum total bilirubin: 20.5 μmol/L (1–22)
Serum unconjugated bilirubin: elevated

Which is the most likely enzyme deficiency?
A. Glucuronosyl transferase/UDP-glucoronyl transferase
B. Glutathione peroxidase
C. Glutathione S-transferase
D. Glucokinase
E. Glucose-6-phosphate dehydrogenase

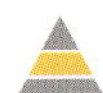 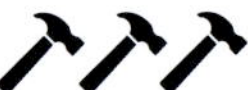

60. A 49-year-old woman is due for a hepatitis B vaccination as her husband was diagnosed with hepatitis B two weeks ago. She is unsure whether she has had a hepatitis B vaccination in the past, as she only moved to the UK 5 years ago.

	HBsAg	Anti-HBs	Anti-HBc
A	Positive	Negative	Positive
B	Negative	Positive	Positive
C	Positive	Positive	Negative
D	Negative	Negative	Negative
E	Negative	Positive	Negative

Which is associated with previous hepatitis B immunisation?
A. A
B. B
C. C
D. D
E. E

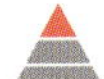 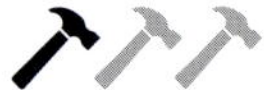

61. A 69-year-old man has had difficulty swallowing solids, bad breath and a feeling of a lump in his throat for 3 months. He has a palpable mass in the neck at the level of the cricoid cartilage.

Which is the most likely diagnosis?
A. Achalasia
B. Boerhaave syndrome
C. Hiatus hernia
D. Oesophageal cancer
E. Pharyngeal pouch

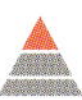 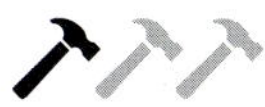

62. A 52-year-old woman has fatigue and itching for 5 months. She has rheumatoid arthritis, managed with methotrexate. She has xanthelasma on her eyelids and hepatomegaly.

Investigations:
Antimitochondrial (AMA) M2 subtype antibodies: positive
Serum IgM: elevated
Liver biopsy: lymphocytic infiltration and destruction of the small bile ducts.

Which is the most likely diagnosis?
A. Acute cholecystitis
B. Ascending cholangitis
C. Autoimmune hepatitis
D. Primary biliary cirrhosis
E. Primary sclerosing cholangitis

63. A 52-year-old man has confusion and increased bowel movements for 1 week, going to the toilet at least four times daily. He has a scaly, erythematous rash on his hands and is not oriented to time, place, or person.

Which is the most likely diagnosis?
A. Vitamin B1 deficiency
B. Vitamin B3 deficiency
C. Vitamin B6 deficiency
D. Vitamin B12 deficiency
E. Vitamin C deficiency

 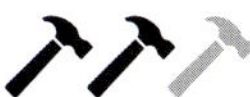

64. A 59-year-old woman with a background of constipation presents for a postcolonoscopy consultation because incidental polyps were found in her colon.

Investigations:
Colonoscopy: abnormal pigmentation of the colon, with periodic acid-Schiff staining showing pigment-laden macrophages within the mucosa.

Which is the most likely cause?
A. Autoimmune
B. Cephalosporin abuse
C. Idiopathic
D. Laxative abuse
E. Premalignancy

 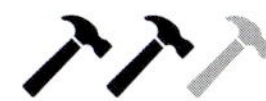 

65. A 40-year-old man has diarrhoea, epigastric pain, and unintentional weight loss of 4 kg for three months. His stools are bulky and malodorous. The man has ankle swelling, and tender hepatomegaly, and his skin has got noticeably darker.

Which is the most appropriate diagnostic investigation?
A. Chest X-ray
B. Colonoscopy
C. CT abdomen
D. Liver US
E. Jejunal biopsy

 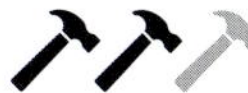

66. A 48-year-old woman has severe right upper quadrant pain and bilious vomiting for 48 hours. She also has not passed stool and has abdominal distension.

Investigations:
AXR: small bowel diameter of 5 cm, air within the biliary system and a calcified gallstone outside the gall bladder.

Which is the most likely diagnosis?
A. Acute cholecystitis
B. Chronic pancreatitis
C. Gallstone ileus
D. Mirizzi syndrome
E. Sigmoid volvulus

67. A 2-year-old girl has severe, cramping abdominal pain, intermittent vomiting and jelly-like blood in her stool for 2 days. She has a tender abdomen with guarding; however, there is no organomegaly.

Investigations:
AXR: mass in the right upper quadrant.

Which is the most appropriate diagnostic investigation?
A. Abdominal US
B. Barium enema
C. CT abdomen
D. Chest X-ray
E. Stool microscopy and culture

 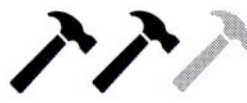 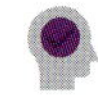

68. A 40-year-old woman has diarrhoea with floating stools for 5 months. She had a laparoscopic cholecystectomy six months ago.

Investigations:
SeHCAT scan: 12% SeHCAT retention after seven days.

Which is the most appropriate management?
A. Cholestyramine
B. Creon
C. Loperamide
D. Senna
E. Ursodeoxycholic Acid

69. A 19-year-old woman has severe muscle weakness and shortness of breath for 2 hours. She has anorexia nervosa, for which she was started on nutritional rehabilitation in the hospital.

Which is the most likely electrolyte abnormality?
A. Hyperkalaemia
B. Hypernatremia
C. Hypocalcemia
D. Hypomagnesaemia
E. Hypophosphataemia

  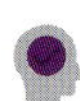

70. A 67-year-old woman has difficulty swallowing, especially with solid food and a feeling of a lump in his throat for 5 months. She has halitosis and a palpable mass in the neck at the level of the cricoid cartilage.

Investigations:
Barium swallow: outpouching of the posterior hypopharyngeal wall.

Which is the most appropriate management?
A. Endoscopic diverticulectomy
B. Ivor-Lewis oesophagectomy
C. Omeprazole
D. Pneumatic dilation
E. Watchful waiting

 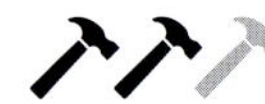

71. A 34-year-old woman has sudden central, tearing chest pain. She had food poisoning for 24 hours, and since then, she has been vomiting every 2 hours. She has dry mucous membranes and chest crepitations on palpation of the chest wall.

Investigations:
CT contrast swallow: rupture distally sited on the left side of the oesophagus.

Which is the most likely diagnosis?
A. Aortic dissection
B. Achalasia
C. Boerhaave syndrome
D. Hiatus hernia
E. Mallory-Weiss tear

72. An 80-year-old woman has severe, sudden right upper quadrant pain and abdominal swelling. She has a palpable mass in the right upper quadrant and generalized abdominal tenderness.

Investigations:
AXR: dilated small bowel loops, pneumobilia, and a radiopaque gallstone.

Which is the most appropriate management?
A. Enterolithotomy
B. IV antibiotics
C. Laparoscopic cholecystectomy
D. Prednisolone
E. Ursodeoxycholic acid

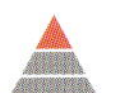 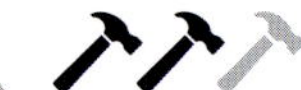 

73. A 36-year-old woman has sudden, severe abdominal pain and abdominal swelling. She has premenstrual syndrome, managed with the combined oral contraceptive pill. She has tender hepatomegaly and shifting dullness on the percussion of her abdomen.

Which is the most appropriate management?
A. Hepatic vein angioplasty
B. Octreotide
C. Percutaneous drainage
D. Surgical resection
E. Venesection

 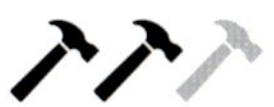 

74. A 42-year-old man has severe chest pain radiating to his back that started after forceful vomiting for 4 hours. He had 20 units of alcohol preceding the vomiting episode. He has crepitations on palpation of the neck and chest.

Investigations:
CT contrast swallow: distally sited rupture on the left side of the oesophagus.

Which is the most appropriate management?
   A. Endoscopic diverticulectomy
   B. Ivor-Lewis oesophagectomy
   C. Oesophageal stent placement
   D. Primary oesophageal repair
   E. Pneumatic dilation

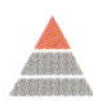 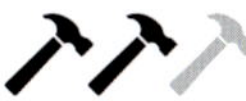

75. A 49-year-old woman has difficulty swallowing and a sensation of food being stuck in her throat for 6 months. She is pale and her tongue appears inflamed.

Investigations:
Blood film: microcytic, hypochromic cells

Which is the most likely diagnosis?
   A. Achalasia
   B. Barrett oesophagus
   C. Chagas disease
   D. Oesophageal stricture
   E. Plummer-Vinson syndrome

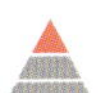 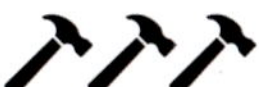 

76. A 45-year-old man has had persistent epigastric pain and diarrhoea for 2 months. He has recurrent peptic ulcers, resistant to proton pump inhibitors treatment. He has yellowing of his sclera and tenderness in the epigastric region.

Which is the appropriate diagnostic investigation?
   A. Chest X-ray
   B. CT abdomen
   C. Fasting gastrin level
   D. Oesophago-gastro-duodenoscopy (OGD):
   E. Stool culture

 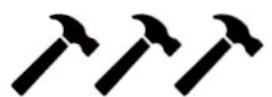

77. A 45-year-old man has right upper quadrant pain and jaundice for 1 week. He has recurrent episodes of pyogenic cholangitis. His temperature is 38.6°C. His liver edge is palpable 3 cm below the costal margin and he has right upper quadrant tenderness.

Investigations:
Liver CT: central, fluid-filled low attenuation lesion is surrounded by a high attenuation inner rim and a low attenuation outer rim

Which is the most likely causative organism?
   A. *Escherichia coli*
   B. *Klebsiella pneumoniae*
   C. *Salmonella typhi*
   D. *Staphylococcus aureus*
   E. *Streptococcus pneumoniae*

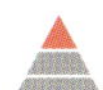 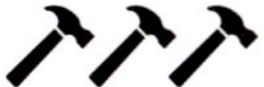 

78. A 52-year-old woman has had diarrhoea and abdominal discomfort every day for 4 months. She has recurrent urinary tract infections (UTIs), managed with broad-spectrum antibiotics. She has abdominal bloating.

Investigations:
Hydrogen Breath Test: positive

Which is the most appropriate management?
   A. Amoxicillin
   B. Ciprofloxacin
   C. Co-trimoxazole
   D. Rifaximin
   E. Vancomycin

 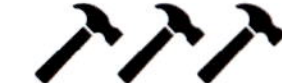

79. A 3-day-old boy has abdominal distension and failure to pass meconium since birth. He has a palpable faecal mass in the lower abdomen and a digital rectal examination shows an empty rectal vault.

What is the pathophysiology of the likely diagnosis?
   A. Abnormal development of the circular and longitudinal colonic muscle layers
   B. Absence of ganglion cells in the myenteric and submucosal plexus
   C. Mutation in the CFTR gene
   D. Hypertrophy of the pyloric sphincter
   E. Intestinal malrotation in utero

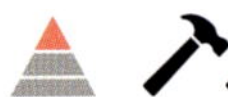 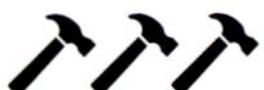 

80. A 42-year-old man has had confusion and malodorous diarrhoea for 1 week. He has asthma managed with salbutamol and beclomethasone inhalers. He has ophthalmoplegia and noticeable hyperpigmentation of his skin.

Investigations:
Jejunal biopsy: deposition of macrophages containing Periodic acid-Schiff granules.

Which is the most appropriate management?

A. Oral amoxicillin
B. Oral ciprofloxacin
C. Oral co-trimoxazole
D. Oral piperacillin-tazobactam
E. Oral vancomycin

Respiratory

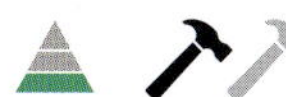

1. A 56-year-old woman with recurrent respiratory infections has had a productive cough with purulent sputum and occasional blood in her sputum for 2 years. She has bilateral finger clubbing and bilateral coarse crepitations on chest auscultation.

Investigations:
CXR: dilated, thickened bronchial walls with tramline markings.

Which is the most likely diagnosis?
A. Asthma
B. Bronchiectasis
C. Extrinsic allergic alveolitis
D. Idiopathic pulmonary fibrosis
E. Psittacosis

 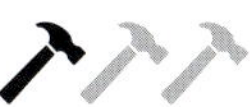

2. A 21-year-old woman has pleuritic chest pain and shortness of breath for 2 hours. She has smoked 20 cigarettes a day for 7 years. She has decreased breath sounds and hyperresonant percussion on her right chest auscultation.

Investigations:
CXR: absence of lung markings on the right chest.

Which is the most likely diagnosis?
A. Chronic obstructive pulmonary disease
B. Lung cancer
C. Obstructive sleep apnoea
D. Pneumonia
E. Pneumothorax

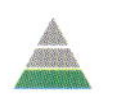 

3. A 33-year-old man has recurrent sudden breathlessness and wheezing, worse in cold weather. He has atopic dermatitis, managed with topical hydrocortisone. He has a bilateral expiratory wheeze on chest auscultation.

Investigations:
FeNO: 45 parts per billion (>40)

Which is the most likely diagnosis?
A. Asthma
B. Bronchiectasis
C. Extrinsic allergic alveolitis
D. Idiopathic pulmonary fibrosis
E. Psittacosis

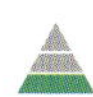 

4. A 62-year-old woman has had worsening breathlessness and a productive cough for 2 years. She has smoked 20 cigarettes a day for 40 years. She has an expiratory bilateral wheeze on chest auscultation.

Which is the most likely diagnosis?
A. Asthma
B. Bronchiectasis
C. Chronic obstructive pulmonary disease
D. COVID-19
E. Influenza

 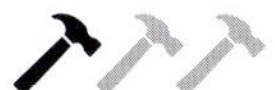 

5. A 21-year-old woman has had breathlessness and cough, worse at night, for 6 months. She has atopic dermatitis, managed with topical betamethasone. She has a bilateral expiratory wheeze on chest auscultation.

Investigations:
PEFR: >20% diurnal variation.

Which is the most appropriate management?
A. Beclomethasone
B. Doxycycline
C. Montelukast
D. Pirfenidone
E. Salbutamol

 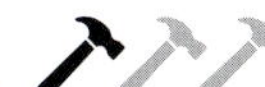 

6. A 29-year-old man has a severe headache and muscle aches for 36 hours. His temperature is 38.9°C. He has mild pharyngeal erythema.

Investigations:
Rapid antigen testing: positive for influenza A respiratory pathogens.

Which is the appropriate management?

A. Amoxicillin
B. Doxycycline
C. Oseltamivir
D. Prednisolone
E. Salbutamol

7. A 54-year-old man has had a fever and shortness of breath for a week. He has no recent foreign travel. He has bilateral crepitations on chest auscultation.

Investigations:
Nasopharyngeal swab PCR testing: positive for severe acute respiratory syndrome coronavirus 2 (SARS-CoV-2).

Which is the most likely diagnosis?

A. Asthma
B. Bronchiectasis
C. Chronic obstructive pulmonary disease
D. COVID-19
E. Influenza

 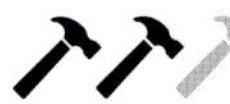 

8. A 41-year-old woman has had a cough producing copious yellow-green sputum for 4 years. He has recurrent respiratory infections, managed with antibiotics. She has bilateral finger clubbing, with bilateral coarse crepitations and an expiratory wheeze on chest auscultation.

Which are the most likely imaging findings?

A. Bilateral hilar lymphadenopathy
B. Bilateral reticular opacities
C. Egg-shell calcification of the hilar lymph nodes
D. Lower zone fibrosis
E. Signet ring sign

9. A 62-year-old woman has progressive shortness of breath and a chronic, productive cough for 2 years. She has smoked 20 cigarettes a day for 45 years. She has a bilateral expiratory wheeze on chest auscultation.

Which is the most appropriate investigation?

A. Chest X-ray
B. CT chest
C. Polysomnography
D. Postbronchodilator spirometry
E. Sputum culture

 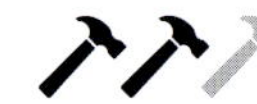

10. A 21-year-old man has severe breathlessness for 30 minutes. He has asthma, managed with salbutamol and beclomethasone inhalers. His pulse is 126 bpm, and respiratory rate 28 breaths per minute. He is unable to complete full sentences and has a bilateral expiratory wheeze on chest auscultation.

Investigations:
CXR: subcutaneous air.

Which is the most likely peak expiratory flow findings?

A. 0%–17%
B. 17%–33%
C. 33%–50%
D. 50%–75%
E. 75%–100%

 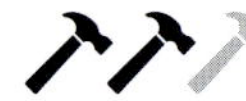 

11. A 32-year-old man has had a persistent cough with purulent sputum and shortness of breath for 9 months. He has bilateral coarse crepitations on chest auscultation.

Investigations:
CT chest: enlarged bronchi with the signet ring sign.

Which is the most appropriate management?

A. Avoid precipitating factors
B. Doxycycline
C. Inspiratory muscle training
D. IV antibiotics
E. Pirfenidone

 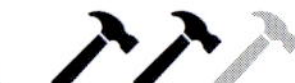 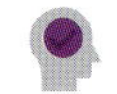

12. A 22-year-old woman with Marfan syndrome has sudden chest pain worse on inspiration and shortness of breath. She has decreased breath sounds and hyperresonance to percussion on her right chest auscultation.

Which is the most appropriate investigation?

A. Chest X-ray
B. CT chest
C. Polysomnography
D. Postbronchodilator spirometry
E. Sputum culture

 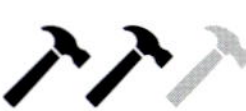 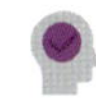

13. A 28-year-old woman has severe shortness of breath and chest tightness for 4 hours. She has asthma, managed with a salbutamol inhaler, which has not improved her symptoms. Her pulse is 90 bpm, and respiratory rate 30 breaths per minute. She has increased work of breathing and a bilateral expiratory wheeze on chest auscultation.

Investigations:
pH: 7.27 (7.35–7.45).
PO_2: 11.8 kPa (11.3–12.6).
PCO_2: 7.1 kPa (4.7–6.0).
Bicarbonate: 26 mmol/L (21–29).

Which is the most appropriate interpretation of her ABG?
A. Metabolic acidosis
B. Metabolic alkalosis
C. Respiratory acidosis
D. Respiratory alkalosis
E. Normal

14. A 16-year-old boy has chest pain after a stab wound in the right chest. He has absent breath sounds and hyperresonance to percussion on the right chest.

Investigations:
CXR: left tracheal deviation and loss of lung markings on the right.

Which is the most likely diagnosis?
A. Bronchiectasis
B. Idiopathic pulmonary fibrosis
C. Pleural effusion
D. Simple pneumothorax
E. Tension pneumothorax

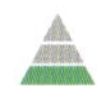 

15. A 42-year-old man has difficulty breathing and chest pain following a laparoscopic cholecystectomy a day ago. He has dullness to percussion and decreased breath sounds over the right base.

Investigations:
CXR: right lower lobe opacification and right-sided tracheal deviation.

Which is the most likely diagnosis?
A. Atelectasis
B. Idiopathic pulmonary fibrosis
C. Pleural effusion
D. Pneumonia
E. Tension pneumothorax

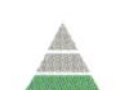 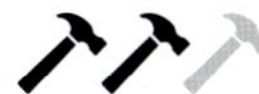

16. A 22-year-old woman has dizziness and difficulty catching her breath as she is worried about an upcoming medical school exam. She has generalized anxiety disorder, managed with sertraline. Her pulse is 120 bpm, respiratory rate 33 breaths per minute and oxygen saturation 98% on room air.

Which would be most likely seen on ABG?
A. pH 7.25, PO_2 11.2 kPa, PCO_2 7.4 kPa and bicarbonate 24 mmol/L
B. pH 7.38, PO_2 12.1 kPa, PCO_2 5.1 kPa and bicarbonate 29 mmol/L
C. pH 7.43, PO_2 10.3 kPa, PCO_2 6.5 kPa and bicarbonate 18 mmol/L
D. pH 7.51, PO_2 11.6 kPa, PCO_2 4.4 kPa and bicarbonate 25 mmol/L
E. pH 7.54, PO_2 10.4 kPa, PCO_2 4.9 kPa and bicarbonate 32 mmol/L

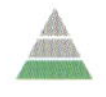  

17. A 61-year-old man has a chronic cough and shortness of breath on exertion. He has smoked 15 cigarettes a day for 30 years. He has decreased breath sounds bilaterally and prolonged expiration.

Investigations:
Spirometry: FEV1/FVC ratio: 0.62.

Which is the most appropriate management?
A. Amoxicillin
B. Doxycycline
C. Ipratropium
D. Pirfenidone
E. Salmeterol

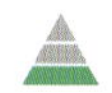 

18. A 25-year-old woman has a productive cough and shortness of breath for 4 days. She has bilateral finger

clubbing and coarse crepitations on chest auscultation.

Investigations:
CXR: thick-walled dilated bronchi.

Which is the most likely causative organism?

A. *Haemophilus influenzae*
B. *Moraxella catarrhalis*
C. *Mycobacterium tuberculosis*
D. *Pseudomonas aeruginosa*
E. *Streptococcus pneumoniae*

19. A 27-year-old man has sudden shortness of breath and pleuritic chest pain. He has had 3 pneumothoraces in the last 3 years. He has decreased breath sounds and hyperresonance to percussion on his left chest auscultation.

Investigations:
CXR: 3 cm rim of air.

Which is the most appropriate management?

A. Aspiration
B. Chest drain
C. Observation
D. Needle decompression
E. Video-assisted thoracoscopic surgery

 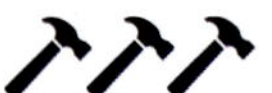 

20. A 72-year-old man has severe breathlessness, worse when exercising for 5 days. He has pitting oedema in the ankles bilaterally and bibasilar fine crepitations on chest auscultation.

Investigations:
CXR: cardiomegaly and Kerley B lines.
He is started on 15 L high-flow oxygen and IV furosemide, but a repeat chest X-ray shows minimal change.

Which is the most appropriate management?

A. Bisoprolol
B. Continuous positive airway pressure (CPAP)
C. Dobutamine
D. IV fluids
E. Ramipril

 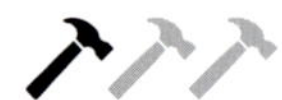

21. A 35-year-old woman has a productive cough and sore throat for a week. She has no fever, chest pain or shortness of breath. She has bilateral scattered wheeze and coarse crepitations on chest auscultation.

Which is the most likely diagnosis?

A. Acute bronchitis
B. Bronchiectasis
C. Chronic obstructive pulmonary disease
D. Influenza
E. Pneumonia

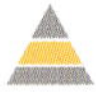 

22. A 31-year-old man with HIV infection has a persistent cough and unintentional weight loss of 5 kg for 2 months. He has enlarged lymph nodes bilaterally in the anterior and posterior cervical chain and right upper lobe crepitations.

Investigations:
CXR: right upper lobe consolidation and right-sided hilar enlargement.

Which is the most likely diagnosis?

A. Asbestosis
B. Psittacosis
C. Sarcoidosis
D. Silicosis
E. Tuberculosis

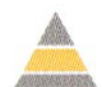 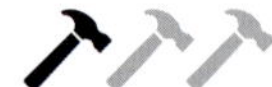

23. A 54-year-old woman has had a worsening productive cough and pleuritic chest pain for 3 days. She has hypertension, managed with ramipril. She has decreased breath sounds and bronchial breathing on the left chest auscultation.

Investigations:
CXR: left lower lobe consolidation

Which is the most likely diagnosis?

A. Asthma
B. Bronchiectasis
C. Chronic obstructive pulmonary disease
D. Influenza
E. Pneumonia

24. A 64-year-old man has had a productive cough and occasional blood-tinged sputum for 2 months. He has enlarged supraclavicular lymph nodes bilaterally and bilateral crepitations on chest auscultation.

Investigations:
CXR: bilateral hilar lymphadenopathy.

Which is the most likely causative organism?
   A. *Haemophilus influenzae*
   B. *Mycoplasma pneumoniae*
   C. *Mycobacterium tuberculosis*
   D. *Pneumocystis jirovecii*
   E. *Streptococcus pneumoniae*

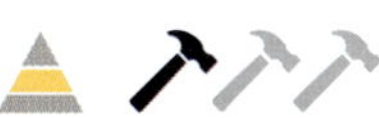

25. A 57-year-old woman has had unintentional weight loss and a nonproductive cough for 3 months. She has rheumatoid arthritis, managed with methotrexate. She has painful red bumps over her shins and a violet rash over her nose.

Investigations:
Serum calcium: 2.78 mmol/L (2.20–2.60).
Serum phosphate: 0.97 mmol/L (0.8–1.4).
CXR: bilateral hilar lymphadenopathy.

Which is the most likely diagnosis?
   A. Cystic fibrosis
   B. Idiopathic pulmonary fibrosis
   C. Lung cancer
   D. Sarcoidosis
   E. Tuberculosis

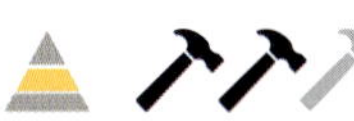

26. A 16-year-old girl with recurrent chest infections has had a productive cough for a year. Her lungs are hyperresonant to percussion, and a bilateral, expiratory wheeze on chest auscultation.

Investigations:
Sweat test: sweat chloride level of 72 mEq/L
CT chest: multiple dilated bronchi.

Which is the most likely diagnosis?
   A. Cystic fibrosis
   B. Idiopathic pulmonary fibrosis
   C. Lung cancer
   D. Sarcoidosis
   E. Tuberculosis

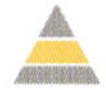 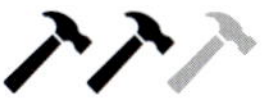

27. A 42-year-old woman with a background of working on her farm has a productive cough and shortness of breath. The symptoms worsen when cleaning hay and get better when she takes a break from work. She has bibasilar inspiratory crepitations on chest auscultation.

Investigations:
Bronchoalveolar lavage: lymphocytosis.

Which is the most likely diagnosis?
   A. Bronchiectasis
   B. Cystic fibrosis
   C. Extrinsic allergic alveolitis
   D. Idiopathic pulmonary fibrosis
   E. Lung abscess

 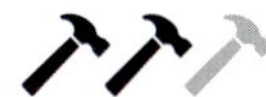

28. A 22-year-old man has shortness of breath and a productive cough. He injects IV heroin recreationally. He has decreased breath sounds and bronchial breathing on right chest auscultation.

Which is the most likely causative organism?
   A. *Chlamydia pneumoniae*
   B. *Haemophilus influenzae*
   C. *Legionella pneumophila*
   D. *Mycoplasma pneumoniae*
   E. *Staphylococcus aureus*

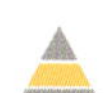 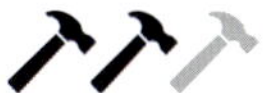 

29. A 29-year-old man has increasing shortness of breath and a dry cough. He has unintentionally lost 2 kg in 6 weeks. She has sensitive, erythematous pretibial nodules and a purple lesion on his nose and cheeks.

Which is the most appropriate histological investigation?
   A. Haemotoxylin and Eosin Stain
   B. Flow cytometry
   C. Lymph node biopsy
   D. Serum angiotensin-converting enzyme (ACE)
   E. Silver stain

 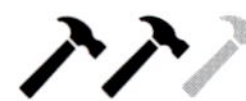

30. A 56-year-old woman has had a persistent, productive cough with a foul smell and unintentional weight loss for 3 months. She has chronic alcohol misuse, managed with acamprosate. She has decreased breath sounds over the left lower lobe.

Investigations:
CXR: left lower cavitary lesion with an air-fluid level.

Which is the most likely diagnosis?
A. Bronchiectasis
B. Lung abscess
C. Lung cancer
D. Pneumonia
E. Psittacosis

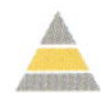 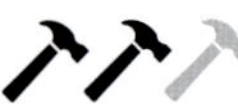

31. A 57-year-old man, who has worked in shipbuilding and insulation installation for 30 years, has gradually worsening exercise tolerance and a dry cough for 2 years. He has finger clubbing bilaterally and bibasal inspiratory crepitations on chest auscultation.

Which of the following findings would most likely be seen on imaging?
A. Bilateral hilar lymphadenopathy
B. Bilateral reticular opacities
C. Egg-shell calcification of the hilar lymph nodes
D. Lower zone fibrosis
E. Signet ring sign

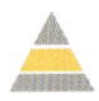  

32. A 48-year-old man has had daytime sleepiness and morning headaches for 4 months. His wife says he snores loudly and often wakes up gasping for breath. His BP is 157/102 mmHg. He has an enlarged neck circumference and tonsils.

Which is the most appropriate investigation?
A. Chest X-ray
B. CT chest
C. Polysomnography
D. Spirometry
E. Sputum culture

 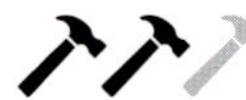

33. A 10-year-old boy with recurrent respiratory infections has a persistent, productive cough and steatorrhoea for a week. He has a barrel-shaped chest and bilateral crepitations on chest auscultation.

Investigations:
Sweat test: sweat chloride level of 74 mmol/L.

Which is the most likely gene affected?
A. CFTR
B. FOXF1
C. SERPINA1
D. SFTPA2
E. TERT

 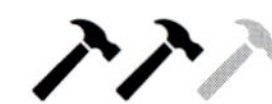

34. A 59-year-old man presents to the intensive care unit after having severe pneumonia. He is cyanotic and diaphoretic and has bilateral coarse crepitations and decreased breath sounds on chest auscultation.

Investigations:
PaO_2/FiO_2 ratio:150 mmHg
CXR: diffuse bilateral infiltrates.

Which is the most likely diagnosis?
A. Acute respiratory distress syndrome (ARDS)
B. Heart failure
C. Lung abscess
D. Pneumothorax
E. Tuberculosis

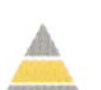  

35. A 34-year-old man has a chronic cough and night sweats for 5 days. He has returned from Asia a week ago. He has decreased breath sounds at the right base on chest auscultation.

Investigations:
CXR: right upper consolidation.
Sputum culture: acid-fast bacilli.

Which is the most appropriate management?
A. Amoxicillin
B. Clarithromycin
C. Doxycycline
D. Prednisolone
E. Rifampicin, isoniazid, pyrazinamide and ethambutol

  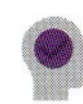

36. A 48-year-old woman, a dockyard worker for 18 years, has had difficulty breathing, made worse by exertion and a dry cough for 6 weeks. She has bibasilar end-inspiratory crepitations on chest auscultation.

Investigations:
CXR: basal opacities obscuring the cardiac borders.

Which are her pulmonary function tests likely to show?
  A. Forced expiratory volume in 1 second (FEV1) = normal, FEV1/forced vital capacity (FVC) = decreased
  B. FEV1 = normal, FEV1/FVC = increased
  C. FEV1 = normal, FEV1/FVC = normal
  D. FEV1 = reduced, FEV1/FVC = decreased
  E. FEV1 = reduced, FEV1/FVC = increased

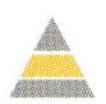 

37. A 5-year-old boy has had difficulty breathing and coughing fits for 30 minutes after playing with some Lego. He has a stridor and reduced air entry on the right chest.

Investigations:
Expiratory CXR: continued expansion of the lungs on the right side.

Where is the most likely area of obstruction?
  A. Left inferior bronchus
  B. Left superior bronchus
  C. Right inferior bronchus
  D. Right superior bronchus
  E. Trachea

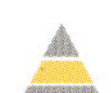  

38. A 69-year-old woman has shortness of breath and a productive cough. Her temperature is 38.7°C, and respiratory rate 36 breaths per minute. She has dull percussion of the right lower lobe and has an abbreviated mental test score of 7/10.

Investigations:
CXR: right lower lobe consolidation.

Which is the most appropriate management?
  A. Discharge home with amoxicillin
  B. Discharge home with doxycycline
  C. Nonurgent assessment at the hospital
  D. No treatment needed
  E. Urgent admission to hospital

  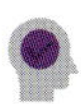

39. A 62-year-old man has blood in his sputum and unintentional weight loss for 4 months. He has bilateral finger clubbing and a fixed, monophonic wheeze on chest auscultation.

Investigations:
CXR: solitary pulmonary nodule in the right middle lobe.

Which is the most appropriate investigation?
  A. Bronchoscopy and endobronchial US-guided transbronchial needle aspiration (EBUS-TBNA)
  B. Peak Flow
  C. Spirometry
  D. Sputum culture
  E. Thoracoscopy and histology

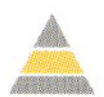 

40. A 51-year-old man has a fever and a productive cough with a red-currant jelly consistency. He has liver cirrhosis secondary to chronic alcohol misuse. He has a dullness to percussion in the right upper lobe.

Investigations:
CXR: cavitating lesion in the right upper lobe.

Which is the most likely causative organism?
  A. *Haemophilus influenzae*
  B. *Klebsiella pneumoniae*
  C. *Mycobacterium tuberculosis*
  D. *Mycoplasma pneumoniae*
  E. *Streptococcus pneumoniae*

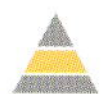 

41. A 49-year-old man has excessive daytime somnolence and relationship issues, which his wife attributes to his excessive snoring during the night. His BP is 174/112 mmHg. His BMI is 47 kg/m^2.

Investigations:
Polysomnography: apnoea-hypopnoea index of 7 episodes per hour.

Which is the most likely diagnosis?
A. Chronic obstructive pulmonary disease
B. Lung cancer
C. Narcolepsy
D. Obstructive sleep apnoea
E. Pneumonia

42. A 52-year-old man has a productive cough and pleuritic chest pain. He has hypertension, type 2 diabetes mellitus, and hypercholesterolemia managed with ramipril, amlodipine, metformin, empagliflozin and atorvastatin. He also has a penicillin allergy. He has bilaterally reduced breath sounds and bronchial breathing, and the medical team started him on treatment for typical community-acquired pneumonia.

Which medications need to be stopped due to this new treatment?
A. Amlodipine
B. Atorvastatin
C. Empagliflozin
D. Metformin
E. Ramipril

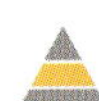 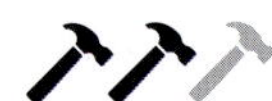 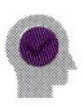

43. A 64-year-old woman has a dry cough and progressively worsening shortness of breath, worse when exercising, for a year. She has bibasilar inspiratory crepitations on chest auscultation.

Investigations:
High-resolution CT: bibasilar reticular opacities.

Which is the most appropriate management?
A. Avoid precipitating factors
B. Doxycycline
C. Inspiratory muscle training
D. Pirfenidone
E. Salbutamol

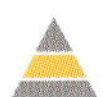 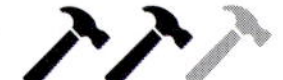 

44. A 42-year-old woman has had a dry cough and shortness of breath for 6 months. She has painful, red eyes and a purple lesion covering her nose and cheeks.

Investigations:
CXR: bilateral hilar lymphadenopathy.

Which of the following would be an indication for steroids in this woman?
A. Absence of erythema nodosum
B. Bilateral hilar lymphadenopathy
C. Lupus pernio
D. Symptoms >6 months
E. Uveitis

 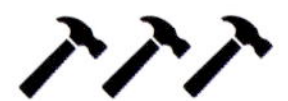 

45. A 62-year-old man has had progressively worsening shortness of breath and a dry cough for 5 months. He has congestive heart failure, managed with ramipril and bisoprolol. He has decreased breath sounds and dullness to percussion on his right chest auscultation.

Investigations:
CXR: large pleural effusion on the right side.

Which of the following is most important in distinguishing between a transudative and exudative effusion?
A. Amylase levels
B. Bacterial count
C. Glucose levels
D. Malignant cells
E. Protein levels

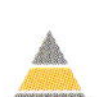  

46. A 57-year-old man, recently diagnosed with tuberculosis, has pain with eye movement and vision loss. He attributes this to the combination of medications he was started on due to his tuberculosis diagnosis. His visual acuity is 6/18 in both eyes when testing his vision, despite being 6/6 when last tested 6 months ago.

Which is the most likely cause of his presentation?
A. Ethambutol
B. Isoniazid
C. Pyrazinamide
D. Pyridoxine
E. Rifampicin

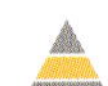 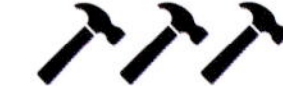

47. A 25-year-old woman has had a dry cough and shortness of breath for 4 days. Her temperature is

38.5°C. She has painful red lesions on the front of both shins and generalized joint pains.

Investigations:
CXR: bilateral hilar lymphadenopathy.

Which is the most likely diagnosis?
A. Heerfordt syndrome
B. Lofgren syndrome
C. Pneumonia
D. Systemic lupus erythematosus
E. Tuberculosis

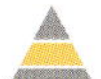 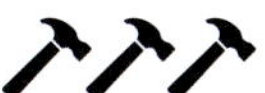

48. A 53-year-old woman has blood in her sputum and unintentional weight loss for 4 months. He has smoked 20 cigarettes a day for 30 years. She has pain in the flank regions.

Investigations:
CXR: multiple well-defined nodules shaped like cannonballs.

Which is the most likely diagnosis?
A. Adenocarcinoma of the lung
B. Pancoast tumour
C. Renal cell carcinoma
D. Small cell lung cancer
E. Squamous cell carcinoma of the lung

49. A 64-year-old man presents to the intensive care unit with shortness of breath after having severe acute pancreatitis. His respiratory rate is 32 breaths per minute. He is cyanotic and has bilateral coarse crepitations on chest auscultation.

Investigations:
PaO_2/FiO_2 ratio: 210 mmHg.
CXR: diffuse bilateral infiltrates.

Which are the most appropriate diagnostic criteria?
A. Berlin criteria
B. Centor criteria
C. Duke criteria
D. Jones criteria
E. Light criteria

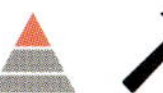 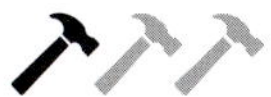

50. A 34-year-old woman has recurrent coughing and shortness of breath after work. She has worked in a car painting shop for 15 years. She has bilateral expiratory wheezes on chest auscultation.

Investigations:
Spirometry: postbronchodilator reversibility present.

Which is the most likely cause?
A. Dust mites
B. Epoxy resins
C. Flour
D. Isocyanates
E. Platinum salts

 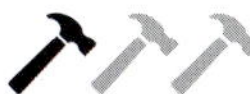

51. A 6-month-old girl has a worsening dry cough and difficulty breathing for 3 days. She had an upper respiratory tract infection a week ago. She has nasal flaring, and diffuse bilateral wheezes are heard on chest auscultation.

Investigations:
Immunofluorescence of nasopharyngeal secretions: respiratory syncytial virus (RSV) present.

Which is the most likely diagnosis?
A. Asthma
B. Bronchiolitis
C. Croup
D. Kartagener syndrome
E. Pneumonia

 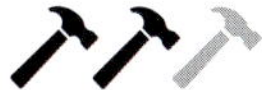 

52. An 81-year-old man has had a productive cough with blood in his sputum and an unintentional weight loss of 5kg over 4 months. He has worked in an insulation factory for 40 years. There is dullness to percussion on the left chest auscultation.

Investigations:
CXR: an opacity that extends around and encases the left lung, causing irregular margins.

Which is the most appropriate investigation?
A. Bronchoscopy and endobronchial US-guided transbronchial needle aspiration (EBUS-TBNA)
B. Peak Flow
C. Spirometry
D. Sputum culture
E. Thoracoscopy and histology

53. A 19-year-old woman has difficulty breathing and a productive cough. She has asthma, managed with salbutamol and beclomethasone inhalers. She has an expiratory wheeze.

Investigations:
Eosinophils: 1.3×10^9/l (0–0.4).
Lymphocytes: 2.6×10^9/L (1.5–4.0).
CXR: multiple dilated bronchi.

Which is the most appropriate management?
A. Itraconazole
B. Pirfenidone
C. Prednisolone
D. Salbutamol
E. Salmeterol

 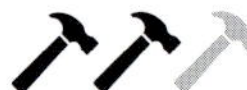 

54. A 58-year-old woman has difficulty breathing. She has COPD, managed with salmeterol. Her chest is barrel-shaped, and an expiratory wheeze on chest auscultation. She is started on nebulized salbutamol, ipratropium bromide and a venturi mask at a FiO_2 of 28%.

Investigations:
pH: 7.29 (7.35–7.45).
PO_2: 8.3 kPa (11.3–12.6).
PCO_2: 7.8 kPa (4.7–6.0).

Which is the most appropriate management?
A. Bilevel-positive airway pressure (BIPAP)
B. Continuous positive airway pressure (CPAP)
C. Intubation and ventilation
D. IV hydrocortisone
E. IV magnesium sulphate

 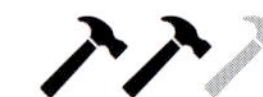

55. A 35-year-old man has chronic shortness of breath. He has hepatocellular carcinoma and is scheduled to have surgery in 2 months. He has decreased breath sounds and a bilateral expiratory wheeze on chest auscultation.

Investigations:
Forced expiratory volume in 1 second (FEV1)/forced vital capacity (FVC) ratio: 0.63.

Which is the most likely diagnosis?
A. Alpha-1 antitrypsin deficiency
B. Asthma
C. Bronchiolitis obliterans
D. Chronic obstructive pulmonary disease
E. Pneumonia

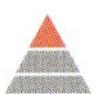 

56. A 52-year-old man has had unintentional weight loss and hoarseness of his voice for 4 months. He has smoked 20 cigarettes a day for 38 years. He has a fixed, monophonic wheeze on chest auscultation and bilateral finger clubbing.

Investigations:
CXR: increased opacification at the apex of the right lung.

Which is the most likely diagnosis?
A. Adenocarcinoma of the lung
B. Pancoast tumour
C. Renal cell carcinoma
D. Small cell lung cancer
E. Squamous cell carcinoma of the lung

57. A 39-year-old woman has had a headache and dry cough for a week after going to a bird sanctuary 2 weeks ago. She has muscle aches and right-sided basilar crepitations on chest auscultation.

Investigations:
CXR: right lower lobe consolidation.

Which is the most appropriate management?
A. Amoxicillin
B. Co-trimoxazole
C. Clarithromycin
D. Doxycycline
E. Piperacillin-tazobactam

 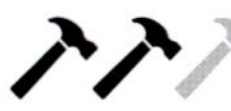 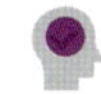

58. A 48-year-old man who has been a miner for 28 years has had a persistent cough and gradually worsening shortness of breath for 2 years. His lips have a blueish discolouration and bibasal end-inspiratory fine crepitations on chest auscultation.

Which of the following findings would most likely be seen on imaging?

A. Bilateral hilar lymphadenopathy
B. Bilateral reticular opacities
C. Egg-shell calcification of the hilar lymph nodes
D. Lower zone fibrosis
E. Signet ring sign

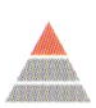 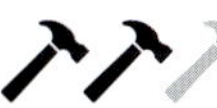

59. A 63-year-old has shortness of breath and a cough progressively worsening for 5 years. He smoked 20 cigarettes daily for 30 years but quit 5 years ago. He has bilateral expiratory wheezes on chest auscultation.

Investigations:
Spirometry: FEV1/FVC ratio: 0.63; a significant increase in FEV1 after bronchodilator administration.

Which is the most likely diagnosis?

A. Asthma
B. Asthma-COPD overlap syndrome
C. Bronchiectasis
D. Chronic obstructive pulmonary disease
E. Lung cancer

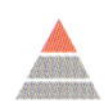  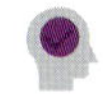

60. A 61-year-old man has excessive coughing on the background of COPD diagnosed 3 years ago. He is a plumber by occupation.

Investigations:
CXR: multiple nodular lesions in the upper lobes bilaterally.

Which is the most appropriate management?

A. No follow-up needed
B. Palliative chemotherapy
C. Routine specialist referral
D. Tiotropium and salmeterol
E. Yearly monitoring

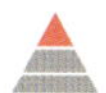 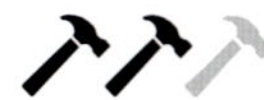

61. A 56-year-old woman has had progressive shortness of breath on exertion for 7 months. Her pulse is 87 bpm, BP 128/84 mmHg and oxygen saturation 96% on room air. She has a loud S2 heart sound and ejection systolic murmur, loudest at the left sternal border on chest auscultation.

Investigations:
ECG: right axis deviation and right ventricular hypertrophy.

Which is the most likely diagnosis?

A. Asthma
B. Bronchiectasis
C. Chronic obstructive pulmonary disease
D. Pulmonary embolism
E. Pulmonary hypertension

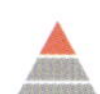 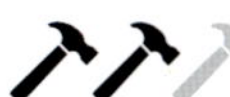

62. A 34-year-old woman has a worsening cough, with occasional blood in her sputum for 6 months. She has had multiple chest infections and has been struggling to conceive. She has widespread coarse crepitations and quiet heart sounds on chest auscultation.

Which is the most likely diagnosis?

A. Cystic fibrosis
B. Kartagener syndrome
C. Lung cancer
D. Sarcoidosis
E. Tuberculosis

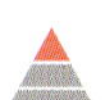  

63. A 34-year-old man has had breathlessness and a dry cough for a week. He has scattered crepitations on chest auscultation.

Investigations:
CXR: bilateral interstitial pulmonary infiltrates.
Bronchoalveolar lavage with a silver stain: ping-pong ball cysts.

Which is the most appropriate management?

A. Amoxicillin
B. Co-trimoxazole
C. Clarithromycin
D. Doxycycline
E. Piperacillin-tazobactam

64. A 43-year-old man has had blood in his sputum and nosebleeds several times for a week. He has a saddle-shaped nose deformity and proptosis of his eyes.

Investigations:
CXR: multiple cavitating, ill-defined lung lesions.
Renal biopsy: epithelial crescents in the Bowman capsule.

Which antibody is most likely to be present in this man?

A. Anticardiolipin
B. Anti-CCP
C. Anti-GBM
D. cANCA
E. pANCA

Renal

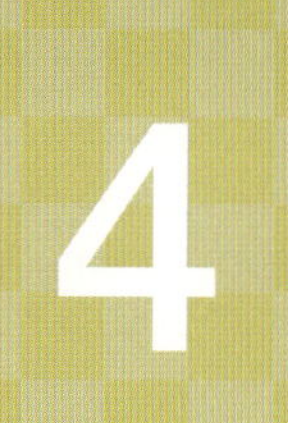

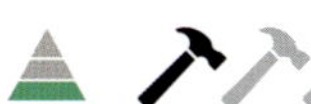

1. A 61-year-old man has fatigue, loss of appetite and leg swelling for 1 month. He has type 2 diabetes mellitus, managed with metformin. His BP is 172/103 mmHg. He has mild pallor and pitting oedema to the knees.

Investigations:
Serum urea: 7.3 mmol/L (2.5–7.0).
Serum creatinine: 128 µmol/L (60–110).
Estimated glomerular filtration rate (eGFR):
58 mL/min/1.73 m^2 (>90).

Which is the most likely cause of his symptoms?
  A. Glomerulonephritis
  B. Hypertension
  C. Polycystic kidney disease
  D. Pyelonephritis
  E. Type 2 diabetes mellitus

2. A 45-year-old woman has generalized leg swelling and a rash over her back for a week. She had tuberculosis 2 weeks ago, managed with rifampicin, isoniazid, pyrazinamide and ethambutol. She has a diffuse maculopapular rash over her back and costovertebral angle tenderness.

Investigations:
Serum urea: 7.9 mmol/L (2.5–7.0).
Serum creatinine: 138 µmol/L (60–110).
Eosinophils: 0.53 × 10^9/L (0–0.40).

Which is the most likely diagnosis?
  A. Acute interstitial nephritis
  B. Acute tubular necrosis
  C. Henoch-Schonlein purpura
  D. IgA nephropathy
  E. Polycystic kidney disease

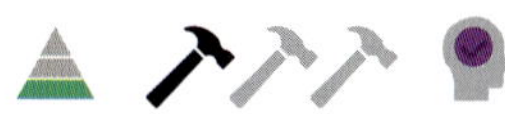

3. A 79-year-old woman has shortness of breath and reduced urine output after elective knee replacement surgery 3 days ago. She was given ibuprofen for postoperative pain relief. She has reduced skin turgor and dry mucous membranes.

Investigations:
Serum urea: 7.8 mmol/L (2.5–7.0).
Serum creatinine: 235 µmol/L (60–110).

Which is the most appropriate management?
  A. 500 mL Hartmann solution
  B. Blood transfusion
  C. Furosemide
  D. Renal replacement therapy
  E. Stop ibuprofen

4. A 61-year-old man has a clinic BP of 165/98 mmHg, and subsequent ambulatory monitoring confirms a daytime average of 158/94 mmHg.

Investigations:
Serum urea: 7.1 mmol/L (2.5–7.0).
Serum creatinine: 131 µmol/L (60–110).
Estimated glomerular filtration rate (eGFR):
54 mL/min/1.73 m^2 (>90).
Urinary albumin creatinine ratio: 43 mg/mmol (<3).

Which is the most appropriate management?
  A. Amlodipine
  B. Dapagliflozin
  C. Lifestyle modification
  D. Ramipril
  E. Refer to nephrologist

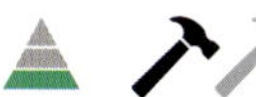

5. A 72-year-old man has had bilateral leg swelling and difficulty breathing for 2 days. He had an inferior STEMI a week ago, managed with contrast-guided percutaneous coronary intervention (PCI) and has had decreased urine output since the PCI was performed. He has pitting oedema to the knees bilaterally and bibasal crepitations on chest auscultation.

Investigations:
Serum urea: 7.6 mmol/L (2.5–7.0).

Serum creatinine: 149 μmol/L (60–110).
Serum sodium: 138 mmol/L (137–144).
Serum potassium: 5.4 mmol/L (3.5–4.9).

Which is the most likely diagnosis?
A. Acute interstitial nephritis
B. Acute tubular necrosis
C. Henoch-Schonlein purpura
D. IgA nephropathy
E. Polycystic kidney disease

 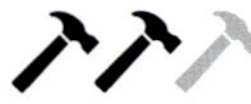 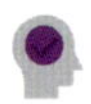

6. A 67-year-old woman has a hypertension review. She takes amlodipine.

Investigations:
Serum urea: 7.2 mmol/L (2.5–7.0).
Serum creatinine: 115 μmol/L (60–110).
Estimated glomerular filtration rate (eGFR): 84 mL/min/1.73 m^2 (>90).

What stage of disease does this woman have?
A. Stage 1
B. Stage 2
C. Stage 3
D. Stage 4
E. Stage 5

 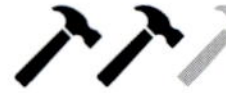 

7. A 30-year-old man has a large rash on his lower back and generalized back aches. He has tonsilitis, managed with amoxicillin 2 days ago. He has a diffuse maculopapular rash and sacrolumbar tenderness.

Investigations:
Serum urea: 8.5 mmol/L (2.5–7.0).
Serum creatinine: 138 μmol/L (60–110).
Eosinophils: 0.46 × 10^9/L (0–0.40).
Urinalysis: urinary casts

Which of the following urinary casts would most likely be seen?
A. Brown granular casts
B. Fatty casts
C. Hyaline casts
D. Red cell casts
E. White cell casts

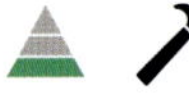 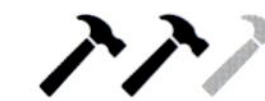

8. A 63-year-old man has confusion, nausea and vomiting after being admitted with AKI secondary to acute urinary retention relating to benign prostatic hyperplasia. His pulse is 112 bpm. He has deep, laboured breathing, with pronounced abdominal and chest movement.

Which is the most likely diagnosis?
A. Acute tubular necrosis
B. Hyperkalaemia
C. Metabolic acidosis
D. Uraemic encephalopathy
E. Volume overload

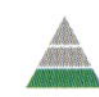 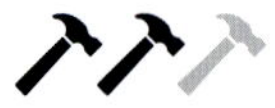 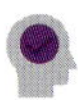

9. A 55-year-old woman has had leg swelling and abdominal discomfort for a week, with decreased urine output. She drinks 20 units of alcohol per week. She has yellowing of her sclera, pitting oedema to the thighs and bibasal crepitations on chest auscultation.

Investigations:
Serum potassium: 5.6 mmol/L (3.5–4.9).
Serum creatinine: 212 μmol/L (60–110).
ECG: normal.

Which is the most appropriate management?
A. 10 mL of 10% calcium gluconate + 10 units of insulin + 50 mL of glucose
B. 500 mL of Hartmann solution
C. Furosemide only
D. Furosemide + 500 mL of Hartmann solution
E. Furosemide + restrict dietary intake of potassium

10. A 76-year-old woman has fatigue and decreased daily urine output. She has hypertension, managed with amlodipine. Her BP is 164/101 mmHg.

Investigations:
Serum creatinine: 215 μmol/L (60–110), which 1 month previously was at 104 μmol/L
Urine output: 0.3 mL/kg/hr for 15 hours.

What stage of AKI does this woman have?
A. Stage 0
B. Stage 1
C. Stage 2
D. Stage 3
E. Stage 4

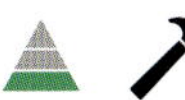
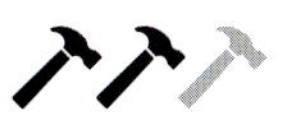

11. A 42-year-old man has severe muscular pain and dark red urine after a weightlifting competition a week ago. He has generalized muscle swelling and tenderness with reduced limb ROM.

Investigations:
Urinalysis: brown granular casts.

Which is the most appropriate investigation?
A. Serum calcium
B. Serum creatine kinase
C. Serum phosphate
D. Serum potassium
E. Serum urea

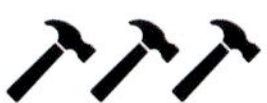

12. A 71-year-old woman has had dizziness and decreased urine output for 3 days. She has congestive heart failure. Her BP is 87/58 mmHg. She has dry mucous membranes and shifting dullness on abdominal percussion.

Investigations:
Serum potassium: 4.4 mmol/L (3.5–4.9).
Serum creatinine: 126 μmol/L (60–110).

Which of the following investigation findings would be associated with the likely diagnosis?
A. Brown granular urinary casts
B. High urinary sodium
C. Low urine osmolality
D. Poor response to fluid challenge
E. Raised serum urea: creatinine ratio

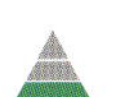
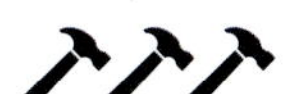

13. An 82-year-old woman has 2 days of worsening shortness of breath. She has an AKI secondary to rhabdomyolysis, managed with IV fluids. She has bi basal crepitations on chest auscultation and pitting oedema to the ankles.

Investigations:
CXR: peri-hilar opacities.

Which is the most appropriate management?
A. Haemodialysis
B. Noninvasive ventilation
C. Peritoneal dialysis
D. Renal transplant
E. Spironolactone

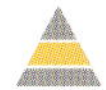
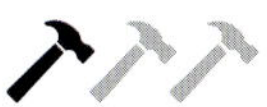

14. A 40-year-old man has had dull abdominal pain for 2 months. He has had three urinary tract infections in the past year, managed with trimethoprim. His BP is 167/101 mmHg. He has bilateral flank masses and hepatomegaly.

Investigations:
Urinalysis: blood +, protein -, glucose -, leucocytes -
Abdominal US: multiple fluid-filled masses on the liver

What is the most likely diagnosis?
A. Acute tubular necrosis
B. IgA nephropathy
C. Minimal change disease
D. Polycystic kidney disease
E. Urinary tract calculi

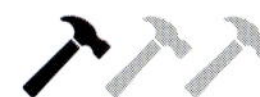

15. A 7-year-old girl has swelling around her eyes and lower limbs and reduced urine output for 3 days. She has hepatomegaly and periorbital oedema.

Investigations:
Urinalysis: protein +, blood -, glucose -, leucocytes - and urinary casts
24-h urinary albumin: 23mg (<30)

Which of the following urinary casts would most likely be seen?
A. Brown granular casts
B. Fatty casts
C. Hyaline casts
D. Red cell casts
E. White cell casts

16. A 52-year-old woman has abdominal pain, bloating and reduced urine output with visible blood in her urine for 1 month. She has a family history of polycystic kidney disease. Her BP is 154/93 mmHg. She has mild abdominal tenderness, and the kidneys are palpable.

Which is the most appropriate investigation?
A. Genetic testing
B. Renal US
C. Serum creatinine
D. Urinalysis
E. Urine culture

 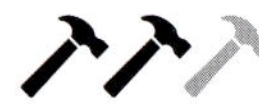

17. A 9-year-old boy has facial and leg swelling and a sore throat for a week. He has bilateral lymphadenopathy in the anterior neck triangle.

Investigations:
Urinalysis: protein +, blood -, glucose -, leucocytes -
24-h urinary albumin: 25mg (<30)
Renal biopsy under electron microscopy: podocyte fusion and effacement of foot processes.

Which is the most likely diagnosis?
A. Anti-glomerular basement membrane disease
B. Focal segmental glomerulosclerosis
C. Membranoproliferative glomerulonephritis
D. Minimal change disease
E. Poststreptococcal glomerulonephritis

 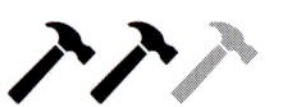 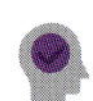

18. A 59-year-old woman has had persistent right flank pain and blood in her urine for 6 months, with 4 kg of unintentional weight loss. She has a right flank mass.

Investigations:
CT abdomen: heterogeneous mass on the right kidney.
Renal biopsy: staged T1N0M0.

Which is the most appropriate management?
A. Alpha-interferon
B. Partial nephrectomy
C. Radical cystectomy
D. Sunitinib
E. Total nephrectomy

 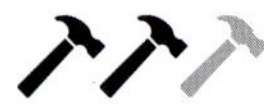

19. A 14-year-old boy has facial swelling and dark urine for a week. He had a sore throat and a fever 2 weeks ago. He has periorbital oedema.

Investigations:
Urinalysis: protein +, blood +, glucose -, leucocytes -
Renal biopsy: endothelial proliferation with neutrophils.

Which is the most likely diagnosis?
A. Antiglomerular basement membrane disease
B. IgA nephropathy
C. Membranoproliferative glomerulonephritis
D. Minimal change disease
E. Poststreptococcal glomerulonephritis

 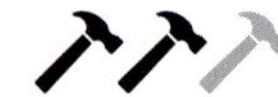

20. A 65-year-old woman has sudden severe shortness of breath with no chest pain. She has hypertension, managed poorly with amlodipine. Her pulse is 114 bpm and BP 168/101 mmHg. She is in acute distress and has bilateral crepitations throughout both lung fields and a bruit to the left of her umbilicus.

Investigations: Figure 4.1 (see Chapter 37).

Which is the most likely cause of her pulmonary oedema?
A. AKI
B. IgA nephropathy
C. Myocardial infarction
D. Pulmonary embolism
E. Renal artery stenosis

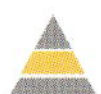 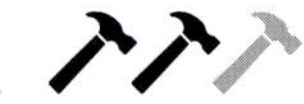

21. A 31-year-old man has blood in his urine and intermittent flank pain for 24 hours. He had an upper respiratory infection that self-resolved 2 days ago. He has pitting oedema in his legs.

Investigations:
Urinalysis: protein +, blood +, glucose -, leucocytes -
Renal biopsy: mesangial hypercellularity.

Which is the most likely diagnosis?
A. Antiglomerular basement membrane disease
B. IgA nephropathy
C. Membranoproliferative glomerulonephritis
D. Minimal change disease
E. Poststreptococcal glomerulonephritis

 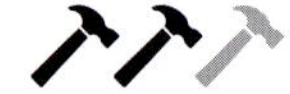 

22. A 76-year-old man has had headaches for a month. He has hyperlipidaemia managed with lifestyle modifications. His BP is 178/101 mmHg. He has a left flank bruit.

Investigations:
Serum creatinine: 90 μmol/L (60–110).
Serum total cholesterol: 7.7 mmol/L (<5.2).
Serum LDL cholesterol: 4.18 mmol/L (<3.36).
Renal duplex US scan: stenosis of left renal artery by >50%.

Which is the most appropriate management?

A. Amlodipine + aspirin
B. Amlodipine + aspirin + statin
C. Amlodipine + statin
D. Aspirin + statin
E. Renal artery stenting

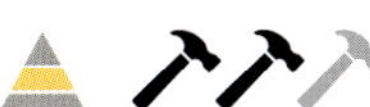

23. A 62-year-old woman has shortness of breath and a persistent cough with occasional blood in her sputum for a week. Her temperature is 38.2°C. She has bilateral crepitations on chest auscultation.

Investigations:
Urinalysis: protein +, blood +, glucose -, leucocytes -
Serum urea: 10.9 mmol/L (2.5–7.0).
Serum creatinine: 191 µmol/L (60–110).

Which is the most likely diagnosis?

A. Antiglomerular basement membrane disease
B. IgA nephropathy
C. Membranoproliferative glomerulonephritis
D. Minimal change disease
E. Poststreptococcal glomerulonephritis

24. A 40-year-old woman has progressively worsening hypertension, managed poorly with ramipril. Her BP is 164/106 mmHg. She has nontender, nonpalpable kidneys and a bruit is heard to the left of her umbilicus.

Investigations:
Renal duplex US scan: multiple outpouchings in both renal arteries.

Which is the most likely diagnosis?

A. Antiglomerular basement membrane disease
B. Fibromuscular dysplasia
C. IgA nephropathy
D. Phaeochromocytoma
E. Polycystic kidney disease

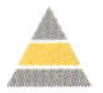 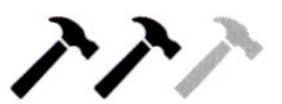 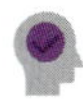

25. A 63-year-old man has had blood in his sputum and urine for a week. He has smoked 30 cigarettes a day for 20 years. His temperature is 38.4°C.

Investigations:
Urinalysis: protein +, blood +, glucose -, leucocytes -
Serum urea: 10.3 mmol/L (2.5–7.0).
Serum creatinine: 174 µmol/L (60–110).
Renal biopsy: linear IgG deposits along the basement membrane.

Which antibody is most associated with the likely diagnosis?

A. Anti-CCP
B. Anti-GBM
C. Anti-dsDNA
D. cANCA
E. pANCA

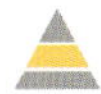 

26. A 12-year-old girl has had swelling in his face and legs and brown urine for 3 days. She had a sore throat a week ago, which self-resolved. She has oedema of the periorbital region and a decreased urine output.

Investigations:
Urinalysis: protein +, blood +, glucose -, leucocytes - and urinary casts.

Which of the following urinary casts would most likely be seen?

A. Brown granular casts
B. Fatty casts
C. Hyaline casts
D. Red cell casts
E. White cell casts

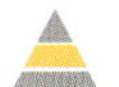 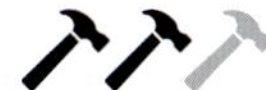 

27. A 26-year-old man has had lower back pain and fatigue for 3 months. He has hypertension, managed with ramipril. He has a family history of kidney disease. His BP is 142/92 mmHg. He has palpable kidneys with tenderness.

Investigations:
Serum creatinine: 159 µmol/L (60–110).
Estimated glomerular filtration rate (eGFR): 51 mL/min/1.73 m^2 (>60).
Renal US scan: Three fluid-filled sacs in his left kidney.

Which is the most appropriate management?

A. Amlodipine
B. IV fluids
C. Peritoneal dialysis
D. Prednisolone
E. Tolvaptan

  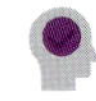

28. A 56-year-old woman has had facial and leg swelling for 4 days. She has gout, managed with ibuprofen. Her BP is 124/83 mmHg. She has oedema in the periorbital region.

Investigations:
Urinalysis: protein +, blood -, glucose -, leucocytes -
24-h urinary albumin: 27mg (<30)

Which would be seen on renal biopsy?

A. Areas of mesangial collapse and sclerosis
B. Focal and segmental sclerosis
C. Kimmelstiel-Wilson nodules
D. Normal glomeruli
E. Spike and dome appearance

 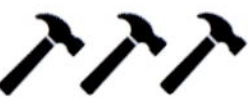 

29. A 27-year-old woman has severe swelling of her face and legs. She has type 1 diabetes mellitus, poorly controlled with a basal-bolus regime. She appears pale and bloated, with pitting oedema to the thighs.

Investigations:
HbA1c: 56 mmol/mol (20–42).
Urinalysis: protein +, blood -, glucose -, leucocytes -
24-h urinary albumin: 20mg (<30)

Which would be seen on renal biopsy?

A. Areas of mesangial collapse and sclerosis
B. Focal and segmental sclerosis
C. Kimmelstiel-Wilson nodules
D. Podocyte effacement
E. Spike and dome appearance

 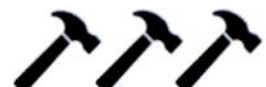

30. A 60-year-old man has intermittent swelling in his legs and face and 2 kg weight gain for 6 months. He has vitiligo, managed with a tacrolimus ointment. He has pitting oedema in his lower extremities and face.

Investigations:
Urinalysis: protein +, blood -, glucose -, leucocytes -
24-h urinary albumin: 22mg (<30)
Renal biopsy: basement membrane thickening with spike and dome appearance.

Which is the most likely diagnosis?

A. Antiglomerular basement membrane disease
B. IgA nephropathy
C. Membranoproliferative glomerulonephritis
D. Membranous glomerulonephritis
E. Polycystic kidney disease

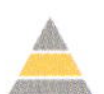 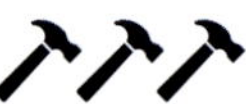 

31. A 23-year-old man has had a cough with occasional red streaks in his sputum and dark urine for a week. He has smoked 20 cigarettes a day for 15 years.

Investigations:
Urinalysis: protein +, blood +, glucose -, leucocytes -
Renal biopsy: linear IgG deposits along the basement membrane.

Which is the most appropriate management?

A. Azathioprine
B. Fluid restriction
C. Furosemide
D. Plasmapheresis
E. Tolvaptan

 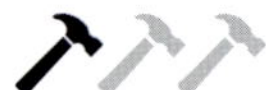

32. A 45-year-old woman had a headache and muscle aches during recovery from a subarachnoid haemorrhage 2 days ago. She has been vomiting frequently during her recovery. She has Addison disease, managed with hydrocortisone and fludrocortisone.

Investigations:
Urinary Na+: 49 mmol/L (20–40 mmol/L).
Urine osmolality: 260 mOsml/kg (>100 mOsm/kg).

Which is the most likely diagnosis?

A. Addison disease
B. Loop diuretic usage
C. Psychogenic polydipsia
D. Syndrome of inappropriate antidiuretic hormone secretion
E. Vasospasm

33. A 45-year-old woman has small, reddish-purple dots on her lower limbs and brown urine for a month. She has asthma and allergic rhinitis, managed with a budesonide/formoterol inhaler and cetirizine.

Investigations:
Urinalysis: protein +, blood +, glucose -, leucocytes -

Which is the most likely diagnosis?
A. Acute interstitial nephritis
B. Eosinophilic granulomatosis with polyangiitis
C. Granulomatosis with polyangiitis
D. Henoch-Schonlein purpura
E. Poststreptococcal glomerulonephritis

 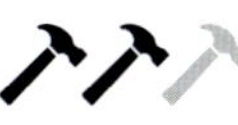 

34. A 59-year-old woman has facial and leg swelling and shortness of breath on minimal exertion for a month. She has hepatitis C. Her BP is 162/104 mmHg. She has pitting oedema to the mid-thigh and facial oedema.

Investigations:
Urinalysis: protein +, blood -, glucose -, leucocytes -
Renal biopsy: subendothelial and mesangial immune deposits.

Which is the most appropriate management?
A. Furosemide
B. IV fluids
C. Prednisolone
D. Ramipril
E. Tolvaptan

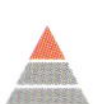 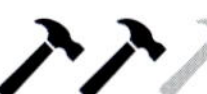

35. A 5-year-old girl has a rash over her legs and buttocks for 4 days. She also has joint pain in the knees and ankles and blood on urination. Her blood pressure is 129/87 mmHg. She has a palpable, purpuric rash over the legs and buttocks and tenderness and swelling over the knees and ankles.

Which is the most likely diagnosis?
A. Acute interstitial nephritis
B. Acute tubular necrosis
C. Henoch-Schonlein purpura
D. IgA nephropathy
E. Poststreptococcal glomerulonephritis

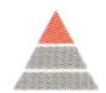 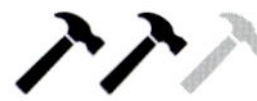

36. A 56-year-old man has had fatigue and ankle swelling for 4 months. He also has a loss of appetite and unintentional weight loss of 4 kg during this time period. His BP is 132/73 mmHg. He has bilateral ankle oedema and hepatomegaly.

Investigations:
Urinalysis: protein +, blood -, glucose -, leucocytes -
Abdominal fat biopsy: apple-green birefringence on Congo red staining.

Which is the most likely diagnosis?
A. Amyloidosis
B. Antiglomerular basement membrane disease
C. Focal segmental glomerulosclerosis
D. Membranoproliferative glomerulonephritis
E. Minimal change disease

 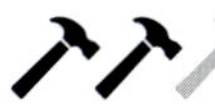

37. A 29-year-old woman has had fatigue and leg swelling for a week. She has had IgA nephropathy 3 months ago, managed conservatively. Her blood pressure is 163/104 mmHg, and she has pitting oedema in both legs.

Investigations:
Renal biopsy: areas of mesangial collapse

Which is the most likely diagnosis?
A. Antiglomerular basement membrane disease
B. Focal segmental glomerulosclerosis
C. Membranoproliferative glomerulonephritis
D. Minimal change disease
E. Poststreptococcal glomerulonephritis

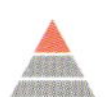 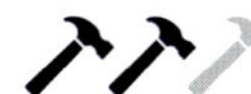

38. A 47-year-old man has abdominal pain. He has end-stage renal failure managed with continuous ambulatory peritoneal dialysis. He has generalized abdominal tenderness and guarding.

Investigations:
Dialysis effluent: cloudy.

Which is the most common causative organism?
A. *Clostridium difficile*
B. *Escherichia coli*
C. *Staphylococcus aureus*
D. *Staphylococcus epidermis*
E. *Streptococcus viridans*

 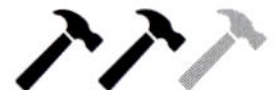 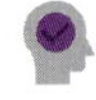

39. A 43-year-old woman has recurrent nosebleeds and nasal stuffiness, causing difficulty breathing. She has had similar episodes for 5 weeks. Her temperature is 38.1°C.

Investigations:
Serum urea: 11.2 mmol/L (2.5–7.0).
Serum creatinine: 197 μmol/L (60–110).

Which antibody is most associated with the likely diagnosis?
A. Anti-CCP
B. Anti-GBM
C. Anti-dsDNA
D. cANCA
E. pANCA

 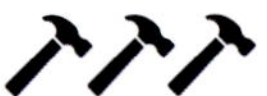

40. A 54-year-old man has had abdominal bloating and fever for 12 hours. He has liver cirrhosis, managed with alcohol abstinence. He has shifting dullness.

Investigations:
Serum creatinine: 98 μmol/L (60–110).
Serum urea: 6.4 mmol/L (2.5–7.0).
Paracentesis: neutrophil count of 340 cells/μL in the ascitic fluid.
Two hours later, while recovering, another set of blood results shows a serum creatinine of 240 μmol/L (60–110) and serum urea of 11 mmol/L (2.5–7.0).

Which is the most likely diagnosis?
A. Diverticulitis
B. Hepatorenal syndrome
C. Hydronephrosis
D. Peritonitis
E. Sepsis

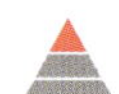 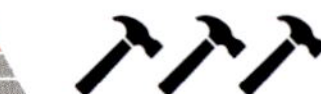

41. A 24-year-old man has had blood in his urine for a week. He has had similar episodes, which would resolve after a day. He has used hearing aids since birth. His abdomen is soft and nontender, whilst his Rinne test was positive in both ears and on Weber test, he hears the sound equally well in both ears.

Investigations:
Serum sodium: 142 mmol/L (137–144).
Serum potassium: 5.4 mmol/L (3.5–4.9).
Serum urea: 10.1 mmol/L (2.5–7.0).
Serum creatinine: 134 μmol/L (60–110).

Which is the mode of inheritance for this likely diagnosis?
A. Autosomal dominant
B. Autosomal recessive
C. Mitochondrial
D. X-linked dominant
E. X-linked recessive

Neurology

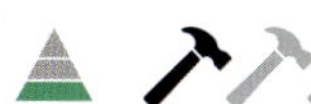

1. A 26-year-old woman has an intermittent, stress-induced headache, described as a dull, tight band around the head. She has no focal neurological signs.

Investigations:
Fundoscopy: unremarkable.

Which is the most likely diagnosis?

A. Brain abscess
B. Cluster headache
C. Idiopathic intracranial hypertension
D. Migraine
E. Tension headache

2. A 35-year-old woman has sudden unconsciousness, with her husband describing stiffening of her body followed by jerking movements of her legs and arms for 2 minutes. She subsequently regained consciousness but felt drowsy.

Which is the most likely diagnosis?

A. Absence seizure
B. Atonic seizure
C. Focal aware seizure
D. Focal impaired seizure
E. Tonic-clonic seizure

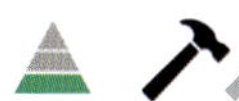

3. A 67-year-old woman has confusion, difficulty finding words and weakness in her right arm and leg. She has hypertension, managed with amlodipine. She speaks in complete sentences; however, the words are unrelated, and the sentences lack meaning. Her right arm and leg have significant weakness and sensory loss.

Which is the most likely diagnosis?

A. Lacunar infarct
B. Lateral medullary syndrome
C. Partial anterior circulation infarct
D. Posterior circulation infarct
E. Total anterior circulation infarct

4. A 32-year-old man has 2 months of an episodic, severe left stabbing headache lasting for 15 minutes, with nasal congestion and left eye redness, which spontaneously resolves. He has smoked 20 cigarettes a day for 15 years.

Which is the most likely diagnosis?

A. Cluster headache
B. Idiopathic intracranial hypertension
C. Migraine
D. Subarachnoid haemorrhage
E. Tension headache

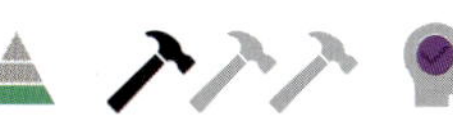

5. A 26-year-old woman has recurrent throbbing right-sided headaches that last for 3 hours, preceded by jagged crescents in her vision. The headaches improve by going to a dark, quiet room and are worsened by stress.

Which is the most appropriate management?

A. High-flow oxygen
B. Metoclopramide
C. Paracetamol
D. Sumatriptan
E. Sumatriptan and paracetamol

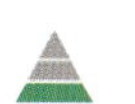

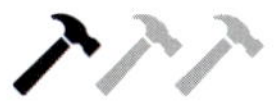

6. A 78-year-old woman has progressively worsening intermittent headaches, confusion and difficulty walking for 3 days. She had a fall at home 2 weeks ago. She has hypertension, managed with amlodipine and mild cognitive impairment on MMSE.

Investigations:
CT head: hypodense crescentic collection.

Which is the most likely diagnosis?

A. Acute subdural haematoma
B. Chronic subdural haematoma
C. Extradural haematoma
D. Normal pressure hydrocephalus
E. Subarachnoid haemorrhage

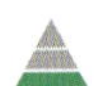  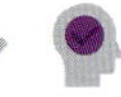

7. A 51-year-old man has 3 hours of difficulty speaking fluently. His comprehension is intact. He has left-sided weakness and homonymous hemianopia.

Investigations:
CT angiography: occlusion of the proximal anterior circulation.

Which is the most appropriate management?
A. Carotid artery endarterectomy
B. Clopidogrel
C. IV thrombolysis
D. IV thrombolysis and thrombectomy
E. Thrombectomy

 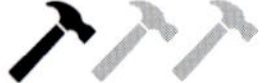 

8. A 72-year-old man has sudden left-sided weakness in his upper and lower limbs and difficulty speaking lasting 30 minutes, which spontaneously resolves. He has hypertension and hypercholesterolaemia, managed with amlodipine and atorvastatin. His BP is 145/100 mmHg.

Which is the most appropriate management?
A. Aspirin
B. Carotid endarterectomy
C. Thrombectomy
D. Thrombolysis
E. Warfarin

 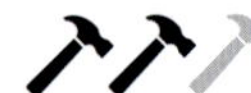 

9. A 53-year-old man had 30 minutes of right arm weakness 3 hours ago, which resolved. He had a pulmonary embolism 3 months ago, managed with apixaban. He has no focal neurological signs.

Which is the most appropriate investigation?
A. Carotid doppler
B. CT angiography head
C. CT head
D. D-dimer
E. MRI head

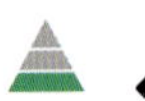 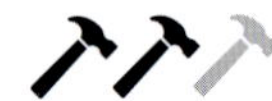

10. A 62-year-old man has a sudden collapse and loss of consciousness for 5 minutes. Upon regaining consciousness, he is dizzy and unsteady on his feet. His speech is slurred with staccato enunciation. He has hypertension, managed with amlodipine. He has nystagmus, past pointing and an unsteady gait.

Which is the most likely diagnosis?
A. Middle cerebral artery infarct
B. Partial anterior circulation infarct
C. Posterior cerebral artery infarct
D. Posterior circulation infarct
E. Total anterior circulation infarct

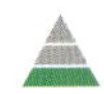 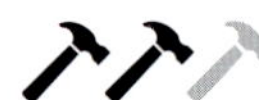

11. A 68-year-old woman has had confusion and disorientation for 3 months. She has fluctuations in alertness throughout the day and regular visual hallucinations. She takes short, shuffling steps and has bilateral resting tremors, which are improved by voluntary movement.

Investigations:
Mini-mental state examination (MMSE): 22 out of 30.

Which is the most likely diagnosis?
A. Alzheimer disease
B. Frontotemporal dementia
C. Lewy body dementia
D. Parkinson disease
E. Vascular dementia

 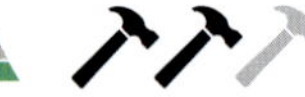

12. A 57-year-old woman has nausea and a headache after a car accident. She has a meningioma and is awaiting surgery. Her pulse is 42 bpm, BP 190/100 mmHg and respiratory rate 7 breaths per minute. Her pupils are dilated and nonreactive to light, and her GCS is 10/15.

Which is the name for the triad of symptoms this woman is presenting with?
A. Charcot triad
B. Cushing triad
C. Gradenigo's triad
D. Horner triad
E. Trotter triad

13. A 72-year-old man has a gradual decline in memory and difficulty with daily activities for a year. He forgets important events, struggles to recall familiar names and frequently misplaces his belongings. His father suffered from a similar decline in cognition. He is disoriented to time and place.

Investigations:
Mini-mental state examination (MMSE): 18 out of 30.

Which is the underlying pathophysiology?
A. Aberrant deposits of alpha-synuclein protein in the primary motor cortex
B. Degeneration of the cholinergic neurons in the basal ganglia striatum
C. Degeneration of dopaminergic neurons in the substantia nigra
D. Loss of neurons in the basal nucleus of Meynert
E. Perisylvian volume loss

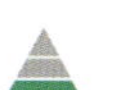 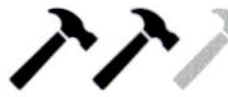 

14. A 52-year-old woman has loss of consciousness, falling onto the floor and stiffening, with tongue biting and incontinence of urine. Upon arrival at the hospital, 20 minutes after the episode started, she was given IV lorazepam. She had not regained consciousness after 10 minutes.

Which is the most appropriate management?
A. IV lorazepam
B. IV phenytoin
C. IV propofol
D. IV sodium valproate
E. Rectal diazepam

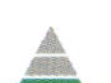  

15. A 40-year-old woman has had severe pain in the back of her head for 3 hours. She has polycystic kidney disease. She has photophobia and neck stiffness.

Investigations:
CT head: normal.

Which is likely to be seen in her cerebrospinal fluid (CSF)?
A. Albuminocytologic dissociation
B. Clear CSF
C. Cloudy CSF
D. Presence of red blood cells
E. Xanthochromia

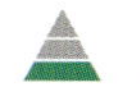 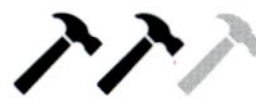

16. A 53-year-old man has sudden right leg weakness. He has laboured, incoherent speech and cannot understand tasks he is asked to do nor repeat words he is asked to repeat.

Which type of aphasia is this man displaying?
A. Anomic aphasia
B. Broca aphasia
C. Conduction aphasia
D. Global aphasia
E. Wernicke aphasia

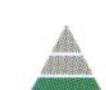 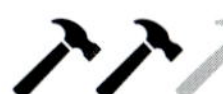

17. A 34-year-old woman has a sudden, severe headache at the back of her head. She has Ehlers-Danlos syndrome. She has neck stiffness and photophobia.

Investigations:
CT head: hyperdensities in the basal cisterns.

Which is the most likely location of the infarct?
A. Basilar artery
B. Bridging veins
C. Circle of Willis
D. Middle meningeal artery
E. Posterior inferior cerebellar artery

 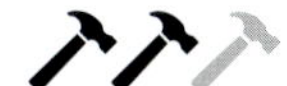 

18. A 47-year-old woman has weakness in her left arm and speech problems for 3 hours. She has hypercholesterolemia, managed with atorvastatin. Her speech is nonfluent, but she can understand what is being said to her. There is an audible carotid bruit on auscultation.

Investigations:
CT head: well-defined area of low density in the right frontoparietal area.

Which is the most appropriate investigation?
A. Chest X-ray
B. CSF sampling
C. CT angiography
D. Duplex US
E. MRI head

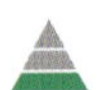 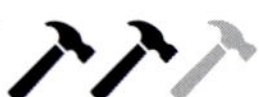 

19. A 32-year-old woman has a severe, stabbing right headache behind her right eye lasting an hour. She has had similar episodes for a month. She has right eyelid swelling and scleral redness and is extremely restless.

Which is the most appropriate management?

A. High-flow oxygen
B. Naproxen
C. Propranolol
D. Topiramate
E. Verapamil

20. A 14-year-old boy lost consciousness after a head collision during a rugby match 3 hours ago. He regained consciousness 2 hours later but subsequently deteriorated to a GCS of 11/15.

Investigations:
CT head: hyperdense, biconvex collection around the surface of the brain.

Which is the most likely location of the infarct?

A. Basilar artery
B. Bridging veins
C. Circle of Willis
D. Middle meningeal artery
E. Posterior inferior cerebellar artery

 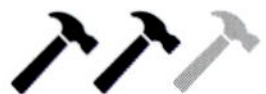 

21. A 52-year-old woman has a severe headache in the occipital region of her head for 2 hours. She has photophobia and neck stiffness.

Investigations:
CT Head: normal
Lumbar Puncture: xanthochromia
She is referred to neurosurgery, where a CT intracranial angiogram confirms an intracranial aneurysm.

Which is the most appropriate management?

A. Aneurysm coiling
B. Ceftriaxone
C. Burr hole evacuation
D. IV alteplase
E. Nimodipine

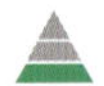 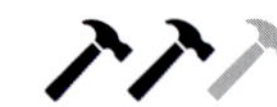

22. A 58-year-old man has become impulsive and shows little empathy towards others over the past year. He frequently makes inappropriate comments in social situations.

Investigations:
Mini-mental state examination (MMSE): 30 out of 30.

Which is the underlying pathophysiology?

A. Aberrant deposits of alpha-synuclein protein in the primary motor cortex
B. Degeneration of the cholinergic neurons in the basal ganglia striatum
C. Degeneration of the dopaminergic neurons in the substantia nigra
D. Loss of neurons in the basal nucleus of Meynert
E. Perisylvian volume loss

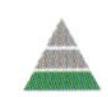 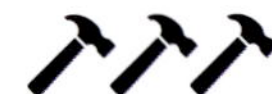

23. A 6-year-old girl has been acting unusually for 2 months. She zones out of conversations, and then her lips start smacking together for a minute. After this event, she is confused and has difficulty communicating with her for about 20 minutes afterwards.

Which structure is most likely affected?

A. Cerebellum
B. Frontal lobe
C. Occipital lobe
D. Parietal lobe
E. Temporal lobe

 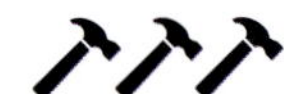 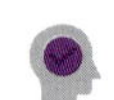

24. A 23-year-old woman has throbbing, left-sided headaches lasting between 6 and 8 hours twice a week. These headaches are preceded by zigzag lines in her vision and are worsened by alcohol. She is on the oral contraceptive pill.

Which is the most appropriate prophylaxis?

A. Naproxen
B. Propranolol
C. Sumatriptan
D. Topiramate
E. Verapamil

 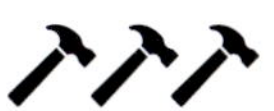 

25. A 78-year-old man has a progressively declining memory, difficulty finding words and following conversations and getting lost in familiar places. He has hypertension, managed with atenolol, experiencing bradycardia as a side effect.

Investigations:
Mini-mental state examination (MMSE): 17 out of 30.

Which is the most appropriate management?
A. Citalopram
B. Donepezil
C. Memantine
D. Risperidone
E. Rivastigmine

 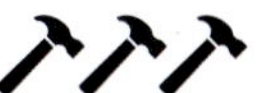 

26. A 35-year-old woman has had a painful rash affecting her skin and oral mucosa and a fever for 6 days. She has generalized tonic-clonic seizures. Her rash is characterized by target lesions, and when rubbed, blisters appear on the skin.

Which is the most likely cause?
A. Carbamazepine
B. Ethosuximide
C. Lamotrigine
D. Levetiracetam
E. Sodium valproate

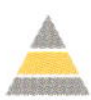 

27. A 35-year-old man has left-sided facial discomfort, postauricular pain and increasing irritability to noise. He has resting facial asymmetry and an inability to raise his left eyebrow. He is also unable to smile or pucker his lips.

Which is the most likely diagnosis?
A. Bell palsy
B. Chronic otitis media
C. Facial nerve schwannoma
D. Lyme disease
E. Ramsay Hunt syndrome

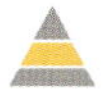 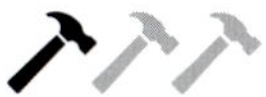

28. A 26-year-old woman has generalized pain around the base of the neck and scapula for a week. She had a total right-sided mastectomy for breast cancer 3 weeks ago. She has a winging of her right scapula.

Which nerve is most likely affected?
A. Axillary
B. Long thoracic
C. Median
D. Radial
E. Ulnar

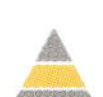 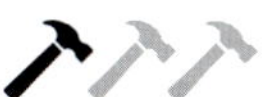 

29. A 57-year-old woman has a progressively worsening tremor in her right hand, affecting her ability to do her job as a waitress. She was diagnosed with Parkinson 3 months ago after presenting with a slow, shuffling gait and demonstrated cogwheel rigidity.

Which is the most appropriate management?
A. Bromocriptine
B. Levodopa
C. Procyclidine
D. Propranolol
E. Riluzole

 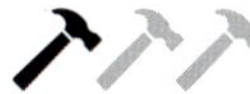

30. A 59-year-old man has increased clumsiness for 2 months, especially stumbling when walking. After examination, he is diagnosed with primary lateral sclerosis, a motor neuron disease that only affects upper motor neurons.

Which symptom is consistent with this diagnosis?
A. Atrophy
B. Fasciculations
C. Hyporeflexia
D. Hypotonia
E. Spasticity

 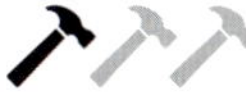

31. A 46-year-old man has weakness in his lower limbs, progressing up his legs for 4 days. He has double vision bilaterally and absent ankle and knee reflexes.

Investigations:
Nerve conduction studies: decreased motor nerve conduction velocity.

Which is the most likely diagnosis?
A. Encephalitis
B. Guillain-Barré syndrome
C. Multiple sclerosis
D. Myasthenia gravis
E. Parkinson disease

 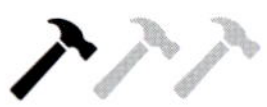

32. A 45-year-old man has right shoulder pain radiating to the right arm, which started after a lymph node biopsy a month earlier. He has drooping of his right shoulder and an inability to shrug his right shoulder against resistance. Furthermore, he has difficulty turning his head to the left when testing the movements of his head.

Which cranial nerve is most likely affected?
A. Accessory
B. Facial
C. Hypoglossal
D. Oculomotor
E. Trigeminal

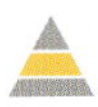 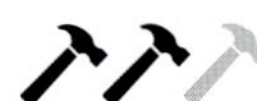

33. A 25-year-old woman has blurred vision and persistent morning headaches for a month. She has acne vulgaris, managed with doxycycline. She has a BMI of 32 kg/m^2.

Investigations:
Fundoscopy: papilloedema.

Which is the most likely diagnosis?
A. Cluster headache
B. Idiopathic intracranial hypertension
C. Medication-overuse headache
D. Migraine
E. Tension headache

 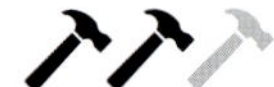

34. A 38-year-old man has increased irritability and neglected his physical appearance for 3 months. His speech is impaired, and his limbs make involuntary jerky movements. He has rapid, ballistic movements of the eyes that abruptly change the point of fixation, and his gait is unsteady on tandem walking.

Which structure is most likely affected?
A. Amygdala
B. Hypothalamus
C. Striatum
D. Substantia nigra
E. Subthalamic nucleus

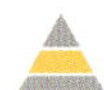 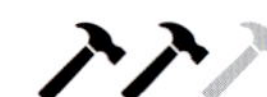

35. A 32-year-old man has had lower leg pain after diarrhoea 4 days ago. The pain has since progressed upwards up to the thighs and developed into bilateral weakness of the lower limbs. He has 5/5 power and present reflexes in the upper limbs but 2/5 power and absent reflexes in the lower limbs, with downgoing plantars.

Which is the most likely cause?
A. *Campylobacter jejuni*
B. Coxsackievirus
C. *Escherichia coli*
D. Herpes simplex virus-1
E. *Neisseria meningitides*

 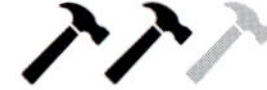 

36. A 38-year-old woman has worsening vision, muscle weakness after exercising and trouble swallowing her meals. She has pernicious anaemia, managed with IM vitamin B12 injections. She has bilateral drooping of her eyelids and double vision on CN III, IV and VI testing.

Which is the most appropriate management?
A. IV aciclovir
B. IV immunoglobulin
C. Prednisolone
D. Pyridostigmine
E. Thymectomy

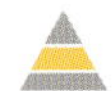 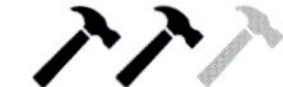

37. A 66-year-old male has sudden problems with his movement. He has Tourette syndrome, managed with haloperidol. He has a slow, shuffling gait and has bilateral tremors in his hands. He shows no signs of cogwheel or lead pipe rigidity.

Which is the most likely diagnosis?

A. Corticobasal degeneration
B. Drug-induced parkinsonism
C. Idiopathic Parkinson disease
D. Multiple system atrophy
E. Progressive supranuclear palsy

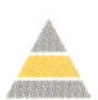 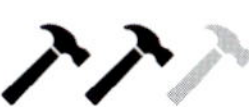 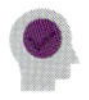

38. A 24-year-old man has a severe headache and fever. He has human immunodeficiency virus (HIV), managed with zidovudine. He has a non-blanching rash on his left arm, photophobia and neck stiffness.

Which is the most appropriate management?

A. Acyclovir
B. Amoxicillin
C. Benzylpenicillin
D. Clarithromycin
E. Gentamicin

 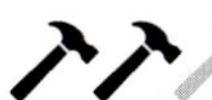

39. A 22-year-old woman presents after a motorcycle accident an hour ago. She is not bleeding severely and has problems with the extension of her right forearm and a right wrist drop.

Investigations:
Humerus X-ray: fracture of the right humeral midshaft.

Which nerve is most likely affected?

A. Axillary
B. Long thoracic
C. Median
D. Radial
E. Ulnar

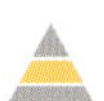  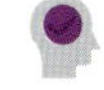

40. A 45-year-old woman has blurred vision and extreme tiredness for a week. She has brisk patellar and ankle reflexes.

Investigations:
MRI head: high-density lesions in the periventricular region of the brain.
A lumbar puncture examines the cerebrospinal fluid's (CSF) composition.

Which is likely to be seen in her CSF?

A. Elevated lymphocytes
B. High protein
C. Low glucose
D. Oligoclonal bands
E. Xanthochromia

 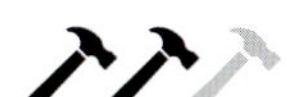

41. A 42-year-old man was hit on the lateral aspect of the left knee by a car. He has problems with dorsiflexion of the left ankle and eversion of the left foot. He also has a loss of sensation over the dorsum of the foot and the lower lateral part of the leg.

Which nerve is most likely affected?

A. Common peroneal
B. Femoral
C. Obturator
D. Superior gluteal
E. Tibial

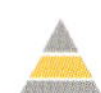 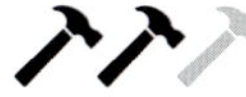 

42. A 23-year-old woman has a high-grade fever, severe headache and stiff neck. Her temperature is 39.5°C and pulse 120 bpm. She has nuchal rigidity and she has pain during extension of her knees beyond 135 degrees.

Investigations:
Viral PCR: *Neisseria meningitides.*

What would be seen in the CSF of this woman?

A. High glucose, high protein, neutrophil predominance
B. High glucose, low protein, lymphocyte predominance
C. High glucose, low protein, neutrophil predominance
D. Low glucose, high protein, neutrophil predominance
E. Low glucose, low protein, lymphocyte predominance

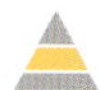 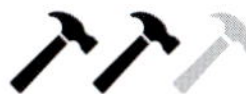

43. A 46-year-old man has a fall when walking down the stairs. He has double vision in the right eye when looking downwards and a deficit when testing his right eye's medial and downward movements.

Which cranial nerve is most likely affected?

A. Abducens
B. Facial
C. Oculomotor
D. Trigeminal
E. Trochlear

 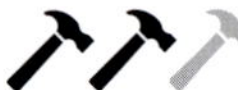

44. A 45-year-old woman has had a tremor for 4 years. She finds difficulty holding things out and needs help completing simple tasks. Her mother had a similar tremor in the past. She has a bilateral tremor appearing when she leaves her arms outstretched.

Which is the most likely diagnosis?
A. Drug-induced parkinsonism
B. Essential tremor
C. Idiopathic Parkinson disease
D. Lewy body dementia
E. Multiple-system atrophy

 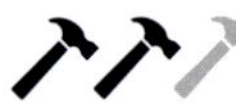 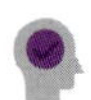

45. A 31-year-old man has had a worsening fever and headache for 3 days. His temperature is 39.2°C. He has nonfluent speech, but his comprehension is intact.

Investigations:
MRI head: increased signal in the right mediotemporal lobe.

Which is the most appropriate management?
A. IM benzylpenicillin
B. IV acyclovir
C. IV ceftriaxone
D. IV dexamethasone
E. IV gentamicin

 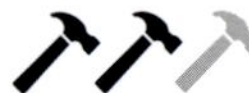 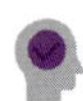

46. A 59-year-old woman has had lower limb weakness for 3 months. She has tongue fasciculations, increased tone in her arms and legs, hyperreflexia when testing the knee and ankle reflexes and atrophy of her tibialis anterior muscle.

Which is the most appropriate management?
A. Bromocriptine
B. Levodopa
C. Procyclidine
D. Propranolol
E. Riluzole

 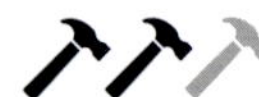

47. A 66-year-old man has a spinning sensation in his right ear lasting for an hour for 2 months. He also has a ringing sensation in the ear and hearing loss during these episodes. He has a positive Romberg's test and rhythmic side-to-side contractions in his right eye.

Investigations:
Rinne's test: air conduction > bone conduction in both ears.

Which is the most likely diagnosis?
A. Acoustic neuroma
B. Acute otitis media
C. Benign paroxysmal positional vertigo
D. Meniere disease
E. Presbycusis

48. A 12-year-old boy has a fall on his outstretched right arm during gymnastics practice. He had bad pain straight after the fall, and his wrist started swelling. He cannot move his thumb away from his index finger.

Investigations:
Radius X-ray: distal radius fracture with dorsal displacement of fragments.

Which nerve is most likely affected?
A. Axillary
B. Long thoracic
C. Median
D. Radial
E. Ulnar

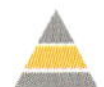 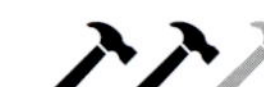

49. A 41-year-old woman has weakness in her lower limbs progressing up her legs and an inability to swallow her food for 3 days. She had gastroenteritis a week ago, which has since resolved. She has double vision and an absent knee reflex.

Which nerve roots correspond to the knee reflex?
A. C5–C6
B. C7–C8
C. L3–L4
D. S1–S2
E. S2–S3

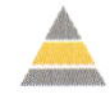 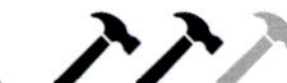

50. A 56-year-old man cannot control the movement of his limbs and has a tremor in his left hand. He has an abnormal heel-to-shin test and staccato speech when asked to repeat phrases.

Where is the most likely location of his lesion?
A. Amygdala
B. Cerebellum
C. Hypothalamus
D. Substantia nigra
E. Subthalamic nucleus

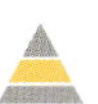  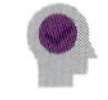

51. A 54-year-old woman has had progressively worsening uncontrollable tremors in her hands and arms for 5 years, affecting her work as a teacher. Her symptoms improve with rest. She has a bilateral tremor that gets worse when her hands are outstretched.

Which is the most appropriate management?
A. Deep brain stimulation
B. Levodopa
C. Propranolol
D. Safinamide
E. Watchful waiting

52. A 61-year-old woman has difficulty walking and numbness in his legs. She started a vegetarian diet 6 months ago. She has impaired vibration and proprioception in the legs. She is Romberg positive and has a wide-based, unsteady gait.

Investigations:
Blood film: megaloblastic anaemia.

Which is the most likely diagnosis?
A. Guillain-Barré syndrome
B. Multiple sclerosis
C. Subacute combined degeneration of the spinal cord
D. Syringomyelia
E. Transverse myelitis

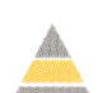  

53. A 72-year-old woman has had a severe temporal headache for a week that is worse in the morning. She has bilateral double vision.

Investigations:
Fundoscopy: swollen pale disc and blurred margins

Which is the most appropriate diagnostic investigation?
A. C-reactive protein (CRP)
B. CT angiography
C. MRI head
D. Skull X-ray
E. Temporal artery biopsy

 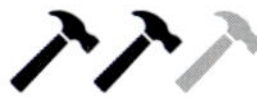

54. A 54-year-old man has muscle weakness in his legs and problems walking. He has small-cell lung cancer, which was successfully treated 5 years ago. He is Romberg's positive, and he has muscular strength improvement after repeated muscle contractions.

Which is the most likely diagnosis?
A. Brain metastases
B. Lambert-Eaton syndrome
C. Motor neuron disease
D. Multiple sclerosis
E. Myasthenia gravis

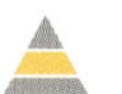  

55. A 41-year-old man has rapidly progressive weakness in his lower extremities, starting from his feet, after resolved gastroenteritis a week ago. He has double vision and absent deep tendon reflexes in his lower limbs.

Which would most likely be seen on lumbar puncture?
A. Albuminocytologic dissociation
B. Lymphocytic pleocytosis
C. Neutrophilic pleocytosis
D. Oligoclonal bands
E. Xanthochromia

 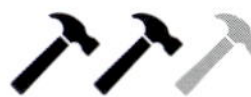 

56. A 63-year-old man has severe right-sided facial pain that he describes as an electric shock lasting for 30 seconds. The pain is precipitated by simple activities such as talking and eating and happens multiple times a day for a week.

Which is the most appropriate management?
A. Carbamazepine
B. Paracetamol
C. Prednisolone
D. Sumatriptan
E. Verapamil

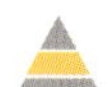 

57. A 34-year-old woman has had weakness in her right arm and double vision for 3 months. She had similar episodes a year ago but did not seek medical assistance since they eventually self-resolved. She has paraesthesia in her arms and legs on neck flexion and hyperreflexia at the knees and ankles.

Which is the most likely pattern of the disease being described?
- A. Cervical spondylosis
- B. Primary progressive disease
- C. Relapse-regressive disease
- D. Relapsing-remitting disease
- E. Secondary progressive disease

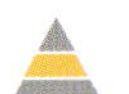 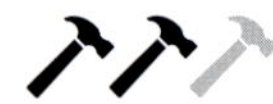

58. A 52-year-old man is confused. He has acute pancreatitis caused by binge drinking problems, as he consumed 40 units of alcohol per week for 10 years. He has bilateral horizontal nystagmus and limited downgaze. He cannot walk in a straight line and is not oriented to time, place or date.

Which is the most likely diagnosis?
- A. Cerebellar infarct
- B. Delirium tremens
- C. Korsakoff syndrome
- D. Parkinson disease
- E. Wernicke encephalopathy

 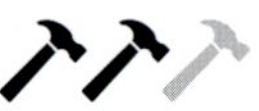 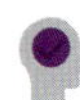

59. A 68-year-old woman had a resting tremor and bradykinesia for 5 months, leading to a diagnosis of Parkinson's disease, for which she was prescribed medication. She also has acute closed-angle glaucoma, managed with acetazolamide. She has become more impulsive, betting large amounts of money on football matches, despite having never bet before the diagnosis. She has also had hallucinations since starting this medication.

Which of the following medications was she prescribed?
- A. Amantadine
- B. Bromocriptine
- C. Entacapone
- D. Levodopa
- E. Selegiline

 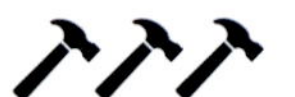 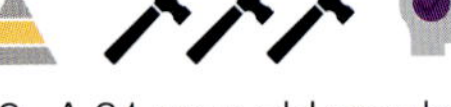

60. A 61-year-old man has struggled with leg stiffness and painful back spasms for 6 months, on the background of multiple sclerosis. He has tried a variety of analgesia for his pain, but nothing has helped for a sustained period.

Investigations:
MRI head: periventricular lesion.

Which is the most appropriate management?
- A. Baclofen
- B. Botox injection
- C. Diazepam
- D. Methylprednisolone
- E. Natalizumab

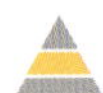 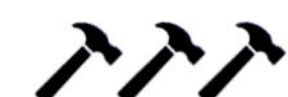

61. A 41-year-old man has bilateral facial drooping. He had a flu-like illness after hiking a month ago, where he had a fever, muscular aches and a rash growing in size in his right axilla, which had a bulls-eye appearance. He cannot puff out both his cheeks or raise either eyebrow.

Which is the most likely cause?
- A. *Borrelia burgdorferi*
- B. *Campylobacter jejuni*
- C. *Escherichia coli*
- D. Herpes simplex virus-1
- E. *Neisseria meningitides*

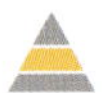 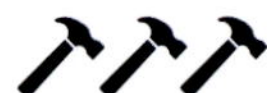

62. A 42-year-old woman has painful blurred vision for a week, which self-resolves and does not return for 6 months. Her visual acuity in her left eye is 3/60 but is normal in her right eye. Her pain is exacerbated when she goes to the sauna or has a hot shower.

What is the name of this clinical feature she is describing?
- A. Brudzinski sign
- B. Internuclear ophthalmoplegia
- C. Kernig sign
- D. Lhermitte's phenomenon
- E. Uhthoff's phenomenon

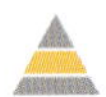 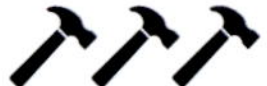

63. A 12-year-old boy has clawing of his right hand and a hyperextended wrist after falling after climbing a tree and attempting to catch onto a branch as he was falling. He has drooping of his upper right eyelid, a constricted right pupil and weakness of finger flexion and extension.

Which is the most likely diagnosis?
- A. Carpal tunnel syndrome
- B. Erb palsy
- C. Humeral midshaft fracture
- D. Humeral neck fracture
- E. Klumpke palsy

64. A 73-year-old man has had multiple falls and erectile dysfunction for a month. His BP is 132/82 mmHg when lying on the bed and 100/70 mmHg standing up. He has a resting tremor in his right hand, has cogwheel rigidity of his limbs and takes short, shuffling steps when testing his gait.

Which is the likely diagnosis?

A. Corticobasal degeneration
B. Drug-induced parkinsonism
C. Idiopathic Parkinson disease
D. Multiple system atrophy
E. Progressive supranuclear palsy

 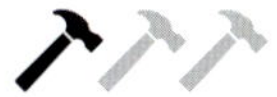

65. A 33-year-old woman has had a persistent, dull headache and visual disturbances for a week. Her temperature is 38.3°C. She has drooping of her right eyelid.

Investigations:
CT head: ring-enhancing lesion on the left frontal lobe.

Which is the likely diagnosis?

A. Brain abscess
B. Brain metastases
C. Cerebral toxoplasmosis
D. Lateral medullary syndrome
E. Tuberculoma

66. A 67-year-old man has had a loss of sensation for 4 hours. He has complete loss of sensation in all the upper and lower limb dermatomes of the left limbs, although the right limb sensation is completely intact.

Investigations:
CT head: small vessel vasculopathy in the basal ganglia

Which is the most likely diagnosis?

A. Lacunar stroke
B. Lateral medullary syndrome
C. Partial anterior circulation stroke
D. Posterior circulation stroke
E. Total anterior circulation stroke

 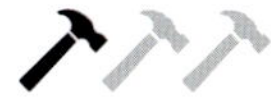

67. A 53-year-old woman has had progressive headaches and cognitive decline for a month. She had an unintentional weight loss of 5 kg.

Investigations:
CT head: multiple well-defined lesions with oedema.

Which is the most likely responsible for her presentation?

A. Breast cancer
B. Colon cancer
C. Lung cancer
D. Melanoma
E. Renal cancer

 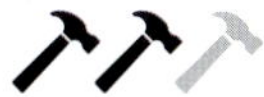

68. An 82-year-old man has been progressively misremembering things and has had urinary incontinence for 4 months. He cannot walk straight and is not orientated to time or place.

Which is the most likely diagnosis?

A. Extradural haematoma
B. Multiple sclerosis
C. Normal pressure hydrocephalus
D. Subarachnoid haemorrhage
E. Subdural haematoma

 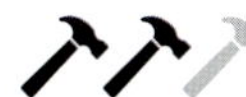

69. A 50-year-old man has left-sided facial numbness and loss of sensation over the right leg. He has trouble walking straight when his gait is tested. He has left-sided miosis and ptosis but no weakness of the limbs.

Which artery is most likely affected?

A. Left posterior cerebral artery
B. Left posterior communicating artery
C. Left posterior inferior cerebellar artery
D. Right posterior cerebral artery
E. Right posterior inferior cerebellar artery

 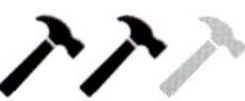

70. A 73-year-old man has had progressively declining hearing in his right ear for 3 years and intermittent vertigo, right-sided headaches and ringing in his right ear. He has an absent corneal reflex, and his Rinne

test shows that air conduction is better than bone conduction bilaterally.

Which is the most likely diagnosis?

A. Acoustic neuroma
B. Acute otitis media
C. Benign paroxysmal positional vertigo
D. Meniere disease
E. Presbycusis

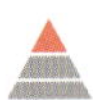 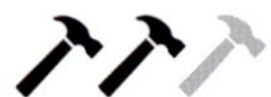 

71. A 62-year-old man has sudden dizziness and a spinning sensation occurring when he moves his head upwards lasting 15 seconds. This has affected his sleep, especially when he rolls over on his bed.

Which is the most appropriate management?

A. Amoxicillin
B. Dix-Hallpike manoeuvre
C. Epley manoeuvre
D. Metoclopramide
E. Stereotactic radiotherapy

 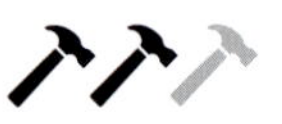 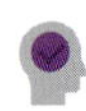

72. A 37-year-old man has a dull headache and high fever for 3 days. He has sinusitis that resolved 3 weeks ago. He has drooping of his right upper eyelid and dilation of the right eye.

Investigations:
Fundoscopy: papilloedema.
MRI head: Ring-enhancing lesion in the right frontal lobe.

Which is the most appropriate management?

A. IV ceftriaxone and benzylpenicillin
B. IV ceftriaxone and metronidazole
C. IV dexamethasone
D. IV pyrimethamine
E. Oral rifampicin

 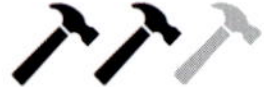

73. A 12-year-old boy has visual problems, fatigue and excessive urination. His mother says that he is short for his age. He has bitemporal hemianopia, which mainly affects the lower quadrants.

Investigations:
CT head: mass in the suprasellar region.

Which is the most likely diagnosis?

A. Craniopharyngioma
B. Occipital cortex lesion
C. Parietal lobe lesion
D. Pituitary adenoma
E. Temporal lobe lesion

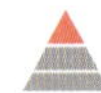 

74. A 3-year-old boy has headaches worse in the morning and vomiting throughout the day.

Investigations:
Fundoscopy: papilloedema.
Histology: rosette pattern of small, blue cells in the cerebellum

Which is the most likely diagnosis?

A. Craniopharyngioma
B. Glioblastoma multiforme
C. Oligodendroma
D. Medulloblastoma
E. Meningioma

 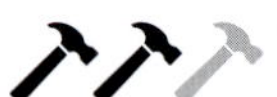

75. A 21-year-old woman has daytime sleepiness, often falling asleep during conversations and a sudden loss of muscle tone whenever she laughs. She has a normal sleep schedule and has an Epworth Sleepiness Scale score of 19 out of 24.

Which is the most appropriate investigation?

A. CT head
B. Lumbar puncture
C. Multiple sleep latency electroencephalography (EEG)
D. Polysomnography
E. Serum ferritin

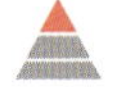 

76. A 5-year-old boy has had difficulty getting up from the floor and climbing stairs for a year. He frequently falls while running and has to use his hands to get up from the floor. He has a waddling gait, calf muscle hypertrophy and diminished tendon reflexes.

Which is the most likely type of inheritance?

A. Autosomal dominant
B. Autosomal recessive
C. Mitochondrial
D. X-linked dominant
E. X-linked recessive

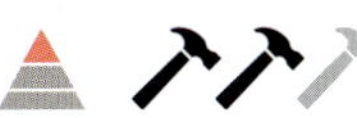

77. A 19-year-old woman has progressive weakness and wasting in her lower legs, often causing her to trip and sprain his ankles. Her older brother had similar issues in the past. She has muscle weakness, particularly in the foot dorsiflexors and ankle plantar flexors. She is only able to feel vibration and proprioception at the level of the ankle and has absent deep tendon reflexes.

Which is the most likely diagnosis?

A. Charcot-Marie-Tooth disease
B. Chronic inflammatory demyelinating polyneuropathy
C. Diabetic neuropathy
D. Hereditary spastic paraplegia
E. Guillain-Barré syndrome

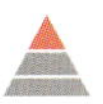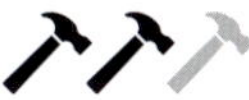

78. A 37-year-old man has shoulder burns after leaning against a radiator despite not feeling the heat at the time. He has Arnold-Chiari malformation, for which he is due for posterior fossa decompression. He has decreased temperature sensation in the neck, shoulders and arms, upgoing plantars and spastic leg weakness.

Which is the most likely diagnosis?

A. Arachnoiditis
B. Brown-Sequard syndrome
C. Guillain-Barré syndrome
D. Syringomyelia
E. Tethered spinal cord syndrome

79. A 33-year-old tennis player has left-sided neck pain and painless weakness in his left hand, most noticeable after training. He has a left rib from the level of C7 found incidentally on a chest X-ray last year. He has wasting and loss of sensation in his left hand.

Which is the most likely diagnosis?

A. Carpal tunnel syndrome
B. Erb palsy
C. Humeral neck fracture
D. Klumpke's palsy
E. Neurogenic thoracic outlet syndrome

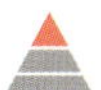

80. A 46-year-old woman has had confusion and agitation for 12 hours. She was diagnosed with schizophrenia a week ago and was given olanzapine. Her temperature is 39.3°C and BP 170/100 mmHg. She has lead-pipe rigidity.

Which is the most appropriate investigation?

A. Electrocardiogram
B. Lumbar puncture
C. Olanzapine level
D. Serum creatine kinase
E. Urea and electrolytes

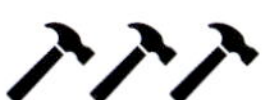

81. A 32-year-old woman has had her hearing progressively worsening for a year. She also has a ringing sensation in both ears and feels a spinning sensation from time to time. Her father suffered from a similar problem when he was younger. She has bilateral sensorineural hearing loss and an absent corneal reflex.

Which is the likely diagnosis?

A. Benign paroxysmal positional vertigo
B. Meniere disease
C. Neurofibromatosis 1
D. Neurofibromatosis 2
E. Otosclerosis

82. A 74-year-old man has confusion and urinary incontinence. He has severe Alzheimer disease, managed with memantine. He cannot recall the date or place he was currently in and has an abnormal gait.

Which is the most appropriate management?

A. Donepezil
B. External ventricular drain
C. Pivmecillinam
D. Repeated large-volume CSF taps
E. Ventriculoperitoneal shunting

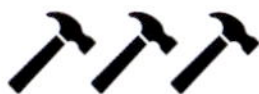

83. A 21-year-old woman has a sudden, severe headache, nausea and vomiting. She had a witnessed seizure 2 days ago. She has left-sided limb weakness.

Investigations:
CT head: Empty delta sign.

Which is the most likely diagnosis?

A. Cavernous sinus thrombosis
B. Lateral sinus thrombosis
C. Sagittal sinus thrombosis
D. Subarachnoid haemorrhage
E. Temporal arteritis

Rheumatology

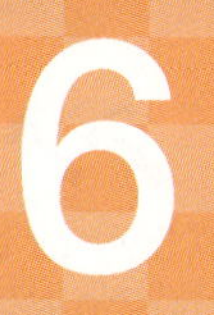

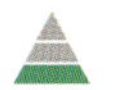 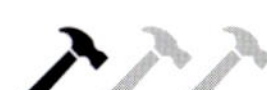

1. A 78-year-old woman has had gradually worsening joint pain and stiffness in her right hip for 6 months, worse with prolonged activity and weight-bearing. She has hypercholesterolaemia, managed with atorvastatin. She has a reduced range of motion in the right hip, with crepitation on passive hip movement.

Which is the most likely diagnosis?
   A. Ankylosing spondylitis
   B. Osteoarthritis
   C. Osteoporosis
   D. Rheumatoid arthritis
   E. Septic arthritis

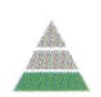 

2. A 43-year-old woman has had bilateral pain and stiffness of the joints in the hands for 3 months. She has type 1 diabetes mellitus, managed with a basal-bolus insulin regime. She has bilateral swelling and tenderness in the proximal interphalangeal joints and wrists, with pain on the metacarpal squeeze.

Which is the most likely diagnosis?
   A. Ankylosing spondylitis
   B. Osteoarthritis
   C. Osteoporosis
   D. Rheumatoid arthritis
   E. Septic arthritis

 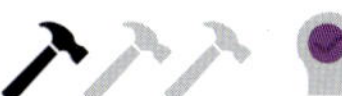

3. A 75-year-old woman has 5 months of right wrist pain that worsens with use and improves with rest. She has hypertension, managed with amlodipine. Her BP is 158/112 mmHg. She has painless nodes on the proximal interphalangeal joints bilaterally.

Which is the most appropriate investigation?
   A. Anti-CCP antibodies
   B. Schirmer test
   C. Synovial fluid analysis
   D. X-ray of the hands
   E. X-ray of the sacroiliac joints

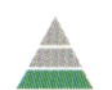 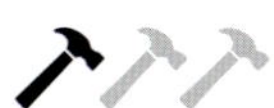

4. A 74-year-old woman has had constant back pain for a year, with recurrent low-energy fractures. She underwent menopause aged 33 and drinks 30 units of alcohol per week. Her mother had back pain for many years. She has lost 3 cm of height since her last check-up and has noticeable forward rounding of her upper back.

Which is the strongest risk factor for this diagnosis?
   A. Alcohol excess
   B. Family history of osteoporosis
   C. Female sex
   D. Premature menopause
   E. Sedentary lifestyle

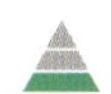 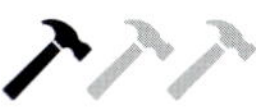 

5. A 62-year-old man has gradually worsening pain and stiffness in his left hip, worse with prolonged activity and weight-bearing. He has type 2 diabetes mellitus, managed with metformin. He has bony enlargements on the distal interphalangeal joints of the hands and a limited range of motion in his left hip.

Which is the most appropriate management?
   A. Colchicine
   B. Exercise and NSAIDs
   C. Methotrexate
   D. Paracetamol
   E. Pilocarpine

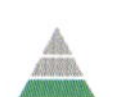 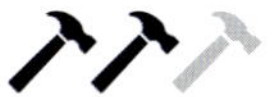 

6. A 64-year-old man has had severe pain and swelling in his right big toe for a day, causing difficulty walking. His temperature is 38.3°C. He has marked erythema and tenderness of his right 1st metatarsophalangeal joint.

Which is the most appropriate investigation?
   A. Anti-CCP antibodies
   B. Dual-energy computed tomography
   C. Schirmer test
   D. Synovial fluid analysis
   E. X-ray of the sacroiliac joints

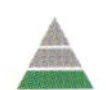  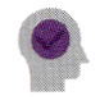

7. A 56-year-old woman has generalized bone pain and muscle weakness for 6 months. She had a right femoral neck fracture, managed with a total hip replacement 3 months ago. She exercises regularly and started a vegan diet 6 months ago. She has generalized rib tenderness and a waddling gait.

Which is the most appropriate management?

A. Cholecalciferol
B. Colchicine
C. Ibuprofen
D. Methotrexate
E. Paracetamol

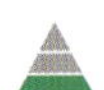 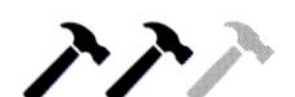 

8. A 69-year-old woman has had bone pain and difficulty mobilizing for 8 months, with multiple falls. She has lost 4 cm of height since her last appointment.

A dual-energy X-ray absorptiometry (DEXA) scan is requested.

Which of the following T score ranges is associated with the diagnosis?

A. >2.5
B. 0.5 to 2.0
C. −1.0 to 0.5
D. −2.5 to −1.0
E. <−2.5

 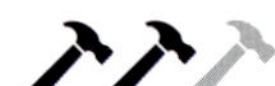 

9. A 49-year-old man has had bilateral intermittent pain and morning stiffness in the hand joints for 5 months. He has Hashimoto thyroiditis, managed with levothyroxine. He has swelling and tenderness in the proximal interphalangeal joints and pain in the metacarpophalangeal squeeze.

Investigations:
X-ray of the hands: joint space narrowing and osteopenia of the proximal interphalangeal joints.

Which is the most appropriate management?

A. Colchicine
B. Exercise and NSAIDs
C. Methotrexate
D. Paracetamol
E. Pilocarpine

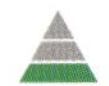 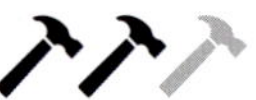 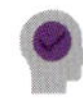

10. A 46-year-old woman has sudden pain and swelling in her left knee. She has haemochromatosis, managed with venesection. Her left knee is erythematous and tender with a reduced range of motion.

Investigations:
Knee X-ray: linear calcifications of the left meniscus.

Which of the following would be seen in synovial fluid analysis?

A. Gram-positive cocci in clusters
B. Negatively birefringent needle-shaped crystals
C. Negatively birefringent rhomboid-shaped crystals
D. Positively birefringent needle-shaped crystals
E. Positively birefringent rhomboid-shaped crystals

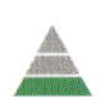  

11. A 91-year-old woman has a fall at her nursing home. She has osteoporosis and Alzheimer disease, managed with Adcal D3 and memantine. Her right leg is shortened and externally rotated.

Bone profile:

	Calcium	Phosphate	ALP	PTH
A	N	N	N	N
B	N	Elevated	N	N
C	Reduced	Elevated	Elevated	Elevated
D	N	N	Elevated	Elevated
E	Elevated	Elevated	Elevated	N

Which is the most appropriate bone profile result?

A. A
B. B
C. C
D. D
E. E

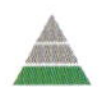  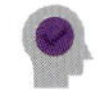

12. A 51-year-old man has sudden severe pain and swelling in his left big toe, worse after consuming alcohol. He has 6 months of similar episodes. He has peptic ulcer disease, managed with omeprazole. His left big toe is erythematous, warm to the touch and extremely tender.

Investigations:
Synovial fluid analysis: negatively birefringent needle-shaped urate crystals.

Which is the most appropriate management?
A. Colchicine
B. Methotrexate
C. Naproxen
D. Paracetamol
E. Physiotherapy

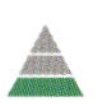 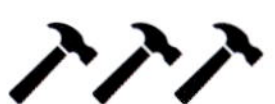

13. A 15-year-old boy has had joint pain and swelling in the knees and wrists for 3 months, with morning stiffness that improves during the day. His temperature has been around 39°C for the past week. He has splenomegaly and a salmon-pink rash is noticed in the axilla.

Investigations:
Antinuclear antibodies: negative

Which is the most likely diagnosis?
A. Osteoarthritis
B. Rheumatoid arthritis
C. Still's disease
D. Systemic sclerosis
E. Systemic lupus erythematosus

 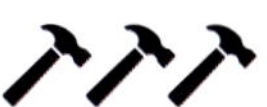

14. A 43-year-old woman presents with joint pain and stiffness in multiple joints for 6 months. Her symptoms are worse in the morning and improve with activity. She has tenderness in the metacarpophalangeal joints and wrists bilaterally.

Investigations:
Anticyclic citrullinated peptide (Anti-CCP) antibodies: elevated.

Which of the following HLA antigens is associated with the likely diagnosis?
A. HLA-B27
B. HLA-B51
C. HLA-DQ2
D. HLA-DR3
E. HLA-DR4

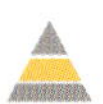 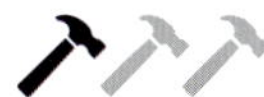

15. A 34-year-old man has had joint pain and fatigue for 3 months. He has Raynaud phenomenon, managed with nifedipine. He has a malar rash, erythematous lesions on his limbs and joint tenderness.

Investigations:
Antibody testing: antinuclear antibody (ANA) positive.

Which is the most likely diagnosis?
A. CREST syndrome
B. Dermatomyositis
C. Polymyositis
D. Sjögren syndrome
E. Systemic lupus erythematosus

 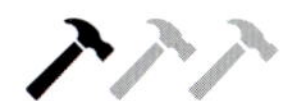

16. A 27-year-old man has had lower back pain and pleuritic chest pain for 6 months. His symptoms are worse in the morning and improve when he exercises. He has reduced lateral and forward flexion and tenderness over the sacroiliac joints.

Investigations:
X-ray of the sacroiliac joints: syndesmophytes.

Which is the most likely diagnosis?
A. Ankylosing spondylitis
B. Axial spondyloarthritis
C. Mechanical back pain
D. Psoriatic arthritis
E. Slipped disc

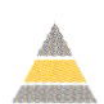 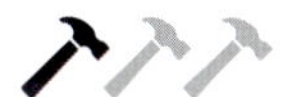 

17. A 28-year-old woman has had bilateral joint pain and swelling in her hands, wrists and knees for 4 months. She also has facial rash. She has tenderness and swelling in multiple joints and has oral ulcers.

Which is the most appropriate management?
A. Hydroxychloroquine
B. Ibuprofen
C. Methotrexate
D. Paracetamol
E. Prednisolone

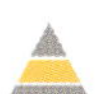 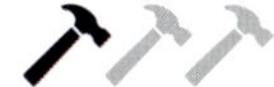

18. A 69-year-old man has had bilateral shoulder and hip pain for 6 weeks. The pain is a dull ache, worse in the morning and stiffness lasting for an hour. He has tenderness and a limited range of motion in his shoulders and hips.

Investigations:
Erythrocyte sedimentation rate (ESR): 54 mm/h (<20).
Temporal artery biopsy: negative.

Which is the most likely diagnosis?
A. Ankylosing spondylitis
B. Chronic Fatigue Syndrome
C. Polymyalgia rheumatica
D. Psoriatic arthritis
E. Shoulder tendinopathy

 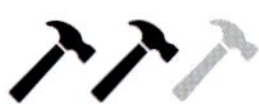

19. A 34-year-old man has had joint pain and stiffness in the right knee and ankle for a week. He had diarrhoea a month ago, which has since self-resolved. He has dysuria, and his eyes are stuck together in the morning. He has purulent discharge from both eyes and tender, swollen knee joints.

Which is the most likely diagnosis?
A. Ankylosing spondylitis
B. Polymyalgia rheumatica
C. Psoriatic arthritis
D. Reactive arthritis
E. Septic arthritis

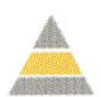  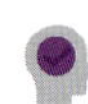

20. A 43-year-old woman has had dryness in her eyes and mouth for 4 months. She had early menopause at the age of 34, managed with combined, continuous HRT. She has sensory polyneuropathy and mild synovitis in multiple joints.

Which of the following antibodies would be raised?
A. Anticardiolipin antibodies
B. Anticentromere antibodies
C. Anti-dsDNA antibodies
D. Anti-Jo-1 antibodies
E. Anti-Ro antibodies

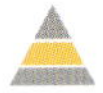 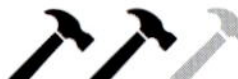

21. A 34-year-old woman has had joint pain and swelling of his fingers for 3 months, with red, scaly patches affecting her knees and elbows. She has tenderness, swelling and erythema of her distal interphalangeal joints bilaterally.

Which is the most likely diagnosis?
A. Ankylosing spondylitis
B. Osteoarthritis
C. Psoriatic arthritis
D. Rheumatoid arthritis
E. Septic arthritis

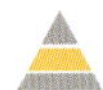 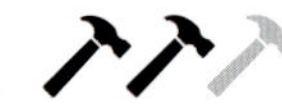 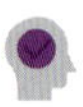

22. A 32-year-old man has lower back pain and stiffness for 5 months. His symptoms are worse in the morning and improve when he plays football. He has anterior uveitis, managed with atropine. He has reduced lumbar spine mobility and tenderness over the sacroiliac joints.

Investigations:
X-ray of the sacroiliac joints: squaring of the lumbar vertebrae.

Which is the most appropriate management?
A. Colchicine
B. Exercise and NSAIDs
C. Flucloxacillin
D. Methotrexate
E. Paracetamol

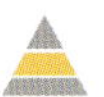  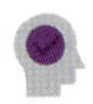

23. A 45-year-old woman has had fatigue and pleuritic chest pain for 2 months. She also has a malar rash worsened by sunlight exposure. She has type 1 diabetes mellitus, managed with a basal-bolus insulin regime. She has mouth ulcers and joint pain.

Investigations:
Erythrocyte sedimentation rate (ESR): 53 mm/h (<20).
Complement levels: low levels of C3 and C4.

Which of the following antibodies would be raised?
A. Anticardiolipin antibodies
B. Anticentromere antibodies
C. Anti-dsDNA antibodies
D. Anti-Jo-1 antibodies
E. Anti-Ro antibodies

 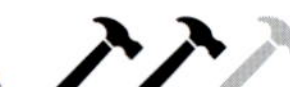 

24. A 46-year-old woman has had dry eyes, causing eye irritation and mouth for 6 months. She has rheumatoid arthritis, managed with methotrexate. She has generalized muscle aches and joint pains throughout the body.

Which is the most appropriate investigation?
A. Anti-CCP antibodies
B. Schirmer's test
C. Synovial fluid analysis
D. X-ray of the hands
E. X-ray of the sacroiliac joints

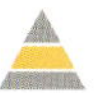 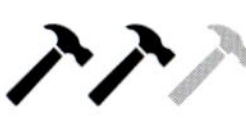 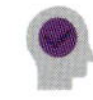

25. A 74-year-old man has had bilateral shoulder and hip pain and stiffness for three weeks. The pain is aching and is worse in the mornings, improving as the day progresses. He has tenderness over the shoulder and hip girdles, with no joint swelling.

Investigations:
C-reactive protein (CRP): 47 mg/L (<10).

Which is the most appropriate management?
   A. Flucloxacillin
   B. Hydroxychloroquine
   C. Ibuprofen
   D. Methotrexate
   E. Prednisolone

 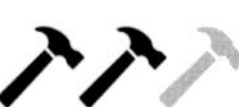

26. A 29-year-old woman has a swollen, painful left knee for a day. She is sexually active with multiple partners. Her left knee is erythematous tender, and she has a limited range of motion.

Investigations:
Erythrocyte sedimentation rate (ESR): 62 mm/h (<20).

Which is the most likely diagnosis?
   A. Ankylosing spondylitis
   B. Osteoarthritis
   C. Reactive arthritis
   D. Rheumatoid arthritis
   E. Septic arthritis

27. A 26-year-old man has had lower back pain and stiffness for 6 months, with the pain and stiffness being worse in the morning and improving with exercise. He has reduced lumbar spine mobility and tenderness over the sacroiliac joints. He also has red eyes bilaterally and complains of intense photophobia.

Which is the most appropriate investigation?
   A. Anti-CCP antibodies
   B. HLA-B27 testing
   C. Schirmer's test
   D. Synovial fluid analysis
   E. X-ray of the sacroiliac joints

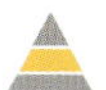 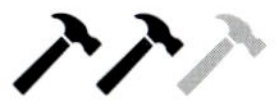 

28. A 59-year-old woman has had persistent dry eyes and mouth for 5 months. She also has difficulty swallowing dry foods and has a decreased sense of taste.

Investigations:
Antibody testing: positive anti-Ro and anti-La antibodies.

Which is the most appropriate management?
   A. Colchicine
   B. Exercise and NSAIDs
   C. Methotrexate
   D. Paracetamol
   E. Pilocarpine

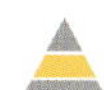 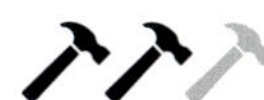 

29. A 24-year-old man has asymmetric arthritis and swelling in his knees and ankles after diarrhoea a month ago. He also has dysuria and purulent eye discharge for a week. He has tenderness and warmth in his knee and ankle joints. Furthermore, he has waxy yellow papules on the soles of his feet.

Which is the most appropriate management?
   A. Flucloxacillin
   B. Hydroxychloroquine
   C. Ibuprofen
   D. Methotrexate
   E. Sulphasalazine

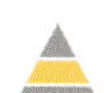  

30. A 67-year-old man has a swollen, red and painful right knee for 1 day. He has type 2 diabetes mellitus, controlled poorly with metformin. He is penicillin allergic. His temperature is 38.5°C. He has a limited range of motion in the right knee.

Investigations:
Blood cultures: *Staphylococcus aureus*.

Which is the most appropriate management?
   A. Clindamycin
   B. Doxycycline
   C. Flucloxacillin
   D. Ibuprofen
   E. Vancomycin

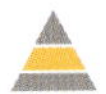 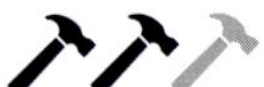 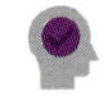

31. A 42-year-old woman has bilateral joint pain, swelling and stiffness. She has tenderness and swelling of the distal interphalangeal joints and red, scaly patches over the extensor surfaces. She also has nail pitting and onycholysis.

Investigations:
X-ray of the hands: periarticular erosions.

Which is the most appropriate management?
A. Flucloxacillin
B. Hydroxychloroquine
C. Ibuprofen
D. Methotrexate
E. Ustekinimab

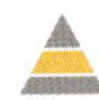 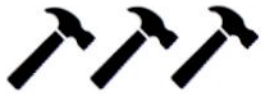 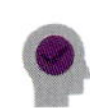

32. A 53-year-old man has had fatigue and chest pain on inspiration for 2 weeks after being started on treatment for tuberculosis 3 months prior. He also has generalized joint pain and a butterfly-shaped facial rash.

Investigations:
Antihistone antibodies: elevated.

Which is the most likely cause of his presentation?
A. Ethambutol
B. Isoniazid
C. Pyrazinamide
D. Pyridoxine
E. Rifampicin

 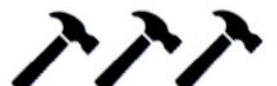 

33. A 12-year-old boy has a severely painful, swollen hip for 1 day. He has sickle cell anaemia, managed with hydroxyurea. His temperature is 38.9°C. His hip has a limited range of motion and cannot bear weight.

Which are the most appropriate criteria to assess the likelihood of this diagnosis?
A. Beighton score
B. FRAX tool
C. Kocher's criteria
D. O'Brien's criteria
E. Oxford Hip score

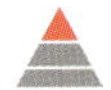 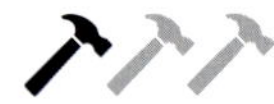

34. A 45-year-old woman has generalized muscular pain, fatigue and difficulty sleeping for 7 months. The pain is present in the neck, shoulders and lower back and is a constant dull ache exacerbated by physical activity. She keeps forgetting the doctor's instructions during the examination.

Investigations:
Erythrocyte sedimentation rate (ESR): 16 mm/h (<20).
C-reactive protein (CRP): 9 mg/L (<10).

Which is the most likely diagnosis?
A. Chronic fatigue syndrome
B. Fibromyalgia
C. Polymyalgia rheumatica
D. Rheumatoid arthritis
E. Systemic lupus erythematosus

 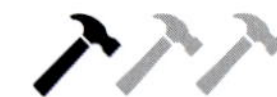

35. A 65-year-old man has 3 years of intermittent back pain, which has worsened recently. He has also had hearing loss and gradual head enlargement for a year. He has tenderness of the lumbar spine with a limited range of motion.

Bone profile:

	Calcium	Phosphate	ALP	PTH
A	N	N	N	N
B	N	N	Elevated	N
C	Reduced	Elevated	Elevated	Elevated
D	N	N	Elevated	Elevated
E	Elevated	Elevated	Elevated	N

Which is the most appropriate bone profile result?
A. A
B. B
C. C
D. D
E. E

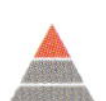 

36. A 59-year-old man has swelling of his fingers and food getting stuck in his throat for 3 months. Her fingers also turn white and numb when exposed to the cold. She has thickened skin on her fingers and visible small blood vessels on her face and hands.

Which is the most likely diagnosis?
A. Dermatomyositis
B. Eosinophilic fasciitis
C. Limited cutaneous systemic sclerosis
D. Scleroedema
E. Systemic lupus erythematosus

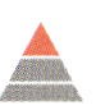  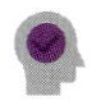

37. A 31-year-old man has had a painful sore on the shaft of his penis and gum ulcers for a week. He has multiple sexual partners, regularly engaging in unprotected sexual intercourse. He has reddening of his eyes with pain and tender, red bumps on his shins bilaterally.

Which is the most appropriate management?
A. Alendronate
B. Amitriptyline
C. Doxycycline
D. Flucloxacillin
E. Triamcinolone

 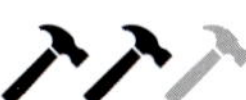

38. A 52-year-old woman has had progressive muscle weakness and a facial rash for 7 weeks. She had ovarian cancer, managed with bilateral salpingo-oopherectomy a year ago. She also has proximal muscle weakness in the hip and shoulder flexors and red bumps on her knuckles bilaterally.

Which is the most likely diagnosis?
A. Cutaneous T-cell lymphoma
B. Dermatomyositis
C. Polymyositis
D. Psoriasis
E. Systemic lupus erythematosus

 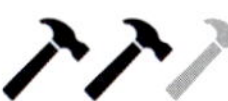

39. A 13-year-old boy has a growing painful lump on his right forearm for a month. The pain worsens at night, and he has lost 2 kg unintentionally this month.

Investigations:
Radial X-ray: multilayered periosteal reaction giving the bone an onion-skin appearance.

Which is the most likely diagnosis?
A. Ewing sarcoma
B. Giant cell tumour
C. Osteochondroma
D. Osteoma
E. Osteosarcoma

 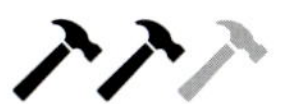 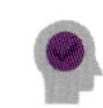

40. A 41-year-old man has progressively worsening weakness in his upper arms and a reddish-purple facial rash. He has Ehlers-Danlos syndrome.

Investigations:
Serum creatinine kinase: 640 U/L (24–195)

Which of the following antibodies would be raised?
A. Anticardiolipin antibodies
B. Anticentromere antibodies
C. Anti-dsDNA antibodies
D. Anti-Jo-1 antibodies
E. Anti-Ro antibodies

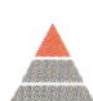 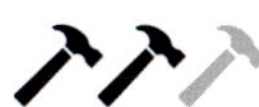

41. A 46-year-old woman has progressive muscle weakness and an inability to do everyday activities for 3 months. She also has fatigue and unintentional weight loss of 4 kg. She has proximal myopathy and an MRC power of 3/5 in the hip flexors and 4/5 in the shoulder abductors.

Investigations:
Serum creatinine kinase: 640 U/L (24–195)
Serum lactate dehydrogenase: 524 U/L (10–250)

Which is the most likely diagnosis?
A. Dermatomyositis
B. Polymyalgia Rheumatica
C. Polymyositis
D. Scleroderma
E. Systemic lupus erythematosus

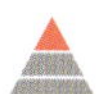  

42. A 41-year-old woman has had widespread muscular pain, a constant dull ache that worsens with physical activity for 6 months. She has difficulty concentrating on what the doctor is telling her to do.

Investigations:
Erythrocyte sedimentation rate (ESR): 18 mm/h (<20).
C-reactive protein (CRP): 7 mg/L (<10).

Which is the most appropriate management?
A. Alendronate
B. Amitriptyline
C. Ibuprofen
D. Paracetamol
E. Prednisolone

43. A 33-year-old woman has persistent fatigue, not improved by rest and generalized muscle pains, worsened by activity for 8 months. She has poor sleep and finds it difficult to concentrate at work.

Investigations:
Serum alanine aminotransferase (ALT): 28U/L (5–35)
Serum aspartate aminotransferase (AST): 23U/L (1–31)
Serum thyroid-stimulating hormone: 3.7mU/L (0.4–5.0)
Serum-free T4: 18.2pmol/L (10.0–22.0)
Antinuclear antibodies: negative.

Which is the most likely diagnosis?
A. Chronic fatigue syndrome
B. Depression
C. Fibromyalgia
D. Rheumatoid arthritis
E. Subclinical hypothyroidism

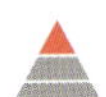 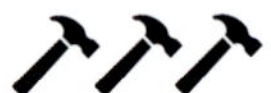

44. A 34-year-old woman has a left-sided, progressively worsening headache. She says the headache feels like something is pressing against her left eyeball. She has Gardner syndrome.

Investigations:
CT head: well-circumscribed, rounded, bony cortical irregularity in the left maxillary sinus.

Which is the most likely diagnosis?
A. Ewing sarcoma
B. Giant cell tumour
C. Osteochondroma
D. Osteoma
E. Osteosarcoma

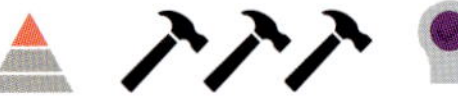

45. A 47-year-old man says his fingers turn white and numb when he walks out into the cold, and he has had difficulty swallowing his food for 3 months. He has rheumatoid arthritis, managed with methotrexate. He has visible small blood vessels on his cheeks.

Which of the following antibodies would be raised?
A. Anticardiolipin antibodies
B. Anticentromere antibodies
C. Anti-dsDNA antibodies
D. Anti-Jo-1 antibodies
E. Anti-Ro antibodies

Endocrine and diabetes

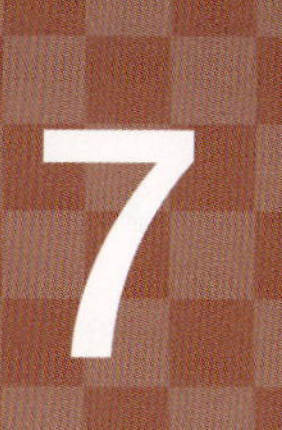

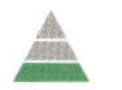 

1. A 29-year-old woman has a smooth swelling in her neck, gradually increasing in size for a year. She has bipolar disorder, managed with lithium three times a day for 2 years.

Which is the most likely diagnosis?
A. Graves disease
B. Hashimoto thyroiditis
C. Iatrogenic goitre
D. Nontoxic multinodular goitre
E. Toxic multinodular goitre

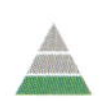 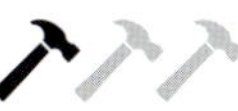

2. A 51-year-old woman is diagnosed with prediabetes following an HbA1c test.

Which HbA1c range is most consistent with a diagnosis of prediabetes?
A. 31–36 mmol/mol
B. 37–41 mmol/mol
C. 42–47 mmol/mol
D. 48–52 mmol/mol
E. 53–58 mmol/mol

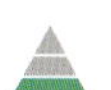 

3. A 34-year-old man has had abdominal pain and vomiting for 4 hours. He has been acting confused and tired since the start of the pain. He has type 1 diabetes mellitus, managed with a basal-bolus insulin regime.

Investigations:
Random blood glucose: 18.4 mmol/L (4.0–7.0).
Urine dipstick: glucose +++, ketones ++, blood -, leucocytes -

Which is the most appropriate management?
A. 0.01 unit/kg/h IV insulin
B. 0.1 unit/kg/h IV insulin
C. IV 5% dextrose
D. IV 0.45% NaCl
E. IV 0.9% NaCl

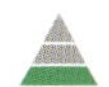  

4. A 52-year-old man was diagnosed with type 2 diabetes mellitus 6 months ago, for which he was recommended lifestyle interventions such as dietary modifications and increased exercise.

Investigations:
HbA1c: 55 mmol/mol (20–42).

Which is the most appropriate management?
A. Empagliflozin
B. Gliclazide
C. Metformin
D. Pioglitazone
E. Sitagliptin

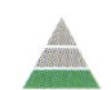 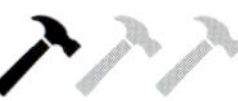 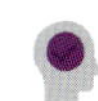

5. A 57-year-old woman has shakiness for 1 hour. She has type 2 diabetes mellitus, managed with metformin. She has not eaten for 12 hours, has had weakness, and is sweating profusely.

Investigations:
Blood sugar level: 2.4 mmol/L (4.0–7.0).

Which is the most appropriate management?
A. IM glucagon
B. IV 10% dextrose
C. IV 20% dextrose
D. IV saline
E. Oral GlucoGel

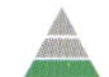 

6. A 43-year-old man has gained 10 kg over 6 months. His recent diet has been purely junk food since his wife passed away 6 months ago. He is diagnosed with obesity stage 2, as per his BMI.

Which of the following BMI ranges is associated with his diagnosis?
A. 18–21 kg/m^2
B. 21–24 kg/m^2
C. 24–30 kg/m^2
D. 30-35 kg/m^2
E. 35-40 kg/m^2

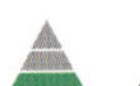 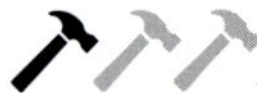

7. A 43-year-old woman has gained weight, despite maintaining a balanced diet and regular exercise for 6 months, with muscle weakness and easy bruising. Her BP is 154/102 mmHg. She has purple stretch marks on her abdomen.

Which is the most likely diagnosis?
   A. Acromegaly
   B. Addison disease
   C. Cushing syndrome
   D. Hashimoto thyroiditis
   E. Polycystic ovarian syndrome

8. A 6-year-old boy has had severe abdominal pain and vomiting for 10 hours. He has type I diabetes mellitus, managed with a basal-bolus insulin. He is breathing very heavily.

Investigations:
Urine dipstick: glucose +++, ketones +++, blood -, nitrites -
He is started on intravenous fluids and a fixed-rate insulin infusion. After 4 hours, he experiences a seizure.

Which of the following is the most likely cause of his seizure?
   A. Acidosis
   B. Cerebral oedema
   C. Hyperglycaemia
   D. Hypoglycaemia
   E. Hypokalaemia

 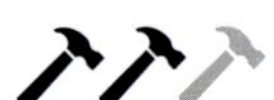 

9. A 32 year-old woman has problems losing weight despite conservative management and orlistat. Her BMI is 38 kg/m^2.

Which is the most appropriate management?
   A. Biliopancreatic diversion with duodenal switch
   B. Laparoscopic sleeve gastrectomy
   C. Naltrexone/bupropion
   D. Roux-en-Y gastric bypass surgery
   E. Semaglutide

10. A 31-year-old woman has had severe abdominal pain for 6 hours. She has type 1 diabetes mellitus, managed with a basal-bolus insulin regime. She has an abnormal breathing pattern.

Arterial Blood Gas (ABG):

	pH	Bicarbonate	pCO_2
A	Reduced	Reduced	Increased
B	Normal	Normal	Normal
C	Increased	Reduced	Increased
D	Reduced	Reduced	Reduced
E	Reduced	Normal	Increased

Which is the most likely ABG interpretation?
   A. A
   B. B
   C. C
   D. D
   E. E

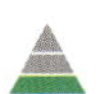 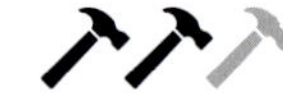 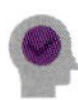

11. A 51-year-old man has muscle weakness and a build-up of fat at the back of the neck. His BP is 152/97 mmHg. He has reduced power in the upper arms and thighs and purple striae on his abdomen.

Which of the following would most likely be seen on arterial blood gas?
   A. Hyperkalaemic metabolic acidosis
   B. Hyperkalaemic metabolic alkalosis
   C. Hypokalaemic metabolic acidosis
   D. Hypokalaemic metabolic alkalosis
   E. Hyperkalaemic respiratory acidosis

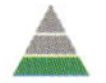 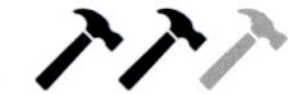 

12. A 53-year-old woman has persistent diarrhoea for a month. She has type 2 diabetes mellitus and was started on medication 2 months ago. She has mild tenderness over the abdomen.

Investigations:
pH: 7.27 (7.35–7.45).
Lactate: 5.9 mmol/L (0.5–1.6).

What is the drug's mechanism of action that has most probably caused his symptoms?

A. Activates PPAR-gamma receptor in adipocytes to promote fatty acid uptake
B. Inhibits glucagon secretion by an incretin mimetic
C. Increases insulin release from beta cells
D. Increases insulin sensitivity
E. Inhibits reabsorption of glucose in the kidney

 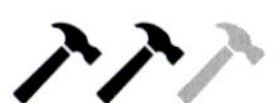 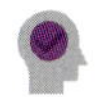

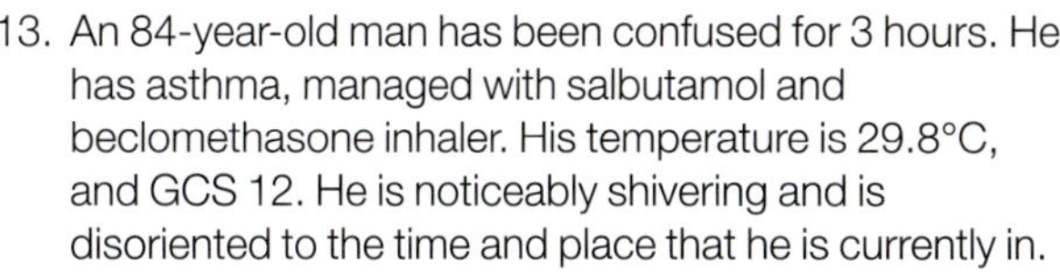

13. An 84-year-old man has been confused for 3 hours. He has asthma, managed with salbutamol and beclomethasone inhaler. His temperature is 29.8°C, and GCS 12. He is noticeably shivering and is disoriented to the time and place that he is currently in.

What is the most likely change seen on this man's ECG?

A. J waves
B. Shortened QT interval
C. ST depression
D. Tented T-waves
E. U waves

14. A 60-year-old man has had weight gain and fatigue for 5 months. His BP is 175/85 mmHg. He has purple striae over his abdomen and a dorso-cervical hump.

What is the likely change you would see on the ECG?

A. Delta wave
B. J waves
C. Prolonged QT interval
D. ST depression
E. Tented T waves

 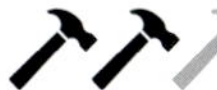

15. A 58-year-old woman has excessive sweating and a tremor in her hands. She has an abnormal protrusion of the eyeballs bilaterally, waxy discolouration of the lower legs and clubbing in both hands.

Investigations:
Thyroid scintigraphy: diffuse, homogenous and increased uptake of radioactive iodine.

Which is the most likely diagnosis?

A. De Quervain thyroiditis
B. Graves disease
C. Primary hyperparathyroidism
D. Toxic adenoma
E. Toxic multinodular goitre

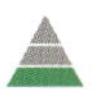 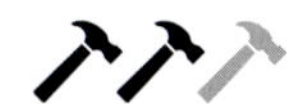 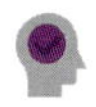

16. A 65-year-old man has had unintentional weight gain and muscle weakness for 5 months. His BP is 168/103 mmHg. He has thin, fragile skin with multiple bruises and purple striae throughout the body and his face is swollen.

Which is the most appropriate investigation?

A. CT adrenals
B. High-dose dexamethasone suppression test
C. Low-dose dexamethasone suppression test
D. Pituitary MRI
E. Short synacthen test

 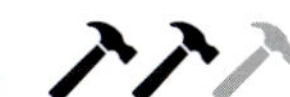

17. A 35-year-old woman has progressively increased fatigue and unintentional weight loss for 3 months.

Investigations:
Serum sodium: 132 mmol/L (137–144).
Serum potassium: 5.7 mmol/L (3.5–4.9).

Which is the most likely diagnosis?

A. Addison disease
B. Cushing syndrome
C. Hashimoto's thyroiditis
D. Polycystic ovarian syndrome
E. Primary hyperaldosteronism

18. A 54-year-old man has a low-grade fever and increased urinary frequency for 2 days. He has type 2 diabetes mellitus and was started on medication 2 months ago. He has hypogastric abdominal pain.

Investigations:
Urine dipstick: positive for nitrites and leucocytes.

What is the drug's mechanism of action that has likely caused his symptoms?

A. Inhibition of alpha-glucosidase
B. Inhibits glucagon secretion by an incretin mimetic
C. Increases insulin release from beta cells
D. Increases insulin sensitivity
E. Inhibits reabsorption of glucose in the kidney

 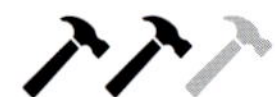 

19. A 42-year-old woman has had unintentional weight loss and weakness for 5 months. She has antiphospholipid syndrome, managed with aspirin and heparin. She has hyperpigmentation of the palmar creases and muscle weakness, worse in the proximal muscles of the limbs.

Investigations:
Serum sodium: 134 mmol/L (137–144).
Serum potassium: 5.9 mmol/L (3.5–4.9).

Which is the most appropriate management?
A. Fludrocortisone and hydrocortisone
B. Ketoconazole
C. Laparoscopic adrenalectomy
D. Spironolactone
E. Trans-sphenoidal surgery

 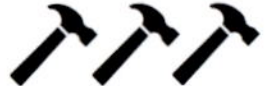 

20. A 73-year-old man has a dry mouth and an increased need to urinate. He has hypertension, GORD and gout managed with amlodipine, ramipril, bendroflumethiazide, omeprazole and allopurinol.

Investigations:
Fasting plasma glucose: 8.2 mmol/L (4.0–7.0).
Oral glucose tolerance test (75 g), 2-hour plasma glucose: 9.6 mmol/L (<7.8).
His general practitioner explains that he has impaired glucose tolerance and believes one of his medications is causing this problem.

Which of his medications is likely to be causing this?
A. Allopurinol
B. Amlodipine
C. Bendroflumethiazide
D. Omeprazole
E. Ramipril

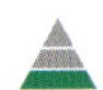 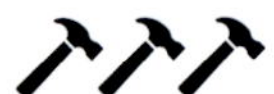 

21. A 58-year-old woman has an unintentional weight loss of 5 kg and haemoptysis for a month. She has smoked 20 cigarettes a day for 30 years and consumes ten units of alcohol a week. She has purple abdominal striae and clubbing of the fingers.

Investigations:
Serum sodium: 128 mmol/L (137–144).
Serum potassium: 3.3 mmol/L (3.5–4.9).

What result would be expected in a high-dose dexamethasone suppression test?
A. High cortisol and high ACTH
B. High cortisol and low ACTH
C. Low cortisol and high ACTH
D. Low cortisol and low ACTH
E. Low cortisol and normal ACTH

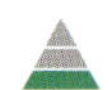 

22. A 19-year-old man has severe headaches for 3 hours. His temperature is 38.7°C, pulse 120 bpm, BP 86/58 mmHg and respiratory rate 22 breaths per minute. He has neck stiffness and a purpuric rash over his torso and limbs.

Investigations:
Serum sodium: 135 mmol/L (137–144).
Serum potassium: 5.1 mmol/L (3.5–4.9).
CT abdomen: bilateral enlargement of his adrenal glands.

Which is the most likely diagnosis?
A. Bilateral idiopathic adrenal hyperplasia
B. Congenital adrenal hyperplasia
C. Cushing syndrome
D. Phaeochromocytoma
E. Waterhouse-Friderichsen syndrome

23. A 49-year-old woman says her shoes no longer fit, and joint pain in her wrists and knees for a year. She has hypertension, managed with ramipril. She has a large tongue, coarse facial appearance and bitemporal hemianopia.

What is the most likely diagnosis?
A. Acromegaly
B. Addison's disease
C. Gigantism
D. McCune-Albright syndrome
E. Primary hyperparathyroidism

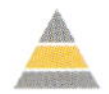 

24. A 31-year-old man has severe loin to groin pain bilaterally and has felt increasingly thirsty for a month. His mother has multiple endocrine neoplasia type 1. He also has generalized bony pain.

What is the most likely diagnosis?
A. De Quervain thyroiditis
B. Hypercalcaemia of malignancy
C. Primary hyperparathyroidism
D. Toxic adenoma
E. Tertiary hyperparathyrodism

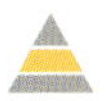  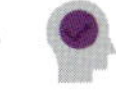

25. A 40-year-old woman has had constant fatigue for 6 months. Her BP is 172/106 mmHg. She has generalized muscular weakness.

Investigations:
Serum sodium: 142 mmol/L (137–144).
Serum potassium: 3.4 mmol/L (3.5–4.9).

Which is the most appropriate investigation?
A. Adrenal vein sampling
B. Low-dose dexamethasone suppression test
C. Plasma aldosterone:renin ratio
D. Short synacthen test
E. Urinary metanephrines

 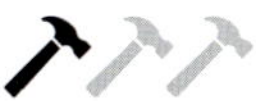

26. A 55-year-old man has excessive thirst and poor sleep due to urinating multiple times during the night. He has bipolar disorder, managed with lithium.

Investigations:
Blood glucose: normal.
Water deprivation test: low urine osmolality originally; after desmopressin, the urine osmolality is still low.

Which is the most likely diagnosis?
A. Cranial diabetes insipidus
B. Nephrogenic diabetes insipidus
C. Psychogenic polydipsia
D. Syndrome of inappropriate antidiuretic hormone secretion
E. Type 2 diabetes mellitus

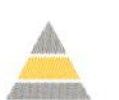  

27. A 64-year-old woman has had fatigue and constipation for 2 weeks. She has breast cancer, managed with her first chemotherapy 2 months ago and has since been in remission. On inspection, she appears pale.

Which is the most appropriate management?
A. Cinacalcet
B. Furosemide
C. Risedronate
D. Total parathyroidectomy
E. IV fluids

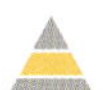 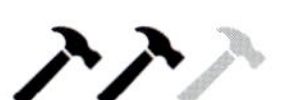 

28. A 60-year-old man has painful swallowing and unintentional weight loss of 5 kg 2 months ago. He had the flu for a week before this, where he was bed-bound and weak.

Investigations:
Serum thyroid-stimulating hormone: 8.1 mU/L (0.4–5.0).
Serum-free T4: 6.4 pmol/L (10.0–22.0).
Thyroid scintigraphy: reduced uptake globally.

Which is the most appropriate management?
A. Levothyroxine
B. Propranolol and carbimazole
C. Radioiodine therapy
D. Subtotal thyroidectomy
E. Total parathyroidectomy

 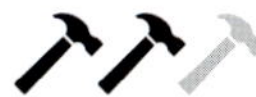

29. A 14-year-old boy of abnormally large stature has breast enlargement. He has small and firm testes, a lack of pubic hair and bilateral gynaecomastia.

Investigations:
Plasma follicle-stimulating hormone: 9.6 U/L (1.0–7.0).
Serum luteinizing hormone: 12.0 U/L (1.0–10.0).
Serum testosterone: 7 nmol/L (9–35).

Which is the most likely diagnosis?
A. Androgen-insensitivity syndrome
B. Kallmann syndrome
C. Klinefelter syndrome
D. Testosterone-secreting tumour
E. Turner syndrome

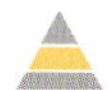 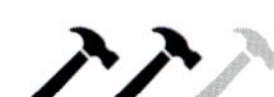 

30. A 60-year-old woman has bone pain and a low mood. She has chronic kidney disease managed with ramipril and alfacalcidol. She has generalized abdominal pain, muscular weakness and constipation.

	PTH	Calcium	Phosphate
A	Increased	Increased	Increased
B	Normal	Increased	Decreased
C	Increased	Increased	Decreased
D	Increased	Increased	Decreased
E	Normal	Increased	Normal

Which blood results is associated with the most likely diagnosis?

A. A
B. B
C. C
D. D
E. E

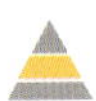 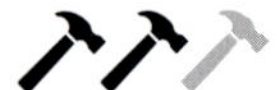 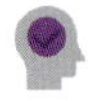

31. A 43-year-old man with episodic headaches and palpitations. His BP is 179/102 mmHg.

Investigations:
24-hour urinary collection of metanephrines: increased.
CT abdomen: right adrenal medulla mass.

Which is the most appropriate initial management?

A. Amlodipine
B. Phenoxybenzamine
C. Propranolol
D. Ramipril
E. Surgical excision

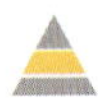  

32. A 32-year-old woman has nocturia and feels thirsty all the time. She had a concussion 3 weeks ago when playing for her local rugby team.

Investigations:
Blood glucose: normal.
A water deprivation test is done as part of her general investigations.

What is her water deprivation test likely to show?

A. High urine osmolality after both water deprivation and desmopressin
B. Low urine osmolality after both water deprivation and desmopressin
C. Low urine osmolality after water deprivation but high urine osmolality after desmopressin
D. Low urine osmolality after water deprivation but normal urine osmolality after desmopressin
E. Normal urine osmolality after both water deprivation and desmopressin

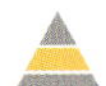 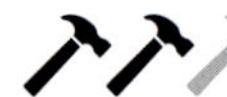 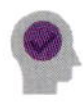

33. A 44-year-old man has had a worsening headache for 3 weeks. He has also been anxious and has a racing heartbeat. He tried paracetamol for his headaches but has since stopped using it. His BP is 178/101 mmHg. He has a bilateral fine tremor.

Investigations:
Serum sodium (Na^+): 143 mmol/L (137–144).
Serum potassium (K^+): 4.2 mmol/L (3.5–4.9).

Which is the most appropriate investigation?

A. Low-dose dexamethasone suppression test
B. Plasma aldosterone:renin ratio
C. Short Synacthen test
D. Urinary catecholamines
E. Urinary metanephrines

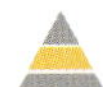 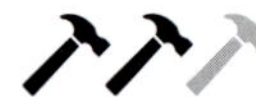

34. A 26-year-old woman has a road traffic accident with a car whilst crossing the road. She has had intermittent headaches and no periods for 4 months. She has a broken femur, bruises and bilateral hemianopia.

Which is the most likely diagnosis?

A. Acromegaly
B. Craniopharyngioma
C. Pituitary apoplexy
D. Prolactinoma
E. Turner syndrome

 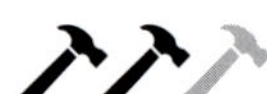

35. A 12-year-old has severe testicular pain for 1 week. He has right subareolar glandular tissue enlargement, but denies any pain. He had pain on eating and muscular pain three months prior to the testicular pain. He has a tender, swollen right testicle but there is some relief of pain on elevation of the scrotum.

Which is the most likely cause of his presentation?

A. Hyperthyroidism
B. Klinfelter syndrome
C. Mumps
D. Pubertal gynaecomastia
E. Testicular cancer

 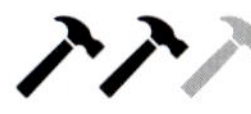

36. A 62-year-old woman has blurred vision and floaters in her right eye for a month. She has type 2 diabetes mellitus, managed poorly with metformin.

Investigations:
Fundoscopy: neovascularization, intraretinal haemorrhages and cotton-wool spots in the right eye.

Which is the most likely diagnosis?
- A. Background retinopathy
- B. Central retinal vein occlusion
- C. Diabetic maculopathy
- D. Preproliferative retinopathy
- E. Proliferative retinopathy

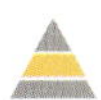 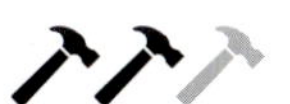 

37. A 34-year-old man has had unintentional weight loss, a racing heartbeat and heat intolerance for 3 months. His pulse is 120 bpm. He has a diffusely enlarged thyroid gland.

Investigations:
Serum thyroid-stimulating hormone: 0.3 mU/L (0.4–5.0).
Serum-free T4: 27.4 pmol/L (10.0–22.0).

Which of the following antibodies would be the most likely to be positive?
- A. Anti-GAD antibodies
- B. Anti-TPO antibodies
- C. Insulin autoantibodies
- D. Thyroglobulin antibodies
- E. TSH receptor-stimulating antibodies

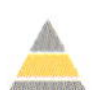 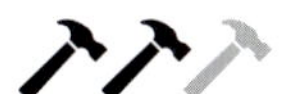 

38. A 39-year-old woman has had progressively enlarging hands and feet and joint pain in his wrists and knees for 2 years, with her facial features coarsening. Her hands and feet are much larger than expected with her height, and she has macroglossia.

Which is the most appropriate management?
- A. Cabergoline
- B. Octreotide
- C. Subtotal thyroidectomy
- D. Total parathyroidectomy
- E. Trans-sphenoidal surgery

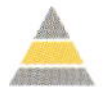 

39. A 32-year-old man has had muscular cramps and facial twitching for 5 months. He has thyroid cancer, managed with a thyroidectomy last year. He has twitching of facial muscles when tapping over the area of the facial nerve.

Investigations:
Serum-corrected calcium: 2.14 mmol/L (2.20–2.60).
Serum phosphate: 1.68 mmol/L (0.8–14).
Plasma parathyroid hormone: 0.71 pmol/L (0.9–5.4).

Which is the most likely diagnosis?
- A. Hypercalcaemia
- B. Hyperparathyroidism
- C. Hypocalcemia of malignancy
- D. Hypoparathyroidism
- E. Hypothyroidism

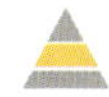 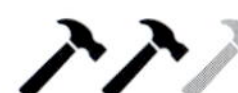

40. A 46-year-old woman has abdominal pain, bloating and frequent vomiting after eating. She has type 2 diabetes mellitus, managed with metformin. However, she has been having erratic blood glucose measures when she measures it daily. She has abdominal distension and generalized abdominal pain.

Investigations:
Urine dipstick: glycosuria.

Which is the most likely diagnosis?
- A. Acute cholecystitis
- B. Acute pancreatitis
- C. Diabetic ketoacidosis
- D. Gastroparesis
- E. Hyperosmolar hyperglycaemic state

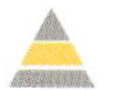 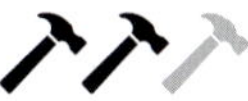 

41. A 54-year-old man has had fatigue and muscle weakness for 3 months. His BP is 162/104 mmHg.

Investigations:
Serum sodium: 141 mmol/L (137–144).
Serum potassium: 3.2 mmol/L (3.5–4.9).

High-resolution CT: adrenal glands' limbs 15mm thick bilaterally

Which is the most appropriate management?

A. Fludrocortisone and hydrocortisone
B. Ketoconazole
C. Laparoscopic adrenalectomy
D. Spironolactone
E. Trans-sphenoidal surgery

 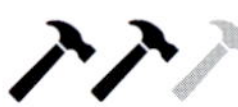

42. A 34-year-old woman has infrequent menstrual periods for 8 months. She has an iodine deficiency. Her temperature is 37.8°C, and pulse 114 bpm. She has an irregular goitre and has bilateral lid lag in her eyes.

Investigations:
Thyroid scintigraphy: patchy uptake.

Which is the most likely diagnosis?

A. De Quervain thyroiditis
B. Graves disease
C. Primary hyperparathyroidism
D. Toxic adenoma
E. Toxic multinodular goitre

 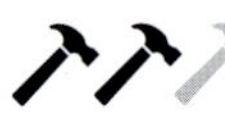 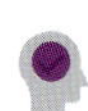

43. A 32-year-old woman, who is 24 weeks pregnant for an oral glucose tolerance test. Her father has type 2 diabetes mellitus.

Investigations:
Fasting plasma glucose: 7.2 mmol/L (<5.6)
Two-hour plasma glucose: 9.2 mmol/L (<7.8)

Which is the most appropriate management?

A. Dietary intervention
B. Glibenclamide
C. Gliclazide
D. Insulin
E. Metformin

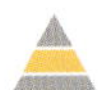 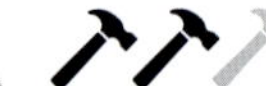 

44. A 54-year-old man has type 2 diabetes, managed poorly with metformin.

Investigations:
Fundoscopy: microaneurysms, blot haemorrhages and hard exudates throughout the retina.

Which is the most appropriate management?

A. Dorzolamide
B. Panretinal laser photocoagulation
C. Ranibizumab
D. Regular observation
E. Vitreoretinal surgery

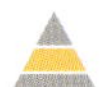 

45. A 63-year-old woman has had confusion for 4 days. She has type 2 diabetes mellitus, managed with metformin. She has been drinking excessive amounts of water during this period.

Investigations:
pH: 7.32 (7.35-7.45)
Blood glucose: 37.5 mmol/L (<11.1).
Serum osmolality: 341 mOsmol/kg (278–300).

Which is the most likely diagnosis?

A. Diabetic ketoacidosis
B. Hyperosmolar hyperglycaemic state
C. Nephrogenic diabetes insipidus
D. Type 2 diabetes mellitus
E. Syndrome of inappropriate antidiuretic hormone secretion

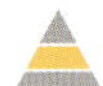 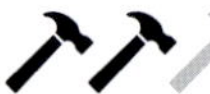 

46. A 42-year-old man has increased sweating and joint pain for a year. His BP is 162/97 mmHg. He has facial features with frontal bossing and hands and feet that are much larger than would be expected, given his height.

Investigations:
Serum IGF-1 level: elevated.

Which is the most common complication?

A. Cardiomyopathy
B. Hypotension
C. Prostate cancer
D. Renal failure
E. Type 1 diabetes mellitus

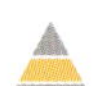 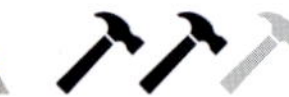 

47. A 31-year-old woman has a check-up at 24 weeks of gestation. She gained more weight during this pregnancy compared to her previous 2 years ago. Both her parents have type 2 diabetes. Her BP is 123/78 mmHg.

Investigations:
Urinalysis: no signs of proteinuria or haematuria.

Which is the most appropriate investigation?
- A. Anticardiolipin antibody assay
- B. Fasting plasma glucose
- C. HbA1c
- D. Oral glucose tolerance test
- E. Random plasma glucose

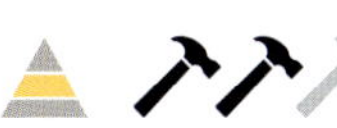
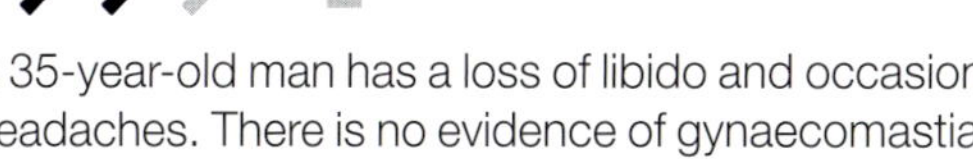

48. A 35-year-old man has a loss of libido and occasional headaches. There is no evidence of gynaecomastia but there is a milky discharge from his nipples present.

Investigations:
Prolactin level: 23,369 mu/L (<360).

Which is the most appropriate management?
- A. Cabergoline
- B. Laparoscopic adrenalectomy
- C. Propranolol and carbimazole
- D. Spironolactone
- E. Trans-sphenoidal surgery

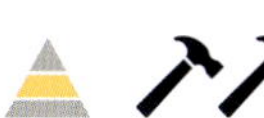

49. A 3-week-old baby girl has been vomiting and poor feeding for a week, and her genitalia appear more male-like. Her BP is 87/58 mmHg. She has fused labia and a mild salt-wasting crisis with hyponatraemia.

Which is the most likely diagnosis?
- A. 5-alpha-reductase deficiency
- B. Androgen insensitivity syndrome
- C. Congenital adrenal hyperplasia
- D. Kallmann syndrome
- E. Turner syndrome

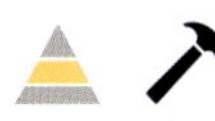
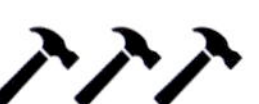

50. A 69-year-old man has had generalized weakness, nausea and vomiting for a week. He has small-cell lung cancer managed with chemotherapy, which started last month. He has orthostatic hypotension, dry mucous membranes and decreased skin turgor.

Investigations:
Serum sodium: 140 mmol/L (137–144).
Serum osmolality: 253 mOsmol/kg (278–300).

Which is the most appropriate management?
- A. Desmopressin
- B. Fluid restriction
- C. Furosemide
- D. Tolvaptan
- E. IV hypertonic saline

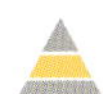
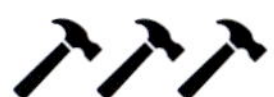

51. A 40-year-old woman has a mass in her neck region growing rapidly for a month. She has had abnormally heavy menstrual periods for 5 months and has felt lethargic. She has a large, tender mass in the neck and problems swallowing.

Investigations:
Serum TSH: 12.3 mU/L (0.4–5.0).
Serum-free T4: 8.6 pmol/L (10.0–22.0).
Anti-TSH receptor stimulating antibodies: negative.
Antithyroid peroxidase (TPO) antibodies: Positive.

Which is the most likely diagnosis?
- A. Anaplastic thyroid cancer
- B. Follicular thyroid cancer
- C. Medullary thyroid cancer
- D. Papillary thyroid cancer
- E. Thyroid lymphoma

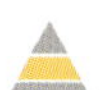

52. A 52-year-old man has had a cough and unintentional weight loss of 6 kg over 3 months. He occasionally brings up blood in his sputum and has a low mood. He has smoked 20 cigarettes a day for 30 years. He has clubbing of his fingers and a fixed, monophonic wheeze.

Investigations:
Serum-corrected calcium: 2.83 mmol/L (2.2–2.6).
Plasma parathyroid hormone: 4.57 pmol/L (0.9–5.4).

Which is the most likely diagnosis?
- A. Primary hyperparathyroidism
- B. Sarcoidosis
- C. Small cell lung cancer
- D. Squamous cell carcinoma
- E. Tertiary hyperparathyroidism

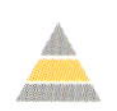

53. A 21-year-old woman has diarrhoea and palpitations. Her mother had cancer that presented very similarly to her current symptoms. Her BP is 172/108 mmHg. She has a

bilateral fine tremor in her hands and a lump in her neck, which she says has grown rapidly over the past month.

Investigations:
Serum-corrected calcium: 3.18 mmol/L (2.2–2.6).
Serum phosphate: 0.69 mmol/L (0.8–1.4).
Plasma parathyroid hormone: 6.71 pmol/L (0.9–5.4).

Which is the most likely diagnosis?
A. Anaplastic thyroid cancer
B. Follicular thyroid cancer
C. Medullary thyroid cancer
D. Papillary thyroid cancer
E. Thyroid lymphoma

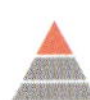 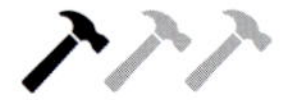 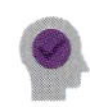

54. A 18-year-old man has left breast enlargement and tenderness for 2 months, causing him to be embarrased to exercise at the gym. He has no discharge from the nipples and he has reduced testicular volume bilaterally.

Which is the most appropriate management?
A. Breast reduction surgery
B. Danazol
C. Reassurance
D. Raloxifene
E. Tamoxifen

 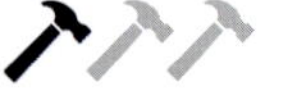 

55. A 39-year-old woman has a consultation posttreatment for thyroid cancer. She has papillary thyroid cancer, which was treated with thyroidectomy followed by radioiodine ablation. She was given levothyroxine to supplement the loss of her thyroid gland.

Which of the following markers should be used to measure the recurrence of her thyroid cancer?
A. Serum AFP
B. Serum CA 19-9
C. Serum calcitonin
D. Serum TSH
E. Serum thyroglobulin

 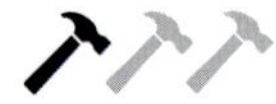

56. A 37-year-old man has eye discomfort and eye protrusion. He has Graves disease, managed poorly with carbimazole and propranolol. He has bilateral eyelid retraction and proptosis; however, visual acuity is normal.

Which of the following is the strongest risk factor for the man's most likely diagnosis?
A. Amiodarone usage
B. Excess alcohol intake
C. Obesity
D. Sedentary lifestyle
E. Smoking

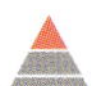 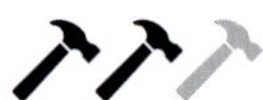 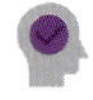

57. A 31-year-old woman has had diarrhoea and abdominal pain for 3 months. Her face has also been increasingly red. Her BP is 86/57 mmHg. She has an ejection systolic murmur best heard at the second left intercostal space.

Which is the most appropriate investigation?
A. Low-dose dexamethasone suppression test
B. Plasma aldosterone:renin ratio
C. Short Synacthen test
D. Urinary 5-HIAA
E. Urinary metanephrines

 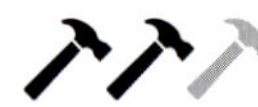 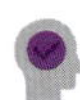

58. A 28-year-old man has a racing heartbeat and headaches. His BP is 184/109 mmHg. He is sweating profusely.

Investigations:
24-hour urinary collection of metanephrines: elevated.
CT abdomen: left adrenal mass.

Which is the most appropriate definitive management?
A. Cabergoline
B. Phenoxybenzamine
C. Propranolol
D. Surgical resection
E. Trans-sphenoidal surgery

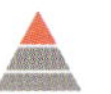 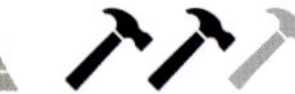

59. A 64-year-old woman has generalized weakness and bilateral loin to groin pain for a year.

Investigations:
Serum-corrected calcium: 2.98 mmol/L (2.2–2.6).
Serum phosphate: 0.71 mmol/L (0.8–1.4).
Plasma parathyroid hormone: 7.02 pmol/L (0.9–5.4).

What is the most likely thing to be seen on an X-ray?

A. Adrenal medulla mass
B. Pepperpot skull
C. Periarticular erosions
D. Raindrop skull
E. Staghorn calculus

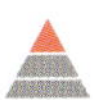 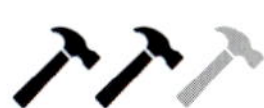

60. A 52-year-old man has a lesion on his left foot after stepping on glass a month ago. He has type 2 diabetes, managed with metformin and empagliflozin. He has been trying to keep the wound clean, but the lesion has increased pain and erythema. He has a deep, necrotic ulcer seen on the plantar surface of the left foot.

Which is the most likely diagnosis?

A. Arterial ulcer
B. Charcot foot
C. Cellulitis
D. Diabetic ulcer
E. Osteomyelitis

61. A 9-year-old girl has muscle cramps and weakness. She has experienced slow growth compared to other children her age. Her BP is 124/87 mmHg.

Investigations:
Serum sodium: 139 mmol/L (137–144).
Serum potassium: 3.1 mmol/L (3.5–4.9).

Which is the most likely diagnosis?

A. Addison disease
B. Bartter syndrome
C. Cushing disease
D. Liddle syndrome
E. Primary hyperaldosteronism

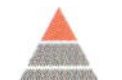  

62. A 44-year-old man has had diarrhoea and flushing for 5 months. His skin is flushed, and a wheeze is heard on his chest auscultation.

Investigations:
Urinary 5-hydroxyindoleacetic acid (5-HIAA): raised.

Which is the most appropriate management?

A. Cabergoline
B. Laparoscopic adrenalectomy
C. Octreotide
D. Propranolol and carbimazole
E. Spironolactone

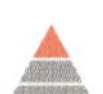 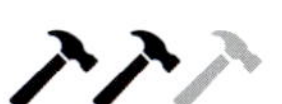 

63. A 21-year-old woman has a lump in her neck after an upper respiratory infection for the third time. The lump usually disappears within 2 weeks of the infection resolving, but this mass has remained for 6 weeks. She has a midline mass found over the anterior neck around 2 cm below the hyoid bone, which is painless and mobile on swallowing.

Which is the most appropriate management?

A. Antibiotics
B. Aspiration and drainage
C. Supportive management
D. Surgical excision
E. Total thyroidectomy

64. A 33-year-old man has recurrent palpitations and bilateral loin to groin pain. His BP is 164/105 mmHg. He has generalized bone pain.

Investigations:
Serum-corrected calcium: 2.99 mmol/L (2.2–2.6).
Serum phosphate: 0.73 mmol/L (0.8–1.4).
Plasma parathyroid hormone: 6.81 pmol/L (0.9–5.4).
Abdominal CT: small, well-defined lesion in the head of the pancreas.

What is the most likely method of inheritance?

A. Autosomal dominant
B. Autosomal recessive
C. Mitochondrial
D. X-linked dominant
E. X-linked recessive

 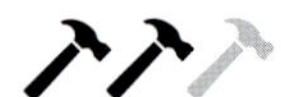 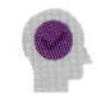

65. A 42-year-old woman has type 2 diabetes, managed with metformin. Her blood glucose level is well controlled at home, with an average blood glucose of 6.6 mmol/L (4.0–7.0).

Investigations:
HbA1c: 51 mmol/mol (<48 mmol/mol)

Which of the following causes can result in a higher-than-expected level of HbA1c?
   A. G6PD deficiency
   B. Haemodialysis
   C. Hereditary spherocytosis
   D. Iron-deficiency anaemia
   E. Sickle-cell anaemia

  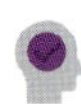

66. A 39-year-old man has redness in his eyes and bilateral eye protrusion. He has Graves disease, managed poorly with carbimazole and propranolol. He has bilateral eyelid retraction and conjunctival injection; however, his visual acuity is normal

Which is the most appropriate management?
   A. Atropine
   B. Prednisolone
   C. Panretinal photocoagulation
   D. Radioactive iodine
   E. Topical lubricants

 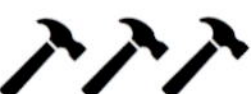

67. A 16-year-old boy has not developed physically like his classmates and has a loss of smell. He has abnormal descent of his testes.

Investigations:
Plasma follicle-stimulating hormone: 0.6 U/L (1.0–7.0).
Serum luteinizing hormone: 0.8 U/L (1.0–10.0).
Serum testosterone: 7 nmol/L (9–35).

What is the most likely mechanism causing this boy's symptoms?
   A. End-organ resistance to testosterone
   B. Failure of gonadotrophin-releasing hormone-secreting neurons to migrate to the hypothalamus
   C. Karyotype 45, XO
   D. Karyotype 47, XXY
   E. Zona reticularis tumour

 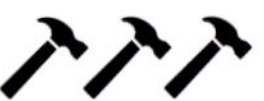

68. A 48-year-old woman has had headaches and a racing heartbeat for 3 weeks. Her mother has medullary thyroid cancer. Her BP is 186/104 mmHg. She appears anxious, but there are no discernible thyroid masses palpable.

Investigations:
Serum calcitonin: elevated.
Thyroid US: multiple thyroid nodules.

Which oncogene is commonly associated with the most likely diagnosis?
   A. BRAF
   B. KRAS
   C. MEN
   D. RET
   E. TP53

 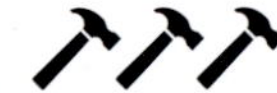 

69. A 22-year-old man has a follow-up appointment after a fasting glucose blood glucose of 10.2 mmol/L picked up on a routine check-up prior to joining the army. His father and paternal grandmother both have type 2 diabetes mellitus and he has a known gene mutation in the HNF1A gene. His BMI is 22.7 kg/m^2 and has no symptoms of polyuria or polydipsia.

Investigations:
Fasting blood glucose: 9.9 mmol/L (3.0–6.0)
Serum C-peptide: 213 pmol/L (180–360)

Which is the most appropriate management?
   A. Conservative management
   B. Empagliflozin
   C. Gliclazide
   D. Insulin
   E. Pancreatic beta-cell replacement

Haematology

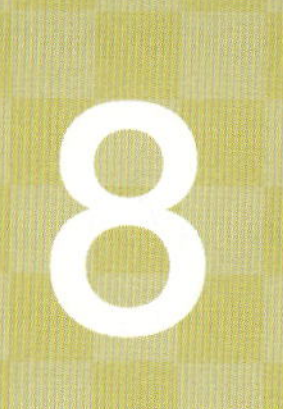

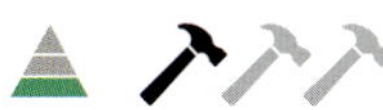

1. A 32-year-old woman has had a painless, enlarged neck lump and severe itching for 2 months. She has human immunodeficiency virus (HIV), managed with an INSTI-based regimen. She has a palpable, rubbery, nontender lymph node in her right neck and small, firm and nontender lymph nodes in her axilla bilaterally.

Investigations:
Haemoglobin: 109 g/L (115–165).
MCV: 87 fL (80–96).
Eosinophils: 0.72×10^9/L (0.0–0.6).
Lymph node biopsy: Reed-Sternberg cells.

Which is the most likely diagnosis?
   A. Acute myeloid leukaemia
   B. Chronic myeloid leukaemia
   C. Hodgkin's lymphoma
   D. Multiple myeloma
   E. Non-Hodgkin lymphoma

2. A 7-year-old boy has had bone pain, fatigue and easy bruising for 4 months. He has multiple petechiae on his skin, palpable lymph nodes in the axilla and neck bilaterally, and hepatosplenomegaly.

Investigations:
Platelets: 123×10^9/L (150–400).
Neutrophils: 1.1×10^9/L (1.5–7.0).

Which is the most likely diagnosis?
   A. Acute lymphoblastic leukaemia
   B. Acute myeloid leukaemia
   C. Hodgkin's lymphoma
   D. Multiple myeloma
   E. Non-Hodgkin lymphoma

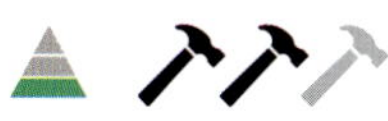

3. A 54-year-old woman has had exertional shortness of breath and fatigue for a year. She has type 1 diabetes mellitus, managed with a basal-bolus insulin regime, with a recent HbA1c of 46 mmol/mol. She has a red, swollen tongue and impaired vibration in the distal lower limbs.

Investigations:
Haemoglobin: 79 g/L (115–165).
Mean cell volume: 113 fL (80–96).

Which of the following antibodies would be raised?
   A. Antihistone antibodies
   B. Antimitochondrial antibodies
   C. Antitissue transglutaminase antibodies
   D. Gastric parietal cell antibodies
   E. Intrinsic factor antibodies

4. A 65-year-old man has had fatigue, unintentional weight loss of 2 kg and shortness of breath for 2 months. He has petechiae on the torso and hepatosplenomegaly.

Investigations:
Haemoglobin: 118 g/L (130–180).
Platelets: 124×10^9/L (150–400).
Neutrophils: 1.3×10^9/L (1.5–7.0).
Blood film: Pleomorphic myeloblasts.

Which is the most likely diagnosis?
   A. Acute myeloid leukaemia
   B. Acute lymphocytic leukaemia
   C. Chronic myeloid leukaemia
   D. Multiple myeloma
   E. Non-Hodgkin lymphoma

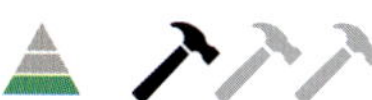

5. An 8-year-old girl has excessive bleeding after minor injuries for a year, with prolonged bleeding after tooth extraction. Her father has haemophilia A. She has multiple minor bruises on her arms and legs but no joint pain.

Which is the mode of inheritance for this likely diagnosis?
   A. Autosomal dominant
   B. Autosomal recessive
   C. Mitochondrial
   D. X-linked dominant
   E. X-linked recessive

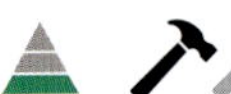

6. A 61-year-old man has had fatigue, night sweats and weakness for 5 months. He has type 2 diabetes mellitus, managed with metformin. He has mild conjunctival pallor with splenomegaly and petechiae.

Investigations:
Haemoglobin: 111 g/L (130–180).
Platelets: 524 × 10^9/L (150–400).
Cytogenetic analysis: t (9;22)

Which is the most likely diagnosis?
- A. Acute myeloid leukaemia
- B. Chronic myeloid leukaemia
- C. Hodgkin lymphoma
- D. Multiple myeloma
- E. Non-Hodgkin lymphoma

 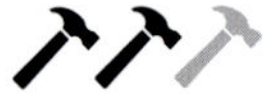 

7. A 14-year-old boy has severe generalized joint pain and difficulty breathing for 2 hours. He has had back pain and breathlessness for 3 months.

Investigations:
Haemoglobin: 122 g/L (130–180).
Reticulocytes: 3.4% (0.5–2.4).
Peripheral blood smear: sickle-shaped red blood cells.

Which is the most appropriate prophylactic management?
- A. Aspirin
- B. Desmopressin
- C. Factor VIII concentrate
- D. Hydroxyurea
- E. Venesection

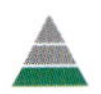  

8. An 8-year-old boy fell whilst playing football and has significant right knee swelling, with prolonged severe bleeding from a laceration on the knee. He has a large effusion in his right knee with a limited ROM due to pain.

Which is the most appropriate investigation?
- A. Activated partial thromboplastin time
- B. Bone marrow biopsy
- C. Glucose-6-phosphate dehydrogenase (G6PD) deficiency enzyme assay
- D. Platelet count
- E. Von Willebrand Factor (vWF) assay

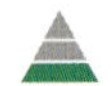 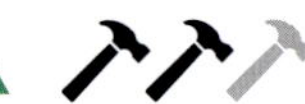 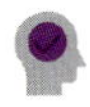

9. A 10-year-old boy has had recurrent severe, generalized bone and joint pain with fatigue and shortness of breath for the past month. He has mild pallor, scleral icterus and generalized joint tenderness.

Investigations:
Haemoglobin: 119 g/L (130–180).
Reticulocytes: 2.7% (0.5–2.4).

Which is the most appropriate investigation?
- A. Activated partial thromboplastin time
- B. Blood film
- C. Bone marrow biopsy
- D. Haemoglobin electrophoresis
- E. Serum ferritin

 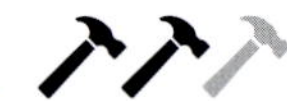 

10. A 5-year-old boy has left elbow swelling with prolonged bleeding from a laceration on the elbow. He has left elbow tenderness and a limited ROM.

Investigations:
Prothrombin time (PT): 14.1 seconds (11.5–15.5).
Activated partial thromboplastin time (aPTT): 47 seconds (30–40).

Which is the most appropriate management?
- A. Blood transfusion and folic acid
- B. Desmopressin
- C. Factor VIII concentrate
- D. Hydroxyurea
- E. Myeloablative stem cell transplant

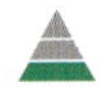  

11. A 52-year-old woman has had fatigue and weakness for 6 months. He also has 5 kg of unintentional weight loss over this period and night sweats. She has type 2 diabetes mellitus, managed with metformin and empagliflozin. She has mild pallor with splenomegaly and petechiae on her arms.

Investigations:
Haemoglobin: 111 g/L (115–165).
Platelets: 465 × 10^9/L (150–400).
Blood film: blast cells.

Which is the most appropriate management?
A. ABVD regimen
B. Aspirin and venesection
C. Hydroxyurea
D. Imatinib
E. Interferon-alpha

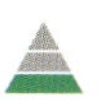 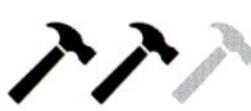

12. A 59-year-old woman has had fatigue, night sweats and an enlarged abdomen for 3 months. She has systemic lupus erythematosus managed with hydroxychloroquine. She has an enlarged liver and spleen and small, firm and tender lymph nodes in her neck and axilla bilaterally.

Investigations:
Haemoglobin: 102 g/L (115–165).
MCV: 91 fL (80–96).
Lymph node biopsy: lymphocyte sheets interspersed with macrophages

Which is the most likely diagnosis?
A. Acute myeloid leukaemia
B. Burkitt's lymphoma
C. Chronic myeloid leukaemia
D. Hodgkin lymphoma
E. Multiple myeloma

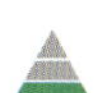  

13. A 22-year-old man has 1 month of a painless, enlarged lymph node in his left neck, that becomes painful when he consumes alcohol. He has night sweats and unintentional weight loss of 3 kg over this period. He has a palpable, rubbery and nontender lymph node in his neck and small, firm and nontender lymph nodes in his axilla and groin bilaterally.

Investigations:
Haemoglobin: 114 g/L (130–180).
MCV: 81 fL (80–96).
Eosinophils: 0.69×10^9/L (0.0–0.6).
Lymph node biopsy: Reed-Sternberg cells.

Which is the most appropriate management?
A. ABVD regimen
B. Bortezomib + stem cell transplant
C. Haematopoietic cell transplantation
D. Prednisolone
E. Ritixumab

 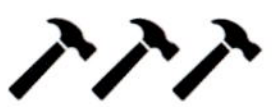

14. A 60-year-old man has night sweats and unintentional weight loss of 2 kg for a week. He has chronic lymphocytic leukaemia, managed with ibrutinib. He has bilaterally enlarged lymph nodes in his neck and axilla and generalized abdominal pain.

Investigations:
Lymph node biopsy: Large atypical lymphoid cells.

Which is the most likely diagnosis?
A. Acute myeloid leukaemia
B. Chronic myeloid leukaemia
C. Hodgkin lymphoma
D. Richter transformation
E. Waldenstrom macroglobulinaemia

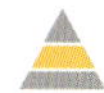 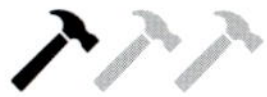

15. A 23-year-old woman has coeliac disease, diagnosed a year ago after chronic diarrhoea and weight loss.

Investigations:
Haemoglobin: 103 g/L (115–165).

Which would be seen on blood film?
A. Howell-Jolly bodies
B. Hypersegmented neutrophils
C. Rouleaux formation
D. Schistocytes
E. Tear-drop poikilocytes

 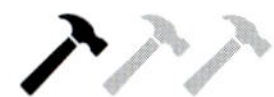 

16. A 37-year-old man has recurrent nosebleeds lasting several minutes a week. He has no history of trauma or bleeding disorders. He has active bleeding from the anterior nasal septum.

Which is the most appropriate management?
A. Cauterization with silver nitrate
B. Direct pressure and nose pinching
C. Nasal packing
D. Nasaseptin
E. Sphenopalatine ligation

 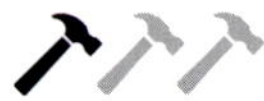

17. A 5-month-old male infant has growth and development issues since birth. He is pale, constantly irritable and tired. He has hepatosplenomegaly.

Investigations:
Blood film: microcytic hypochromic cells.
Haemoglobin electrophoresis: raised HbA2 and HbF.

Which is the most likely diagnosis?
A. Alpha-thalassaemia
B. Beta-thalassaemia
C. Glucose-6-phosphate dehydrogenase (G6PD) deficiency
D. Hereditary spherocytosis
E. Sickle cell anaemia

 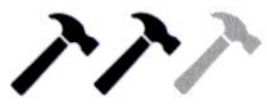

18. A 34-year-old woman has had pain and swelling in her left leg for 2 hours. She has had it multiple times in the past two years, managed each time with rivaroxaban. Her mother had a pulmonary embolism at age 40. She denies recent immobilisation or surgery. She has tenderness in her left calf.

Investigations:
D-dimer: 0.8 mg/L (<0.5)

Which is the most likely cause?
A. Antithrombin III deficiency
B. Factor V Leiden
C. Protein C deficiency
D. Protein S deficiency
E. Prothrombin G20210A mutation

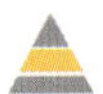 

19. A 60-year-old man has gradually worsening fatigue and shortness of breath on exertion for five months, He has rheumatoid arthritis, managed with methotrexate. He has conjunctival pallor.

Investigations:
Haemoglobin: 102 g/L (130–180).
MCV: 86 fL (80–96).
Serum ferritin: 345 μg/L (15–300)
Serum total iron-binding capacity: 37 μmol/L (45–75)

Which is the most likely diagnosis?
A. Anaemia of chronic disease
B. Autoimmune haemolytic anaemia
C. Chronic myeloid leukaemia
D. Iron deficiency anaemia
E. Vitamin B12 deficiency

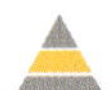 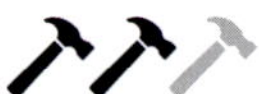 

20. A 4-month-old girl presents after concerns about her growth and fatigue since birth. She has a poor appetite and has constant loose stool. She has pale conjunctiva, yellowing of the skin and hepatosplenomegaly.

Investigation:
Haemoglobin electrophoresis: elevated HbF and HbA2.

Which is the most appropriate management?
A. Ferrous sulfate
B. Lifelong blood transfusion
C. Piperacillin-tazobactam
D. Splenectomy
E. Watchful waiting

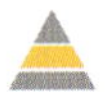 

21. A 38-year-old woman has had recurrent nosebleeds and heavy menstrual bleeding for 6 months. She has multiple petechiae and bruises over the arms and legs.

Investigations:
Haemoglobin: 95 g/L (115–165).
White cell count: 2.2×10^9/L (3.0–10.0).
Platelets: 34×10^9/L (150–400).
Bone marrow biopsy: Hypocellular marrow with fatty infiltrates.

Which is the most likely diagnosis?
A. Aplastic anaemia
B. Glucose-6-phosphate dehydrogenase deficiency
C. Fanconi anaemia
D. Iron-deficiency anaemia
E. Myelodysplasia

 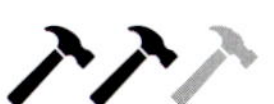 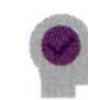

22. An 11-year-old girl has had pallor and yellowing of her skin for a month. She has acute cholecystitis with black-pigmented gallstones. She has splenomegaly and yellowing of her sclera.

Investigations:
Haemoglobin: 93 g/L (115–165).
Reticulocytes: 0.2% (0.5–2.4).
Mean corpuscular haemoglobin concentration (MCHC): 38 g/dL (32–35).

Which is the most appropriate definitive management?
A. Fresh frozen plasma
B. Lifelong blood transfusion
C. Piperacillin-tazobactam
D. Prednisolone
E. Splenectomy

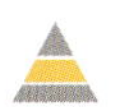 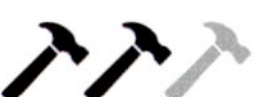 

23. A 57-year-old woman has easy bruising, nosebleeds and bleeding of her gums for 2 weeks. She has multiple petechiae and ecchymoses on her legs but no lymphadenopathy or organomegaly.

Investigations:
Haemoglobin: 149 g/L (115–165).
Platelets: 117 × 10^9/L (150–400).

Which is the most appropriate management?
A. ABVD regimen
B. Bortezomib and stem cell transplant
C. Imatinib
D. Nasal packing
E. Prednisolone

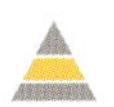 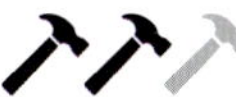

24. A 62-year-old man has had bone pain, worse in the spine and the ribs, for 3 months. His mother passed away from lung cancer at the age of 67. He has mild pallor and multiple bruises all over his body.

Investigations:
Haemoglobin: 110 g/L (130–175).
Serum calcium: 2.84 mmol/L (2.20–2.60).
Blood film: Stacking of red blood cells into coins

Which is the most likely diagnosis?
A. Bone metastasis
B. Chronic myeloid leukaemia
C. Hodgkin lymphoma
D. Non-Hodgkin lymphoma
E. Multiple myeloma

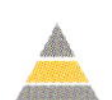 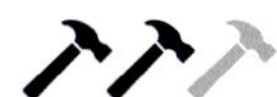 

25. A 51-year-old woman has had fatigue and a worsening headache for 5 months, with itching worse after hot showers. Her BP is 165/106 mmHg. She has an enlarged spleen and excoriations all over the body.

Investigations:
Haemoglobin: 179 g/L (115–165).
Platelets: 425 × 10^9/L (150–400).

Which is the most appropriate management?
A. ABVD regimen
B. Aspirin and venesection
C. Clopidogrel
D. Imatinib
E. Warfarin

26. A 3-year-old boy has bloody diarrhoea and decreased urine output for 2 days. His temperature is 38.4°C. She has diffuse abdominal pain and multiple petechiae on his torso and limbs.

Investigations:
Serum urea: 12.2 mmol/L (2.5–7.0).
Serum creatinine: 134 μmol/L (60–110).
Platelets: 117 × 10^9/L (150–400).
Blood film: schistocytes.

Which is the most likely diagnosis?
A. Haemolytic uraemic syndrome
B. Henoch-Schonlein purpura
C. Immune thrombocytopenic purpura
D. Sickle cell anaemia
E. Thrombotic thrombocytopenic purpura

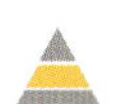 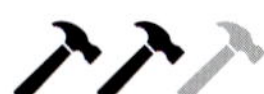 

27. A 22-year-old woman has severe menstrual bleeding. She has had similar bleeding episodes in her previous

menstrual cycles. Her mother and maternal aunt both experienced heavy bleeding during their menstrual cycles.

Investigations:
Platelets: 232 × 10^9/L (150–400).
Prothrombin time: 12.8 seconds (11.5–14.5).

Which is the most appropriate investigation?
A. Activated partial thromboplastin time
B. Blood film
C. Glucose-6-phosphate dehydrogenase (G6PD) deficiency enzyme assay
D. Haemoglobin electrophoresis
E. Von Willebrand Factor (vWF) assay

28. A 10-year-old girl had bloody diarrhoea for 1 day after eating at a street food stall 4 days ago, with fatigue and decreased fluid output despite good fluid intake. Her temperature is 38.1°C. She has oedema in her hands and feet and generalized abdominal pain.

Investigations:
Serum urea: 10.5 mmol/L (2.5–7.0).
Serum creatinine: 127 µmol/L (60–110).
Platelets: 114 × 10^9/L (150–400).

Which is the most likely causative organism?
A. *Bacillus cereus*
B. *Campylobacter jejuni*
C. *Escherichia coli* 0157:H7
D. *Salmonella enterica*
E. *Taenia solium*

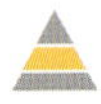 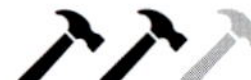 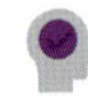

29. A 43-year-old man has prolonged bleeding from a surgical site whilst recovering from an elective hernia repair. His mother suffered from recurrent heavy menstrual bleeding.

Investigations:
Platelets: 324 × 10^9/L (150–400).
Prothrombin time: 12.9 seconds (11.5–14.5).
Von Willebrand Factor: decreased.

Which is the most appropriate management?
A. Blood transfusion and folic acid
B. Cryoprecipitate
C. Desmopressin
D. Factor VIII concentrate
E. Myeloablative stem cell transplant

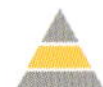 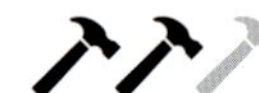 

30. A 72-year-old man has dysuria and confusion after a right hemiarthroplasty a day ago. He has type 2 diabetes mellitus, managed with metformin. His pulse is 132 bpm, and BP 86/51 mmHg. He has petechial bruising over his arms and bleeding from his peripheral cannula.

Investigations:
Platelets: 114 × 10^9/L (150–400).
Prothrombin time (PT): 15.1 seconds (11.5–14.5).
Activated partial thromboplastin time (aPTT): 43 seconds (30–40).

Which is the most appropriate management?
A. Fresh frozen plasma
B. Piperacillin-tazobactam
C. Platelet transfusion
D. Rivaroxaban
E. Vincristine

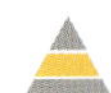 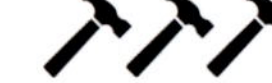 

31. A 54-year-old woman has fatigue, generalized weakness and decreased urine output for a day. She has Burkitt lymphoma, for which she completed her first chemotherapy cycle 2 weeks ago. She has confusion and lethargy.

Investigations:
Serum potassium: 5.2 mmol/L (3.5–4.9).
Serum calcium: 2.15 mmol/L (2.20–2.60).
Serum urate: 0.49 mmol/L (0.19–0.36).
Serum creatinine: 119 µmol/L (60–110).

Which can be given to prevent this complication?
A. Allopurinol
B. Ceftriaxone
C. Furosemide
D. Piperacillin-tazobactam
E. Vincristine

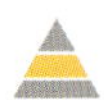 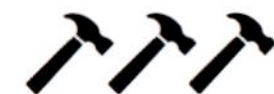

32. A 59-year-old man has a worsening headache and itching after a hot bath for 4 months. He had a pulmonary embolism 3 years ago. His BP is 172/103 mmHg. He has an enlarged spleen and multiple excoriations on the arms and torso.

Investigations:
Haemoglobin: 183 g/L (130–160).
Platelets: 445 × 10^9/L (150–400).

Which is the mutation associated with the most likely diagnosis?

A. BCR-AB1
B. CALR
C. EPOR
D. JAK2
E. MPL

  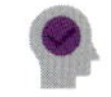

33. A 65-year-old man has had polyuria and bone pain in his back for 4 months. He has had recurrent upper respiratory tract infections, managed conservatively. He has mild pallor and generalized bone tenderness.

Investigations:
Serum calcium: 2.88 mmol/L (2.20–2.60).
Serum urea: 9.2 mmol/L (2.5–7.0).
Serum creatinine: 157 µmol/L (60–110).

Which is the most appropriate management?

A. ABVD regimen
B. Aspirin and venesection
C. Bortezomib + stem cell transplant
D. Dexamethasone
E. Total parathyroidectomy

 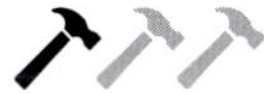

34. A 62-year-old man has chills, a high-grade fever and generalized weakness. He has acute myeloid leukaemia, managed with a chemotherapy cycle a week ago. His temperature is 39.2°C, and pulse 120 bpm. He has mild pallor and weakness over the body.

Which is the most likely diagnosis?

A. Disseminated intravascular coagulation
B. Neutropenic sepsis
C. Transfusion-related acute lung injury
D. Tuberculosis
E. Tumour lysis syndrome

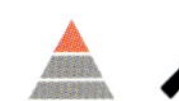  

35. A 75-year-old woman has shortness of breath, worse when lying flat whilst receiving a blood transfusion for anaemia caused by peptic ulcer bleeding. Her pulse is 114 bpm, and BP 165/94 mmHg. She has bibasal crepitations on chest auscultation and a raised JVP.

Which is the most appropriate management?

A. Fresh frozen plasma
B. Lifelong blood transfusion
C. Piperacillin-tazobactam
D. Splenectomy
E. Stop blood transfusion

 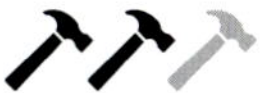 

36. A 63-year-old man has had fatigue and unintentional weight loss for 6 months. He also has early satiety and night sweats. He has polycythaemia vera, managed with regular phlebotomies. His spleen is palpable 6cm below the left costal margin.

Investigations:
Peripheral blood smear: tear-drop poikilocytes.

Which is the most appropriate investigation?

A. Activated partial thromboplastin time
B. Bone marrow biopsy
C. Glucose-6-phosphate dehydrogenase (G6PD) deficiency enzyme assay
D. Haemoglobin electrophoresis
E. Von Willebrand Factor (vWF) assay

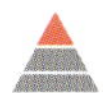 

37. A 51-year-old woman has worsening shortness of breath while receiving a blood transfusion. She has sickle cell anaemia, managed with regular blood transfusions. Her pulse is 120 bpm, temperature 38.2°C and BP 83/57 mmHg. She had bilateral crepitations on chest auscultation.

Investigations:
CXR: bilateral pulmonary infiltrates.

Which is the most likely diagnosis?

A. Acute chest syndrome
B. Anaphylaxis
C. Heart failure
D. Transfusion-associated circulatory overload
E. Transfusion-related acute lung injury

 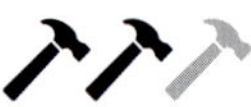 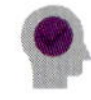

38. A 26-year-old man presents with sudden dark urine and fatigue after taking malaria prophylaxis before a trip to Kenya next week. He has yellowing of his sclera and splenomegaly.

Investigations:
Peripheral blood smear: Heinz bodies.

Which is the most appropriate management?
   A. Blood transfusion and folic acid
   B. Desmopressin
   C. Factor VIII concentrate
   D. Hydroxyurea
   E. Nonmyeloablative stem cell transplant

 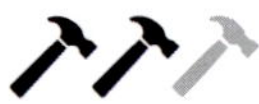

39. A 74-year-old man has night sweats and unintentional weight loss of 10 kg over 3 months. He has recurrent upper respiratory tract infections, often managed with antivirals. She has hepatosplenomegaly and palpable lymph nodes in the neck and axilla bilaterally.

Investigations:
Bone marrow biopsy: lymphoplasmacytoid lymphoma cells.

Which is the most likely diagnosis?
   A. Acute lymphocytic leukaemia
   B. Chronic myeloid leukaemia
   C. Multiple myeloma
   D. Non-Hodgkin's lymphoma
   E. Waldenstrom's macroglobulinaemia

 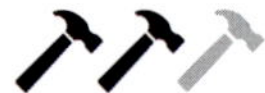 

40. A 68-year-old woman has had severe abdominal pain and high-grade fever for 2 days. She has breast cancer, for which she completed a course of chemotherapy a week ago. Her temperature is 39.1°C, and pulse 114 bpm. She has mild pallor and confusion.

Investigations:
Neutrophils: 0.24×10^9/L (1.5–7.0).

Which is the most appropriate management?
   A. Amoxicillin
   B. Fresh frozen plasma
   C. Peginterferon-alfa
   D. Piperacillin-tazobactam
   E. Splenectomy

 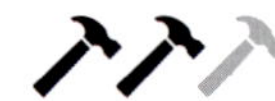

41. A 41-year-old woman has recurrent abdominal pain and fever for a week, with weakness and fatigue. She has systemic lupus erythematosus, managed with hydroxychloroquine. She has multiple petechiae and bruises on her torso.

Investigations:
Platelets: 97×10^9/L (150–400).
Peripheral blood smear: schistocytes.

Which deficiency is associated with the likely diagnosis?
   A. ADAMTS13
   B. Antithrombin III
   C. Factor V Leiden
   D. Protein C
   E. Protein S

 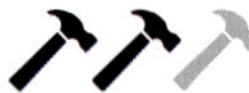 

42. A 31-year-old man has dark urine and generalized weakness for 2 days. His mother had symptoms of haemolytic anaemia in the past. He has yellowing of his eyes and splenomegaly.

Investigations:
Peripheral blood smear: small round inclusions within the RBC

Which is the most appropriate investigation?
   A. Activated partial thromboplastin time
   B. Bone marrow biopsy
   C. Glucose-6-phosphate dehydrogenase (G6PD) deficiency enzyme assay
   D. Haemoglobin electrophoresis
   E. Von Willebrand Factor (vWF) assay

43. A 69-year-old woman has had fatigue, bleeding gums and easy bruising for 5 months. She has multiple petechiae and bruises on her arms and torso.

Investigations:
Haemoglobin: 102 g/L (115–165).
White cell count: 2.6 × 10^9/L (3.0–10.0).
Platelets: 134 × 10^9/L (150–400).
Cytogenetic analysis: 5q deletion

Which is the most likely diagnosis?

A. Aplastic anaemia
B. Chronic lymphocytic leukaemia
C. Immune thrombocytopenia purpura
D. Myelodysplasia
E. Polycythaemia vera

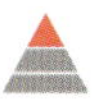 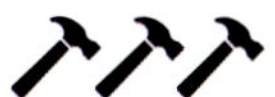

44. A 43-year-old woman has a high-grade fever and generalized weakness for 2 days. She has acute lymphoblastic leukaemia, for which she has received induction chemotherapy. Her temperature is 39.2°C, and pulse 108 bpm. She has mild pallor and is not oriented to time or place.

Investigations:
Neutrophils: 0.18 × 10^9/L (1.5–7.0).

Which is the most likely cause?

A. *Escherichia coli*
B. *Klebsiella pneumoniae*
C. *Listeria monocytogenes*
D. *Staphylococcus aureus*
E. *Staphylococcus epidermidis*

45. A 68-year-old man has had abdominal fullness and night sweats for 6 months. His father has polycythaemia vera. He has massive splenomegaly and multiple bruises all over his body.

Investigations:
Haemoglobin: 95 g/L (130–175)
Blood film: tear-drop poikilocytes >1%.
Bone marrow biopsy: dry tap.

Which is the most appropriate management?

A. Blood transfusion and folic acid
B. Desmopressin
C. Factor VIII concentrate
D. Nonmyeloablative stem cell transplant
E. Peginteferon alfa

Section 2
SURGERY QUESTIONS

Trauma and surgical emergencies

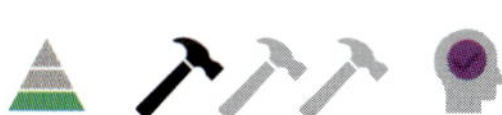

1. A 33-year-old man has severe pain and bruising over the left chest wall after a motorcycle accident.
   His temperature is 37.2°C, pulse 133 bpm, BP 82/61 mmHg, respiratory rate 32 breaths per minute and oxygen saturation 91% on breathing air. He has reduced breath sounds and chest expansion on the left, hyper-resonant percussion and tracheal deviation to the right.

Which is the most appropriate management?
   A. Chest drain placement
   B. Finger thoracostomy
   C. Mechanical ventilation
   D. Needle decompression in the 2nd intercostal space
   E. Thoracotomy

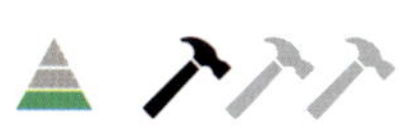

2. A 75-year-old woman has a headache, confusion and an ataxic gait following a fall. There are no long bone injuries. She has hypertension, managed with amlodipine and losartan, and a history of alcohol excess.

Which is the most likely diagnosis?
   A. Diffuse axonal injury
   B. Ischaemic stroke
   C. Intracerebral haemorrhage
   D. Subdural haematoma
   E. Wernicke's encephalopathy

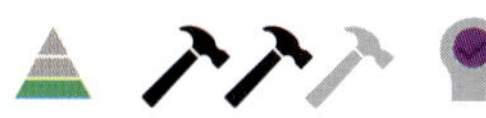

3. A 25-year-old man has a blow to the head and a short period of unconsciousness. He is now alert.

Investigations:
CT scan of head: convex opacity in the temporal area.

Which is the most appropriate management?
   A. Burr hole surgery
   B. External ventricular drain placement
   C. Haematoma evacuation
   D. Mannitol infusion
   E. Tranexamic acid

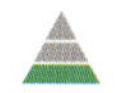  

4. A 22-year-old has a severe headache, worse when bending forward, lying down or coughing, which came on suddenly 1 hour ago. Her temperature is 37.8°C, pulse 132 bpm and BP 115/81 mmHg. She is photophobic, with a stiff neck.

Investigations:
CT scan of head: nil acute intracranial abnormality.

Which is the most appropriate investigation?
   A. CT angiography of head
   B. Digital subtraction angiography
   C. Lumbar puncture
   D. MR angiography
   E. MR scan of brain

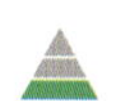 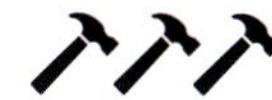 

5. A woman is unconscious after a mountaineering accident. Her temperature is 37.1°C, pulse 56 bpm, BP 102/83 mmHg, respiratory rate 8 breaths per minute and oxygen saturation 93% on breathing air. She has an open left femoral fracture, abdominal and chest wall bruising and a large occipital laceration.

Which is the most important immediate investigation?
   A. Chest X-ray
   B. CT of abdomen
   C. CT scan of head
   D. Point-of-care FAST scan
   E. X-ray of pelvis

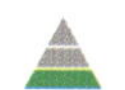 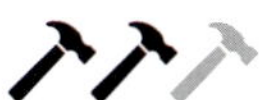 

6. A 25-year-old man has severe left leg pain after a road traffic accident. His temperature is 37.2°C, pulse 87 bpm and BP 128/94 mmHg. His left leg is exquisitely tender, firm, swollen, cool and pale, with absent pedal pulses.

Which is the most appropriate management?

A. Antibiotic therapy
B. Fasciotomy
C. Intravenous fluids
D. Reduction and stabilization
E. Revascularization

7. A 28-year-old man has abdominal and chest pain after a road traffic accident.

Investigations:
Point-of-care FAST scan: massive haemothorax and haemoperitoneum.
Following blood transfusion, his temperature is 36.8°C, pulse 118 bpm, BP 162/109 mmHg, respiratory rate 28 breaths per minute and oxygen saturation 93% on breathing air. His JVP is elevated 5 cm above the sternal angle, and there is pitting oedema to mid-shin.

Which is the most likely diagnosis?

A. Acute heart failure
B. Acute haemolytic transfusion reaction
C. Acute respiratory distress syndrome
D. Transfusion-related acute lung injury
E. Transfusion-related circulatory overload

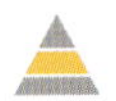 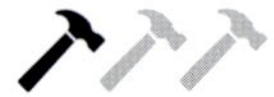

8. A 60-year-old man has chest pain after a road traffic accident. His temperature is 36.8°C, pulse 120 bpm, BP 120/60 mmHg, respiratory rate 45 breaths per minute and oxygen saturation 89% on breathing air. He has right-sided chest wall tenderness, palpable crepitus and paradoxical chest wall movement during respiration.

Which is the most likely diagnosis?

A. Cardiac contusion
B. Flail chest
C. Haemothorax
D. Pericardial effusion
E. Tension pneumothorax

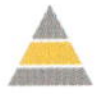 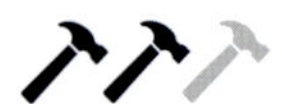 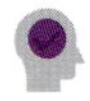

9. A 26-year-old man has abdominal pain after a stabbing. His temperature is 37.9°C, pulse 127 bpm, BP 90/69 mmHg, respiratory rate 28 breaths per minute and oxygen saturation 97% on breathing air. He has a 3 cm laceration in the left upper quadrant, diffuse abdominal pain radiating to the shoulder tip, guarding and dull percussion on the left.

Which is the most appropriate management?

A. Abdominal packing
B. Arterial embolization
C. Nephrectomy
D. Splenectomy
E. Transfusion with blood products

 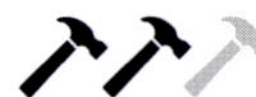 

10. A 19-year-old boy has nonblanching erythema and mottling of his chest wall and upper limbs after spilling hot oil. His temperature is 36.8°C, pulse 102 bpm and BP 85/71 mmHg. Multiple attempts at IV access fail.

Which is the most appropriate management?

A. Arterial line
B. Central line
C. Intraosseous access in the proximal tibia
D. PICC line insertion
E. Subcutaneous fluids

 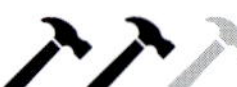 

11. A 32-year-old man is trapped under concrete at a building site. His temperature is 37.1°C, pulse 129 bpm and BP 92/71 mmHg. He is catheterized and fluid resuscitation is started. Observation of his catheter bag reveals:

Figure 9.1 (see Chapter 37).

Which is the most appropriate management?

A. Dialysis
B. Furosemide infusion
C. Large volume fluid resuscitation
D. Mannitol infusion
E. Urinary alkalinization

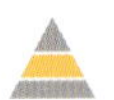 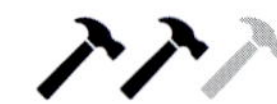 

12. A 28-year-old man has abdominal pain after a road traffic accident. His temperature is 37.1°C, pulse 144 bpm, BP 90/67 mmHg, respiratory rate 23 breaths per minute and oxygen saturation 95% on breathing air. He has diffuse abdominal pain and bruising, guarding and reduced bowel sounds.

Which is the most appropriate investigation?

A. Abdominal X-ray
B. CT of abdomen
C. Diagnostic peritoneal lavage
D. Full blood count
E. Point-of-care FAST scan

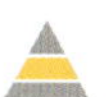 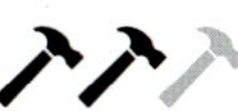 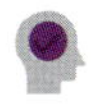

13. An 83-year-old woman has a burn on her left thigh after falling and being trapped next to a radiator. The burn is painless and nonblanching. Appropriate first aid is performed.

Figure 9.2 (see Chapter 37).

Which is the most appropriate management?

A. Antiseptic ointment
B. Debridement and skin graft
C. Escharotomy
D. Silver dressings
E. Topical moisturizer

  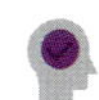

14. A 29-year-old is trapped under a car during a road traffic accident.

Investigations:
Haemoglobin 87 g/L (115–165)
Platelet count 78 × 10^9/L (150–400)
Haematocrit 19% (36–48)
PT 23 (11.5–15.5)
APTT 62 (30–40)
Fibrinogen 627 mg/dL (200–400)
D dimer 1.81 (<0.50)
FAST scan: haemoperitoneum.

Which is the most likely diagnosis?

A. Acute haemolytic anaemia
B. Dilutional coagulopathy
C. Disseminated intravascular coagulation
D. Haemolytic uraemic syndrome
E. Massive haemorrhage

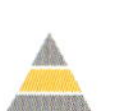 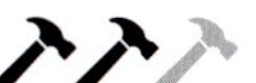 

15. A 32-year-old man is stabbed in the chest. His pulse is 127 bpm, BP 132/92 mmHg, respiratory rate 32 breaths per minute and oxygen saturation 88% on breathing air. He has reduced breath sounds and dull percussion on the right.

Investigations:
Chest X-ray: complete whiteout and meniscal level on the right.

Which is the most appropriate management?

A. Chest drain insertion
B. Needle decompression in the second intercostal space
C. High-flow oxygen therapy
D. Thoracentesis
E. Thoracotomy

 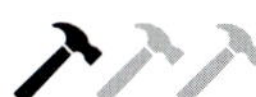

16. A 23-year-old woman is stabbed in the back. Her temperature is 37.1°C, pulse 96 bpm, BP 132/92 mmHg, respiratory rate 12 breaths per minute and oxygen saturation 98% on breathing air. She has reduced power and abnormal proprioception in the right leg, and loss of pain and temperature sensation on the left.

Which is the most likely diagnosis?

A. Central cord syndrome
B. Hemisection of the spinal cord
C. Spinal shock
D. Subacute combined degeneration of the cord
E. Syringomyelia

 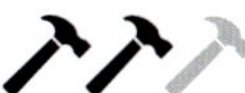 

17. A 52-year-old man has chest pain following a road traffic accident. His temperature is 37.4°C, pulse 144 bpm, BP 112/98 mmHg, respiratory rate 28 breaths per minute and oxygen saturation 91% on breathing air. He has bruising and tenderness on the right chest wall, with palpable crepitus and paradoxical movement during respiration.

Which is the most appropriate immediate management?

A. Analgesia
B. Chest drain insertion
C. Needle decompression in the second intercostal space
D. Pericardiocentesis
E. Thoracotomy

  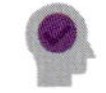

18. A 78-year-old woman has back pain after a fall. Her temperature is 36.8°C, pulse 86 bpm, BP 107/92 mmHg, respiratory rate 12 breaths per minute and oxygen saturation 97% on breathing air. She has focal tenderness over L3/L4, reduced power in the legs and paraesthesia over the anterior thigh bilaterally.

Which is the most appropriate management?

A. Analgesia
B. Decompressive laminectomy
C. Vertebral fusion
D. Vertebroplasty
E. Spondylodesis

 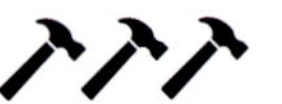 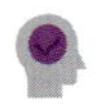

19. A 32-year-old man has 50% burns to the upper and lower limbs, chest and face, after a house fire. He is initially stable but deteriorates after several days. His temperature is 38.3°C, pulse 144 bpm and BP 160/117 mmHg, respiratory rate 23 breaths per minute and oxygen saturation 95% on breathing air. He has lost 10 kg of weight following the injury.

Investigations:
Haemoglobin 125 g/L (130–180).
Platelet count 229 × 10^9/L (150–400).
Urea 18.2 mmol/L (2.5–7.0).
Creatinine 389 μmol/L (60–110).
Bilirubin μmol/L 109 (1–22).
Alanine aminotransferase 671 U/L (5–35).
Alkaline phosphatase 160 U/L (45–105).

Which is the most likely diagnosis?

A. Acute liver injury
B. Acute tubular necrosis
C. Postburn hypermetabolism
D. Rhabdomyolysis
E. Severe dehydration

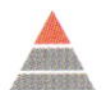 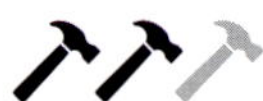

20. A 23-year-old man is stabbed in the chest. He has a respiratory rate of 37 breaths per minute and oxygen saturation 91% on breathing air. He has a 2 cm laceration on the left anterior chest wall and audible bowel sounds in the chest.

Investigations:
Figure 9.3 (see Chapter 37).

Which is the most likely diagnosis?

A. Diaphragmatic rupture
B. Flail chest
C. Haemothorax
D. Pulmonary contusion
E. Tension pneumothorax

Perioperative care

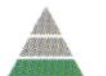 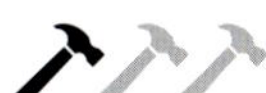

1. A 52-year-old man is 1 day post elective inguinal hernia repair. The surgical site is soft, with no warmth or erythema, but his pain is uncontrolled with regular paracetamol. He has high cholesterol and peptic ulcer disease, managed with atorvastatin and omeprazole.

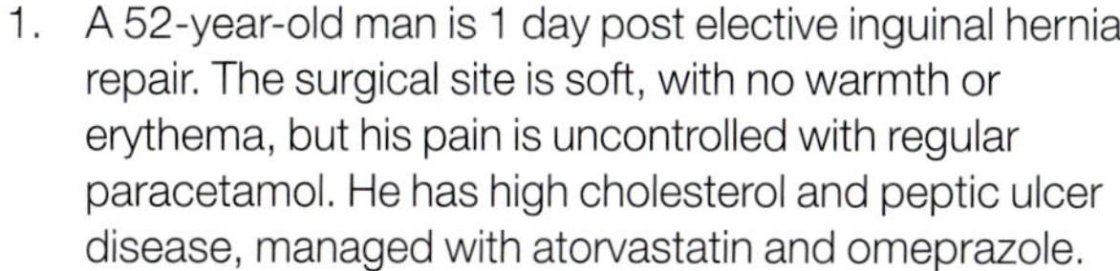

Which is the most appropriate management?

A. Co-codamol
B. Codeine
C. Ibuprofen
D. Morphine
E. PCA pump

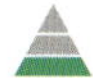 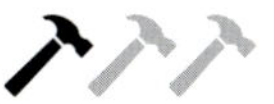 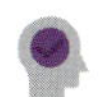

2. A 73-year-old man 1 day post left hemicolectomy for sigmoid carcinoma has chest pain and becomes unresponsive. He has ischaemic heart disease, hypertension and high cholesterol, managed with aspirin, ramipril, amlodipine and atorvastatin. His BP and oxygen saturations are unrecordable.

Which is the most appropriate management?

A. Aspirin
B. CPR
C. Clopidogrel
D. GTN spray
E. Morphine

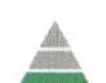  

3. A 62-year-old woman 7 days post hysterectomy for endometrial cancer has right leg pain. She has hypertension and CKD Stage 3 managed with ramipril. Her temperature is 37.5°C, pulse 83 bpm and BP 109/81 mmHg. She has a tender, swollen, warm and erythematous right calf.

Which is the most appropriate management?

A. Apixaban
B. Compression stockings
C. Flucloxacillin
D. Oral analgesia
E. Treatment dose low-molecular-weight heparin

 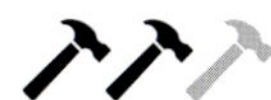 

4. A 63-year-old man 3 days post cholecystectomy has generalized abdominal discomfort, nausea and vomiting. He has not opened his bowels in 5 days. He has a distended, tympanic abdomen, with absent bowel sounds.

Which is the most appropriate management?

A. Endoscopic decompression
B. IV antibiotics
C. Laparotomy
D. Laxatives
E. NG tube and IV fluids

 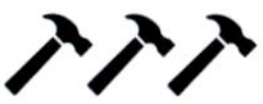 

5. A 78-year-old woman becomes drowsy while awaiting elective femoral hernia repair. She has type 1 diabetes mellitus, managed with insulin. She has deep laboured breathing and has vomited twice. Her temperature is 36.7°C, pulse 128 bpm, BP 102/78 mmHg, respiratory rate 28 breaths per minute and oxygen saturation 99% on breathing air.

Investigations:
ABG:
PO_2: 12.3 kPa (11.3–12.6).
PCO_2: 3.3 kPa (4.7–6.0).
pH: 7.29 (7.35–7.45).
Bicarbonate: 16 mmol/L (21–29).
Base excess: –6 mmol/L (±2).
Lactate: 1.1 mmol/L (0.5–1.6).

Which is the most appropriate management?

A. Fixed-rate insulin infusion
B. IV cyclizine
C. IV sodium bicarbonate
D. 1L IV 0.9% sodium chloride
E. 100 mL IV dextrose

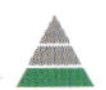  

6. A 22-year-old woman is having a laparoscopic appendectomy for appendicitis. During induction of anaesthesia, the skin surrounding the cannula site becomes warm, itchy and erythematous. Induction is stopped.

Figure 10.1 (see Chapter 37).

Which is the most appropriate management?
   A. Chlorphenamine
   B. High-flow oxygen therapy
   C. IM adrenaline 1:1000
   D. Paracetamol
   E. 1 L IV 0.9% sodium chloride

 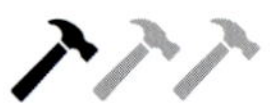

7. A 73-year-old woman 5 days post right total hip replacement has worsening hip pain. Her temperature is 38.4°C, pulse 104 bpm, BP 108/83 mmHg, respiratory rate 18 breaths per minute and oxygen saturation 99% on breathing air.

Which is the most likely cause of her temperature?
   A. Adverse drug reaction
   B. Lower respiratory tract infection
   C. Surgical site infection
   D. Urinary tract infection
   E. Venous thromboembolism

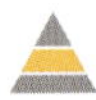 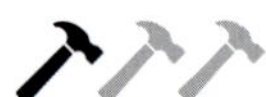

8. A 54-year-old woman 2 days post appendectomy has worsening abdominal pain. Her temperature is 38.2°C, pulse 123 bpm, BP 92/73 mmHg, respiratory rate 29 breaths per minute and oxygen saturation 98% on breathing air. She has diffuse abdominal tenderness, guarding and rigidity.

Investigations:
Haemoglobin: 107 g/L (115–165).
WBC: 18.2×10^9/L (4.0–11.0).
Neutrophil count: 12.7×10^9/L (1.5–7.0).
CRP: 154 mg/L (<10).

Which is the most likely diagnosis?
   A. Anaphylactic shock
   B. Cardiogenic shock
   C. Hypovolemic shock
   D. Obstructive shock
   E. Septic shock

 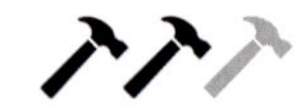 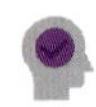

9. A 52-year-old man is drowsy and disoriented following elective inguinal hernia repair. He has type 1 diabetes mellitus, CKD 3 and hypertension, managed with insulin and ramipril. His temperature is 36.7°C, pulse 108 bpm, BP 137/94 mmHg, respiratory rate 23 breaths per minute and oxygen saturation 99% on breathing air. He opens his eyes to pain.

Which is the most appropriate investigation?
   A. Abdominal X-ray
   B. Blood cultures
   C. Capillary blood glucose
   D. CT scan of head
   E. ECG

10. A 63-year-old woman is 1 day post right superficial femoral artery angioplasty for critical limb ischaemia. She has peripheral arterial disease, hypertension and CKD 4, managed with ramipril, amlodipine, aspirin and atorvastatin.

Investigations:
On admission:
Urea: 14.2 mmol/L (2.5–7.0).
Creatinine: 156 µmol/L (60–110).

Postoperatively:
Urea: 33.7 mmol/L (2.5–7.0).
Creatinine: 397 µmol/L (60–110).

Which is the most likely cause of the blood results?
   A. Acute tubular necrosis
   B. Bladder outflow obstruction
   C. Contrast nephropathy
   D. Hypovolaemia
   E. Interstitial nephritis

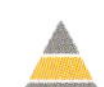 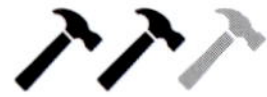

11. An 83-year-old woman 1 day post laparotomy for a bleeding duodenal ulcer has a cough. Her temperature is 37.8°C, pulse 110 bpm, BP 128/93 mmHg, respiratory rate 20 breaths per minute and oxygen saturation 90% on 2 L of oxygen via nasal cannula. She has decreased breath sounds in the right lung base.

Which is the most likely diagnosis?

A. Acute respiratory distress syndrome
B. Atelectasis
C. Lower respiratory tract infection
D. Pneumothorax
E. Pulmonary embolism

  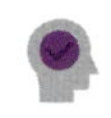

12. A 72-year-old woman 4 days post anterior resection of the rectum has sudden, severe abdominal pain. Her temperature is 38.2°C, pulse 106 bpm, BP 102/81 mmHg, respiratory rate 21 breaths per minute and oxygen saturation 97% on breathing air. Her abdomen is distended, with guarding and rebound tenderness.

Which is the most appropriate investigation?

A. Abdominal X-ray
B. Blood cultures
C. Chest X-ray
D. CT of abdomen
E. Peritoneal fluid analysis

 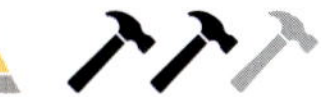 

13. A 72-year-old woman is awaiting for a mastectomy. She has hypertension, managed with amlodipine. She has intermittent palpitations but is otherwise well. She has an ejection systolic murmur in the aortic area.

Which is the most appropriate additional assessment?

A. Chest X-ray
B. Echocardiogram
C. Electrocardiogram
D. Serial troponins
E. 24-hour Holter monitoring

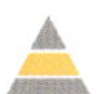 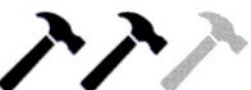 

14. A 72-year-old woman 3 days post elective total knee replacement has haemoptysis and chest pain. Her temperature is 36.7°C, pulse 123 bpm, BP 115/88 mmHg, respiratory rate 24 breaths per minute and oxygen saturation 90% on breathing air.

Which is the most appropriate investigation?

A. Chest X-ray
B. CT scan of pulmonary arteries
C. Echocardiogram
D. ECG
E. Lateral flow test

 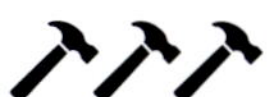 

15. A 52-year-old man is unresponsive 1 day post elective cholecystectomy. His pain is controlled with a PCA pump. His respiratory rate is 7 breaths per minute and oxygen saturation 91% on breathing air. He is unresponsive to pain, with pinpoint pupils, and a high-pitched rattling during respiration.

Which is the most appropriate management?

A. High-flow oxygen therapy
B. Intubation and ventilation
C. IM adrenaline 1:1000
D. 100 mL IV dextrose
E. Naloxone

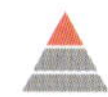 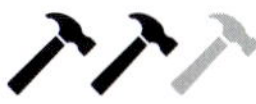 

16. A 62-year-old man has a cough following NG tube placement for acute bowel obstruction. His temperature is 37.8°C, pulse 76 bpm, BP 122/84 mmHg, respiratory rate 26 breaths per minute and oxygen saturation 93% on breathing air.

Investigations:
Figure 10.2 (see Chapter 37).

Which is the most likely diagnosis?

A. Atelectasis
B. Aspiration pneumonia
C. Pleural effusion
D. Pneumothorax
E. Pulmonary embolism

 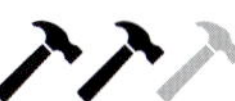 

17. A 78-year-old man is 1 day post elective total hip replacement.

Investigations:
Hb: 78 g/L (130–180).
During blood transfusion, his temperature is 38.1°C, pulse 108 bpm and BP 124/83 mmHg. The transfusion is stopped.

Which is the most appropriate management?

A. Chlorphenamine
B. IM adrenaline 1:000
C. IV furosemide
D. Paracetamol
E. 1 L IV 0.9% sodium chloride

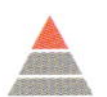 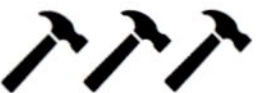 

18. A 38-year-old woman is having IV fluids, NG tube and enteral feeding for acute pancreatitis. She is cachexic and unkempt, with a history of alcohol excess. She becomes tremulous and delirious. Her temperature is 36.7°C, pulse 128 bpm, BP 158/94 mmHg, respiratory rate 28 breaths per minute and oxygen saturation 97% on breathing air. She has pitting oedema to the midshin.

Investigations:
Haemoglobin: 108 g/L (115–165).
WBC: 8.2×10^9/L (4.0–11.0).

Urea and electrolytes:
Na: 131 mmol/L (137–144).
K: 2.8 mmol/L (3.5–4.9).
Urea: 12.3 mmol/L (2.5–7.0).
Creatinine: 163 µmol/L (60–110).
Phosphate: 2.1 mg/dL (2.8-4.5).
Magnesium: 1.3 mg/dL (1.7-2.2).

Liver function tests:
Albumin: 28 g/L (37–49).
Bilirubin: 47 µmol/L (1–22).
Alanine aminotransferase: 289 U/L (5–35).
Alkaline phosphatase: 89 U/L (45–105).
Gamma-glutamyl transferase: 89 U/L (<50).

Which is the most likely diagnosis?

A. Alcohol withdrawal
B. Hepatic encephalopathy
C. Pulmonary oedema
D. Refeeding syndrome
E. Sepsis

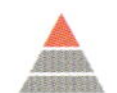 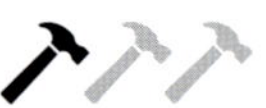

19. A 28-year-old woman detained under the Mental Health Act for psychosis is admitted for elective tonsillectomy. At preoperative assessment, she states that she no longer wants the procedure. She explains she understands she is at risk of further episodes of tonsillitis without having the procedure and would prefer antibiotics if this occurs.

Which is the most appropriate management?

A. Accept her decision and cancel the surgery
B. Administer diazepam 10mg and proceed with surgery
C. Call hospital security
D. Give her a patient information leaflet and attempt to persuade her to have surgery
E. Inform her that as she is detained under the Mental Health Act, she must have the procedure

 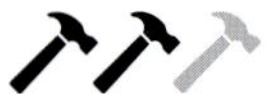 

20. A 68-year-old woman becomes confused following an elective right hemicolectomy for caecal carcinoma. Her temperature is 36.9°C, pulse 117 bpm, BP 80/61 mmHg, respiratory rate 22 breaths per minute and oxygen saturation 99% on breathing air. Her surgical wound is oozing fresh red blood, and there is a diffuse, violaceous lower limb rash.

Figure 10.3 (see Chapter 37).

Which is the most appropriate investigation?

A. Blood cultures
B. Coagulation screen
C. Colonoscopy
D. CT of abdomen
E. Lumbar puncture

Gastrointestinal surgery

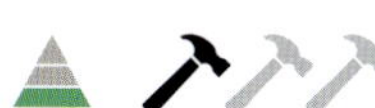

1. A 25-year-old woman has 1 month of upper abdominal pain worse after eating, nausea, reflux and 3 kg of weight loss. She has anxiety, managed with sertraline, and drinks 21 units of alcohol a week. She appears underweight, and has mild epigastric tenderness.

Which is the most likely diagnosis?
   A. Achalasia
   B. Gastroesophageal reflux disease
   C. Gastric cancer
   D. Oesophagitis
   E. Peptic ulcer disease

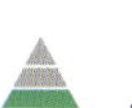 

2. A 52-year-old man has sudden, profuse frank haematemesis. His temperature is 36.9°C, pulse 121 bpm and BP 92/70 mmHg. He has abdominal distention and epigastric tenderness, with dilated veins and excoriations over the abdominal wall, and marked scleral icterus.

Which is the most likely diagnosis?
   A. Bleeding oesophageal varices
   B. Mallory Weiss tear
   C. Oesophageal rupture
   D. Oesophagitis
   E. Peptic ulcer disease

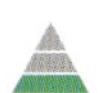 

3. A 64-year-old woman has 3 months of abdominal discomfort and constipation. She has hypothyroidism, managed with levothyroxine, and has smoked 20 cigarettes a day for 30 years. She has mild left lower quadrant tenderness, with sluggish bowel sounds.

Figure 11.1 (see Chapter 37).

Which is the most likely diagnosis?
   A. Colorectal carcinoma
   B. Colorectal polyposis
   C. Crohn disease
   D. Diverticular disease
   E. Irritable bowel syndrome

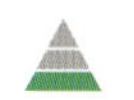  

4. A 54-year-old woman has sudden onset severe upper abdominal pain radiating to the back, nausea and vomiting, after 3 weeks of intermittent upper abdominal pain after meals. Her temperature is 37.8°C, pulse 121 bpm and BP 112/82 mmHg. She has epigastric tenderness and guarding.

Which is the most appropriate management?
   A. Diclofenac
   B. Intravenous antibiotics
   C. Intravenous cyclizine
   D. Intravenous fluids
   E. Intravenous morphine

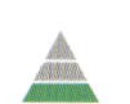 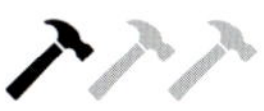 

5. A 23-year-old woman has 2 months of central burning chest pain, nausea and swallowing discomfort, with occasional regurgitation of food, worse when eating large, fatty meals and at night.

Which is the most appropriate management?
   A. Calcium carbonate
   B. Famotidine
   C. Omeprazole
   D. Omeprazole, amoxicillin and clarithromycin
   E. Peptac liquid

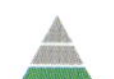 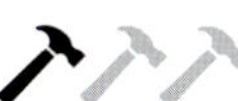 

6. A 19-year-old boy has 1 day of mild diffuse abdominal pain which is now severe and localized to the right lower quadrant, with vomiting, loose stool and loss of appetite. His temperature is 37.9°C, pulse 106 bpm and BP 122/81 mmHg. He has right lower quadrant tenderness, worse on palpation of the left-hand side.

Which is the most appropriate management?
   A. Broad-spectrum antibiotics
   B. Emergency appendectomy
   C. Interval appendectomy
   D. Intravenous fluids
   E. Percutaneous drainage

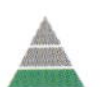 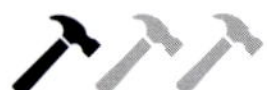 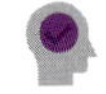

7. A 45-year-old man has 3 months of dull epigastric pain relieved by eating, nausea and indigestion. He takes ibuprofen for knee pain, and has smoked 10 cigarettes a day for 20 years. He has mild epigastric tenderness.

Which is the most appropriate investigation?
- A. Barium swallow
- B. CLO test
- C. Endoscopy
- D. Gastrin levels
- E. Urea breath test

 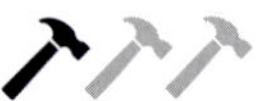

8. A 44-year-old woman has sudden onset abdominal pain radiating to the back and vomiting after an alcoholic binge. Her temperature is 38.2°C, pulse 103 bpm and BP 112/82 mmHg. She has marked epigastric tenderness and guarding.

Which is the most likely diagnosis?
- A. Acute cholecystitis
- B. Acute pancreatitis
- C. Ascending cholangitis
- D. Gallstone ileus
- E. Peptic ulcer perforation

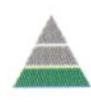 

9. A 72-year-old woman has severe abdominal pain and vomiting after 1 week of intermittent, mild lower abdominal pain relieved by defecation. She had a previous elective cholecystectomy and two caesarean sections. Her temperature is 37.3°C, pulse 126 bpm and BP 90/62 mmHg. She has generalized abdominal tenderness, gross distention and tympanic abdomen, with high-pitched bowel sounds.

Which is the most likely diagnosis?
- A. Caecal volvulus
- B. Large bowel obstruction
- C. Paralytic ileus
- D. Sigmoid volvulus
- E. Small bowel obstruction

10. A 42-year-old woman has three episodes of frank, small-volume haematemesis, with nausea and retrosternal chest discomfort. She has gastroesophageal reflux disease, managed with famotidine. Her temperature is 37.1°C, pulse 87 bpm and BP 132/96 mmHg. She has mild epigastric tenderness.

Which is the most likely diagnosis?
- A. Bleeding peptic ulcer
- B. Mallory-Weiss tear
- C. Oesophagitis
- D. Oesophageal rupture
- E. Oesophageal varices

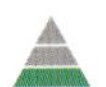 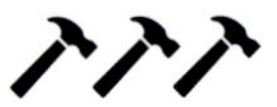 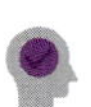

11. A 21-year-old woman has 1 day of central abdominal pain that has become severe and localized to the right lower quadrant, with vomiting and loss of appetite. Her temperature is 37.8°C, pulse 127 bpm and BP 102/81 mmHg. She has severe pain in the right iliac fossa, guarding and rebound tenderness.

Which is the most appropriate investigation?
- A. Abdominal X-ray
- B. Pregnancy test
- C. Ultrasound of abdomen
- D. Urinalysis
- E. Venous blood gas

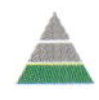 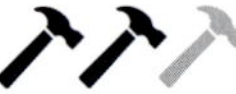

12. A 46-year-old woman has 3 days of worsening upper abdominal pain. Her temperature is 38.2°C, pulse 103 bpm, BP 108/78 mmHg, respiratory rate 22 breaths per minute and oxygen saturation 98% on breathing air. She has severe right upper quadrant tenderness and scleral icterus.

Which is the most likely diagnosis?
- A. Acute cholecystitis
- B. Acute pancreatitis
- C. Ascending cholangitis
- D. Biliary colic
- E. Choledocholithiasis

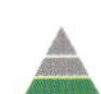 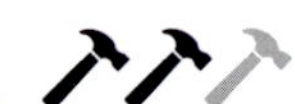 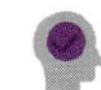

13. A 65-year-old man has 3 days of severe abdominal pain, vomiting and inability to open his bowels or pass gas. He has chronic lower back pain, managed with co-codamol. His temperature is 37.9°C, pulse 106 bpm

and BP 119/72 mmHg. He has generalized abdominal distention and tenderness, a tympanic abdomen and absent bowel sounds.

Which is the most appropriate management?
- A. Emergency laparotomy
- B. Flexible sigmoidoscopy decompression
- C. Laxatives
- D. Manual stool disimpaction
- E. Nasogastric tube insertion and IV fluids

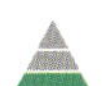 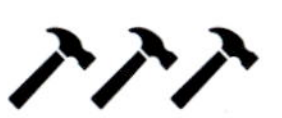 

14. An 82-year-old woman has three episodes of dark, granular vomiting after 2 days of upper abdominal discomfort and black, offensive stools. She has osteoarthritis, managed with naproxen. Her temperature is 37.1°C, pulse 113 bpm and BP 106/74 mmHg. She is pale, with epigastric tenderness, and black stool per rectum.

Investigations:
Hb 112 g/dL (115–165).

Which is the most appropriate immediate management?
- A. Blood transfusion
- B. Intravenous antibiotics
- C. Intravenous fluids
- D. Intravenous proton-pump inhibitors
- E. Terlipressin

 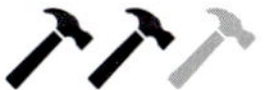 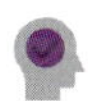

15. A 48-year-old woman has intermittent upper abdominal pain worse after meals, nausea and flatulent dyspepsia. Her temperature is 37.1°C, pulse 66 bpm and BP 121/92 mmHg. Her abdomen is soft and nontender.

Which is the most appropriate investigation?
- A. Abdominal X-ray
- B. CT of abdomen
- C. Endoscopic retrograde cholangiopancreatography
- D. Magnetic retrograde cholangiopancreatography
- E. Ultrasound of abdomen

16. A 67-year-old man has 2 weeks of a painless groin lump. He has a right-sided lump superomedial to the pubic tubercle that does not transilluminate, is reducible but reappears on coughing.

Which is the most likely diagnosis?
- A. Direct inguinal hernia
- B. Femoral hernia
- C. Hydrocele
- D. Indirect inguinal hernia
- E. Varicocele

 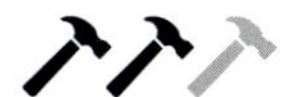 

17. A 42-year-old woman has 6 hours of worsening upper abdominal pain and vomiting, after 2 months of intermittent dull upper abdominal pain after meals. Her temperature is 38.1°C, pulse 107 bpm and BP 123/75 mmHg. She has severe right upper quadrant pain and scleral icterus.

Which is the most appropriate long-term management?
- A. Cholecystectomy
- B. Cholecystostomy
- C. Endoscopic retrograde cholangiopancreatography
- D. Endoscopic ultrasound-guided biliary drainage
- E. Percutaneous transhepatic biliary drainage

 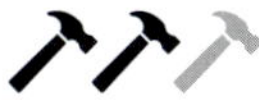 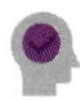

18. An 82-year-old woman has severe abdominal pain, after 3 weeks of intermittent pain and vomiting which resolve after explosive passage of stool and gas. Her temperature is 37.2°C, pulse 126 bpm and BP 81/59 mmHg. She has generalized abdominal tenderness, gross abdominal distention and absent bowel sounds.

Investigations:
Figure 11.2 (see Chapter 37).

Which is the most appropriate management?
- A. Broad-spectrum IV antibiotics
- B. Colonoscopy
- C. Flexible sigmoidoscopy
- D. Nasogastric tube insertion and IV fluids
- E. Sigmoid colectomy

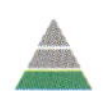 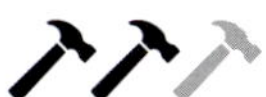 

19. A 65-year-old man has 3 months of fatigue. He has hypertension, managed with amlodipine, and has smoked 20 cigarettes a day for 40 years.

Investigations:
Haemoglobin 87 g/L (130–180).
Platelet count 257 × 109/L (150–400).
Haematocrit 12% (36–48).

Which is the most appropriate investigation?
A. Capillary blood glucose
B. Colonoscopy
C. Chest X-ray
D. CT scan of thorax, abdomen, pelvis
E. Thyroid function tests

 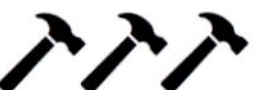 

20. A 69-year-old woman has 3 days of worsening lower abdominal pain, nausea and malaise. She has diverticular disease, managed with laxatives, and typically opens her bowels once a week. Her temperature is 38.9°C, pulse 129 bpm and BP 90/71 mmHg. She has severe generalized abdominal pain, guarding and rebound tenderness.

Which is the most appropriate management?
A. CT-guided drainage
B. Emergency colectomy
C. Intravenous antibiotics
D. Laxatives
E. Oral antibiotics

 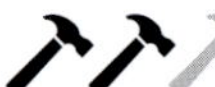

21. A 52-year-old man has 5 years of retrosternal chest pain and nausea, worse when eating and at night. He has type 2 diabetes mellitus and high cholesterol, managed with metformin, gliclazide and atorvastatin. He is overweight, with mild epigastric tenderness.

Investigations:
Endoscopy: erythema and oedema of the lower oesophagus, with superficial erosions and ulcerations.
Histopathology: columnar epithelial and goblet cells.

Which is the most likely diagnosis?
A. Barrett oesophagus
B. Gastroesophageal reflux disease
C. Hiatus hernia
D. Oesophageal carcinoma
E. Oesophagitis

 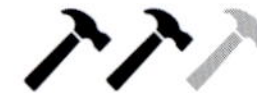 

22. A 44-year-old woman has sudden severe upper abdominal pain and vomiting. She has type 2 diabetes mellitus, managed with metformin, and takes the oral contraceptive pill. Her temperature is 38.2°C, pulse 98 bpm and BP 123/63 mmHg. She has severe right upper quadrant tenderness, worse on inspiration during palpation.

Which is the most appropriate investigation?
A. Abdominal X-ray
B. Amylase
C. Endoscopic retrograde cholangiopancreatography
D. Liver function tests
E. Ultrasound of abdomen

 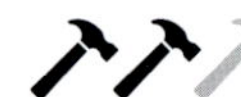

23. An 82-year-old man has sudden abdominal pain and vomiting. He last opened his bowels 10 days ago, and cannot remember passing gas. He has osteoarthritis, managed with codeine. His temperature is 36.9°C, pulse 108 bpm and BP 102/68 mmHg. He has generalized abdominal tenderness and distention, with hyperactive bowel sounds.

Investigations:
Figure 11.3 (see Chapter 37).

Which is the most likely diagnosis?
A. Faecal loading
B. Large bowel obstruction
C. Paralytic ileus
D. Sigmoid volvulus
E. Small bowel obstruction

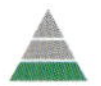 

24. An 18-year-old girl has 2 days of worsening abdominal pain, nausea and loss of appetite. She is normally well. Her temperature is 37.8°C, pulse 102 bpm and BP 113/81 mmHg. She has tenderness in the right lower quadrant, worse on palpation of the left lower quadrant.

Investigations:
Urinalysis: 2+ leucocytosis, + blood, β-hCG negative.

Which is the most likely diagnosis?
A. Appendicitis
B. Ectopic pregnancy
C. Ovarian torsion
D. Pyelonephritis
E. Urinary tract infection

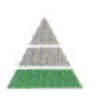  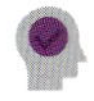

25. A 75-year-old man has 2 months of mild intermittent abdominal pain and increased frequency of loose stool, with occasional streaks of blood.

Investigations:
Colonoscopy: T2N1M0 tumour of the distal transverse colon.

Which is the most appropriate management?
A. Anterior resection
B. Left hemicolectomy
C. Radiochemotherapy
D. Sigmoid colectomy
E. Subtotal colectomy

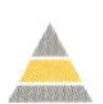 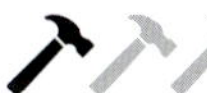 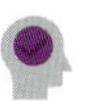

26. A 75-year-old woman has 3 weeks of a mildly tender groin lump. She has a soft, reducible left groin lump, below and lateral to the left pubic tubercle.

Which is the most appropriate management?
A. Analgesia
B. Drainage
C. Elective mesh repair
D. Emergency laparotomy
E. Watchful waiting

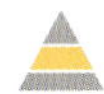 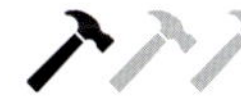 

27. A 54-year-old man has three episodes of frank haematemesis and two episodes of dark, foul stools. He drinks three bottles of rum a week and is an intravenous drug user. His temperature is 36.9°C, pulse 113 bpm and BP 98/69 mmHg. He has generalized abdominal tenderness and distention, with dilated superficial umbilical veins and excoriations over the abdomen, and dark, foul stool per rectum.

Which is the most appropriate scoring system?
A. Alvarado score
B. Child-Pugh score
C. Glasgow-Blatchford score
D. Glasgow-Imrie score
E. Rockall score

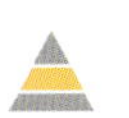 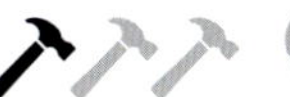 

28. A 62-year-old man has 2 weeks of intermittent bright red blood mixed with his stools. He typically opens his bowels twice a week. He has hypertension, type 2 diabetes mellitus and high cholesterol, managed with ramipril, metformin and atorvastatin, and has smoked 20 cigarettes a day for 40 years.

Investigations:
Colonoscopy with biopsy: multiple pedunculated polyps <10 mm in the sigmoid colon.
Histology: tubular adenomas.

Which is the most appropriate management?
A. Endoscopic mucosal resection
B. Left hemicolectomy
C. Polypectomy
D. Reassure and discharge
E. Surveillance colonoscopy

 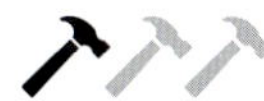 

29. A 32-year-old woman has 2 months of retrosternal chest pain, worse during meals and at night, with nausea and flatulence. She is 7 months pregnant with her first child. Her abdomen is soft and nontender.

Which is the most important immediate investigation?
A. ECG
B. Endoscopy
C. Oesophageal barium swallow
D. Oesophageal manometry
E. Urea breath test

 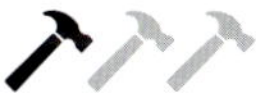 

30. A 50-year-old man has 6 months of abdominal pain and vomiting after meals, with 10 kg of weight loss. He has drunk half a bottle of vodka a day for 10 years. He is cachexic, with marked epigastric tenderness, and a palpable lymph node in the left supraclavicular fossa.

Which is the most appropriate investigation?
A. Abdominal X-ray
B. Colonoscopy
C. CT of abdomen
D. Endoscopy
E. Ultrasound of abdomen

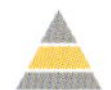  

31. A 25-year-old man has 2 weeks of a painless groin lump, which appeared suddenly after lifting heavy boxes. There is a soft, reducible groin lump

superomedial to the right pubic tubercle, which reappears on coughing while being reduced, with negative transillumination.

Which is the most appropriate management?

A. Drainage
B. Mesh repair
C. Watchful waiting
D. Surgical resection
E. Suspensory truss

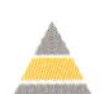  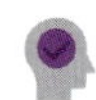

32. A 68-year-old male has 6 months of intermittent abdominal pain, diarrhoea and 5 kg of weight loss. He has mild right lower quadrant discomfort and conjunctival pallor.

Which is the most appropriate investigation?

A. Colonoscopy
B. CT of thorax, abdomen, pelvis
C. Full blood count
D. Gastroscopy
E. Ultrasound abdomen

 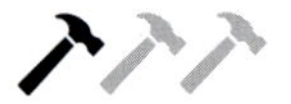 

33. A 23-year-old woman has 6 months of intermittent abdominal pain, bloating and flatulence, relieved by defecation, with alternating diarrhoea and constipation. There is no weight loss, rectal bleeding or nighttime symptoms. She has anxiety, managed with sertraline. Her abdomen is soft, nontender and bowel sounds are present.

Which is the most appropriate management?

A. Azathioprine
B. Dietary modifications
C. Loperamide
D. Prednisolone
E. Sulphasalazine

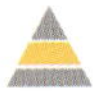 

34. A 65-year-old man has 2 months of abdominal pain, nausea and fatigue. He had a left hemicolectomy for colorectal cancer 2 years ago. He is pale, cachexic, with abdominal distention and mild generalized tenderness. There is bilateral dullness to percussion in the flanks that becomes localized to one side when he lies on that side.

Which is the most likely diagnosis?

A. Cirrhosis
B. Colorectal cancer
C. Hypoalbuminemia
D. Peritoneal carcinomatosis
E. Spontaneous bacterial peritonitis

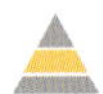 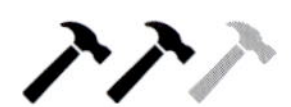 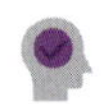

35. A 28-year-old girl presents following a mixed overdose of venlafaxine. She is delirious, with slurred speech, and vomiting. She has right upper quadrant tenderness, abdominal distention and asterixis.

Investigations:
INR 4.7.
Bilirubin 21.9 μmol/L (1–22).

Which is the most appropriate management?

A. Empiric antiviral therapy
B. Intravenous methylprednisolone
C. Liver transplant
D. N-acetylcysteine
E. Spironolactone

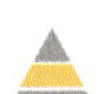  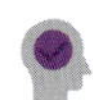

36. An 80-year-old woman has 3 months of weight loss, fatigue, nausea and reduced appetite. She has type 2 diabetes mellitus, managed with metformin, and drinks four bottles of wine a week. She is cachexic, with scleral icterus.

Which is the most appropriate investigation?

A. Abdominal X-ray
B. Chest X-ray
C. CT of abdomen
D. Colonoscopy
E. Liver function tests

 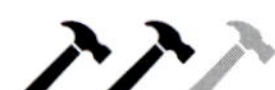 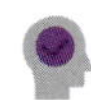

37. A 76-year-old woman has 6 months of intermittent colicky abdominal discomfort and constipation. She has hypothyroidism, managed with levothyroxine, and has smoked 20 cigarettes a day for 50 years.

Which is the most appropriate investigation?

A. Abdominal X-ray
B. Barium swallow
C. Colonoscopy
D. CT of abdomen
E. Ultrasound of abdomen

 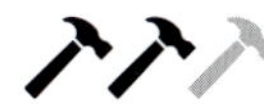

38. A 32-year-old man has severe abdominal pain, after 3 months of intermittent upper abdominal pain relieved by eating, and three stones of weight gain. He has lower back pain, managed with ibuprofen, drinks a crate of beers a week and has smoked 20 cigarettes a day for 10 years. His temperature is 38.4°C, pulse 133 bpm and BP 101/83 mmHg. He has diffuse abdominal pain radiating to the left shoulder, guarding and rigidity.

Which is the most likely diagnosis?
A. Acute cholecystitis
B. Acute pancreatitis
C. Bowel obstruction
D. Perforated peptic ulcer
E. Ruptured abdominal aortic aneurysm

 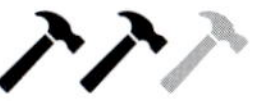 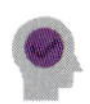

39. A 70-year-old man has sudden onset abdominal pain and bloody diarrhoea. He has atrial fibrillation and peripheral arterial disease, managed with bisoprolol, clopidogrel and atorvastatin. His temperature is 38.2°C, pulse 127 bpm and BP 80/63 mmHg. He has severe periumbilical tenderness, guarding and abdominal rigidity, and fresh red blood per rectum.

Which is the most appropriate management?
A. Angioplasty and stenting
B. Antibiotics
C. Anticoagulation
D. Blood transfusion
E. Emergency laparotomy

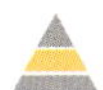 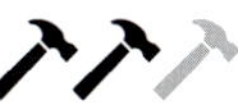 

40. A 28-year-old woman has 1 month of difficulty swallowing both solids and liquids, with painless regurgitation and 3 kg of weight loss.

Which is the most appropriate management?
A. Avoidance of hot and cold foods
B. Botox injections
C. Calcium channel blockers
D. Endoscopic stapling
E. Pneumatic dilation

41. A 70-year-old woman has 2 days of lower abdominal pain and profuse rectal bleeding, after 6 months of alternating diarrhoea and constipation. Her temperature is 37.3°C, pulse 82 bpm and BP 114/82 mmHg. She has left iliac fossa tenderness and bright red bleeding per rectum.

Which is the most likely diagnosis?
A. Acute mesenteric ischaemia
B. Angiodysplasia
C. Colorectal carcinoma
D. Diverticular bleed
E. Haemorrhoids

 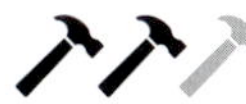 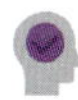

42. A 27-year-old man has 12 hours of constant vomiting with recent streaks of blood after an alcoholic binge. His temperature is 37.1°C, pulse 92 bpm and BP 118/72 mmHg. He is pale, with reduced skin turgor and epigastric tenderness.

Which is the most appropriate management?
A. Blood transfusion
B. Endoscopy
C. Intravenous antibiotics
D. Intravenous cyclizine
E. Intravenous proton pump inhibitors

43. A 23-year-old boy has 1 day of profuse bloody diarrhoea and abdominal pain. He has ulcerative colitis, managed with mesalamine. His temperature is 38.9°C, pulse 123 bpm and BP 94/73 mmHg. He has generalized abdominal tenderness and guarding, with absent bowel sounds.

Investigations:
Venous blood gas:
pH 7.23 (7.35–7.45).
Bicarbonate 8 mmol/L (21–29).
base excess –6 mmol/L (±2).
Sodium 151 nmol/L (135–145).
Potassium 2.9 nmol/L (3.5–5).
Lactate 2.2 mmol/L (0.5–1.6).

Which is the most appropriate management?
A. Azathioprine
B. Emergency colectomy
C. Infliximab
D. Intravenous steroids
E. Oral and rectal mesalamine

 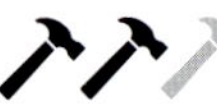 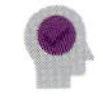

44. A 55-year-old man has severe upper abdominal pain, nausea and dyspepsia, after 3 months of intermittent colicky abdominal pain after meals which can last hours. He has type 2 diabetes mellitus and high cholesterol, managed with metformin and atorvastatin. He has mild right upper quadrant tenderness.

Which is the most appropriate management?
A. Buscopan
B. Cholestyramine
C. Diclofenac
D. Morphine
E. Ursodeoxycholic acid

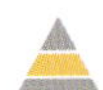 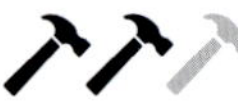 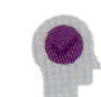

45. A 43-year-old man has 2 days of severe upper abdominal pain, after 6 months of intermittent abdominal pain and dyspepsia after meals. His temperature is 38.3°C, pulse 106 bpm and BP 124/72 mmHg. He has severe tenderness and guarding in the right upper quadrant.

Which is the most appropriate immediate management?
A. Cholecystectomy
B. Cholecystostomy
C. Endoscopic retrograde cholangiopancreatography
D. Intravenous antibiotics
E. Intravenous fluids

 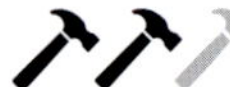 

46. A 46-year-old woman has 2 months of loose, watery stools, up to three times a day, with occasional streaks of blood. Her abdomen is soft, nontender and bowel sounds are present.

Which is the most appropriate management?
A. Dietary modifications
B. Loperamide
C. Oral rehydration solution
D. Reassurance and discharge
E. Urgent 2-week wait referral

 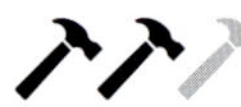

47. A 78-year-old woman has sudden onset abdominal pain and bloody diarrhoea. She has atrial fibrillation, managed with bisoprolol. Her temperature is 38.1°C, pulse 122 bpm and BP 92/71 mmHg. She has generalized abdominal pain, rebound tenderness and fresh red blood per rectum.

Which is the most likely diagnosis?
A. Acute mesenteric ischaemia
B. Angiodysplasia
C. Colorectal carcinoma
D. Ischaemic colitis
E. Ulcerative colitis

 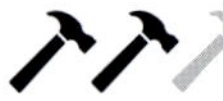 

48. A 45-year-old woman has 3 months of constant, cramping upper abdominal discomfort with increased frequency of loose, foul stools. She drinks two bottles of vodka a week. She is underweight, with conjunctival pallor and mild epigastric tenderness.

Which is the most appropriate investigation?
A. Amylase
B. Antitissue transglutaminase antibodies
C. Faecal calprotectin
D. Faecal elastase
E. Lipase

 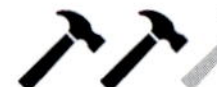 

49. A 65-year-old man has 3 months of difficulty swallowing, initially affecting solids, but now affecting liquids, with painful regurgitation, nausea, with three stones of weight loss. He takes over-the-counter antacids for indigestion, and has smoked 20 cigarettes a day for 30 years. He is underweight, with marked conjunctival pallor.

Which is the most appropriate investigation?
A. Barium swallow
B. Bronchoscopy
C. CT of thorax abdomen
D. Endoscopy
E. Transoesophageal endoscopic ultrasound

 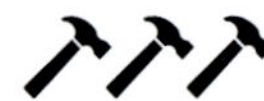 

50. A 41-year-old man has 6 months of constant, cramping abdominal pain, nausea and frequent, loose, foul

stools. He has recurrent episodes of severe epigastric pain and vomiting requiring hospital admissions and drinks a bottle of rum a day. He is cachexic, with mild conjunctival pallor and epigastric tenderness.

Which is the most appropriate management?
A. Alcohol abstinence therapies
B. Empirical antibiotics
C. Enteral nutrition
D. Intravenous fluids
E. Pancreatic enzyme replacement

 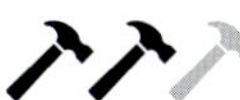

51. A 32-year-old man has 3 months of pain and discharge when passing stool. He has Crohn disease, managed with azathioprine. Digital rectal exam shows circular granulation tissue in the anal canal and perianal discharge.

Which is the most likely diagnosis?
A. Anal fissure
B. Haemorrhoids
C. Perianal abscess
D. Perianal fistula
E. Pilonidal sinus

 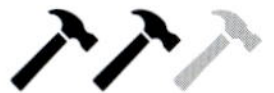 

52. A 19-year-old boy has 7 days of profuse bloody, watery diarrhoea with several abdominal pain and nausea since returning from holiday. His temperature is 37.9°C, pulse 121 bpm and BP 82/63 mmHg. He has reduced skin turgor, generalized abdominal tenderness and hyperactive bowel sounds.

Which is the most appropriate management?
A. Antiemetics
B. Empirical antibiotics
C. Intravenous fluids
D. Intravenous hydrocortisone
E. Loperamide

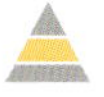 

53. A 72-year-old man has 2 months of increased frequency of foul watery stools, poor appetite and two stones of weight loss. He has type 2 diabetes mellitus, managed with metformin, and has smoked 30 cigarettes a day for 40 years. He has a palpable mass in the right upper quadrant and scleral icterus.

Which is the most likely diagnosis?
A. Cholangiocarcinoma
B. Chronic pancreatitis
C. Colorectal carcinoma
D. Pancreatic cancer
E. Pancreatic pseudocyst

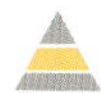 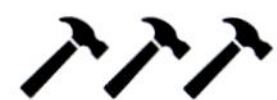

54. A 63-year-old man has 6 months of intermittent chest discomfort when swallowing. He has gastroesophageal reflux disease, managed with omeprazole, and has smoked 20 cigarettes a day for 40 years.

Which is the most likely diagnosis?
A. Achalasia
B. Oesophageal adenocarcinoma
C. Oesophageal candidiasis
D. Oesophagitis
E. Pharyngeal pouch

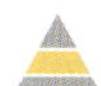 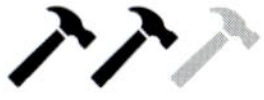 

55. A 28-year-old man has 1 month of increased frequency of pale stools, dark, concentrated urine, fatigue and generalized itch. He has ulcerative colitis, managed with mesalamine. He has mild scleral icterus and excoriations over the arms and abdomen.

Which is the most appropriate investigation?
A. Autoantibody screening
B. Endoscopic retrograde cholangiopancreatography
C. Liver biopsy
D. Liver function tests
E. Ultrasound of abdomen

 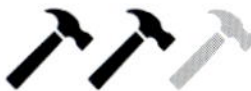

56. A 44-year-old woman has 2 months of upper abdominal pain after meals, nausea, increased frequency of pale stools and darkening of her urine. Her temperature is 36.8°C, pulse 62 bpm and BP 128/91 mmHg. She has mild scleral icterus.

Which is the most likely diagnosis?
A. Biliary colic
B. Cholangitis
C. Cholangiocarcinoma
D. Cholecystitis
E. Choledocholithiasis

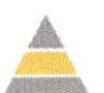
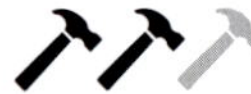

57. A 72-year-old woman has 2 weeks of a mildly tender left groin lump. She has chronic obstructive pulmonary disease, managed with salmeterol and tiotropium inhalers.

Figure 11.4 (see Chapter 37).

Which is the most likely diagnosis?
   A. Femoral hernia
   B. Inguinal hernia
   C. Lipoma
   D. Lymphadenopathy
   E. Saphenous varix

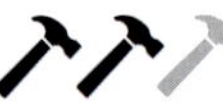

58. A 64-year-old man has 4 days of generalized abdominal tenderness and distention, nausea, vomiting and fevers. He has cirrhosis, managed with propranolol, lactulose and spironolactone. His temperature is 37.9°C, pulse 102 bpm and BP 108/72 mmHg. He has gross tense abdominal distention, generalized abdominal pain, with dullness to percussion, and quiet bowel sounds.

Which is the most appropriate investigation?
   A. Abdominal X-ray
   B. Blood cultures
   C. Liver function tests
   D. Peritoneal fluid analysis
   E. Ultrasound abdomen

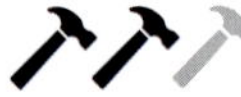
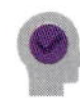

59. A 35-year-old man has severe chest pain radiating to the back after 12 hours of constant vomiting after an undercooked meal. His temperature is 38.1°C, pulse 133 bpm, BP 108/72 mmHg, respiratory rate 26 breaths per minute and oxygen saturation 92% on breathing air. He has palpable suprasternal crepitus and diffuse crepitations in the lung fields.

Which is the most appropriate investigation?
   A. Barium swallow
   B. Chest X-ray
   C. CT of thorax
   D. Contrast oesophagography
   E. Endoscopy

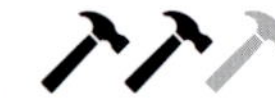
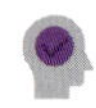

60. A 70-year-old woman has 1 month of abdominal discomfort and 2 kg of weight loss. She has chronic hepatitis B. She has mild right upper quadrant tenderness, a palpable liver border and mild scleral icterus.

Which is the most appropriate investigation?
   A. CT of abdomen
   B. Fibroscan
   C. Liver function tests
   D. Serum alpha-fetoprotein
   E. Ultrasound abdomen

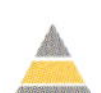

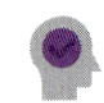

61. An 85-year-old woman has 2 days of abdominal pain and nausea. She last opened her bowels 5 days ago. She has hypothyroidism and osteoarthritis, managed with levothyroxine and codeine. Her temperature is 37.9°C, pulse 76 bpm, BP 118/75 mmHg, respiratory rate 18 breaths per minute and oxygen saturation 98% on breathing air. She has left iliac fossa pain and a palpable mass.

Which is the most appropriate management?
   A. Emergency laparotomy
   B. Intravenous antibiotics
   C. Laxatives
   D. Oral antibiotics
   E. Percutaneous drainage

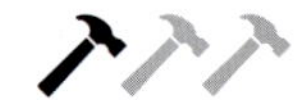

62. A 52-year-old man has 3 months of nausea, poor appetite and 5 kg of weight loss. He manages indigestion symptoms with over-the-counter antacids, and has smoked 30 cigarettes a day for 30 years. He is cachexic, with conjunctival pallor.

Which is the most likely diagnosis?
   A. Gastric cancer
   B. Gastroesophageal reflux disease
   C. Oesophageal cancer
   D. Oesophageal stricture
   E. Peptic ulcer disease

 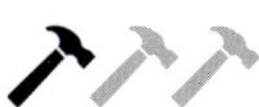 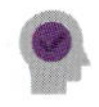

63. A 72-year-old lady has 2 weeks of stool incontinence, with anal itching and a palpable mass. She typically opens her bowels twice a week. She has chronic obstructive pulmonary disease, managed with salmeterol and fluticasone inhalers. Her abdomen is soft, with sluggish bowel sounds.

Figure 11.5 (see Chapter 37).

Which is the most appropriate management?
A. Digital repositioning
B. Haemorrhoidectomy
C. Increase laxatives
D. Injection sclerotherapy
E. Rectopexy

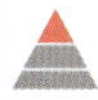 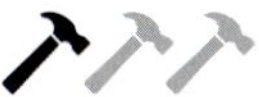 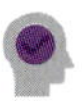

64. A 32-year-old woman has 2 months of fatigue, cold intolerance and pins and needles in her feet. She has Crohn disease, managed with azathioprine. She is pale, and has symmetrical numbness to the mid shin.

Investigations:
Hb 97 (115–165 g/dL).
MCV 108 fL (80–96).

Which is the most appropriate management?
A. Intramuscular hydroxocobalamin
B. Monofer infusion
C. Oral ferrous sulphate
D. Oral folic acid
E. Vitamin B complex

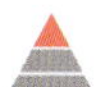  

65. A 32-year-old woman who is 33 weeks pregnant has 1 week of minimal fresh rectal bleeding on defecation. There is a palpable mass in the anal canal that protrudes on coughing.

Which is the most appropriate management?
A. Haemorrhoidectomy
B. Increase dietary fibre
C. Local anaesthetic and steroid cream
D. Reassure and discharge
E. Rubber band ligation

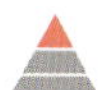  

66. A 23-year-old woman has 3 months of swallowing discomfort and painless regurgitation of food when she lies down, with 4 kg of weight loss. She is pale and appears underweight.

Which is the most appropriate investigation?
A. Chest X-ray
B. CT scan of head
C. Endoscopy
D. H. pylori testing
E. Oesophageal manometry

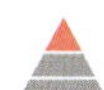 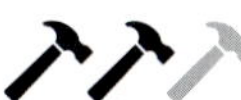

67. A 55-year-old man has sudden severe anorectal pain after opening his bowels. He has diverticular disease, managed with over-the-counter laxatives. He has a 2 cm painful blue swelling in the perianal margin.

Which is the most likely diagnosis?
A. Anal fissure
B. Anal fistula
C. Perianal haematoma
D. Rectal prolapse
E. Thrombosed haemorrhoid

 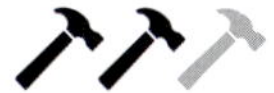 

68. An 82-year-old man has 6 months of cramping abdominal pain after meals, with 5 kg of weight loss. He has ischaemic heart disease, high cholesterol and hypertension, managed with aspirin, ramipril, amlodipine, atorvastatin and GTN spray. He has mild central abdominal tenderness and an audible bruit.

Which is the most appropriate investigation?
A. Abdominal X-ray
B. Colonoscopy
C. CT angiogram
D. Duplex ultrasound abdomen
E. Venous blood gas

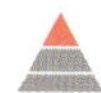  

69. A 72-year-old woman has 2 days of crampy abdominal pain and bloody diarrhoea. She has type 2 diabetes mellitus, hypertension and high cholesterol, managed with metformin, gliclazide, ramipril and atorvastatin. Her

temperature is 37.1°C, pulse 67 bpm and BP 113/83 mmHg. She has tenderness in the left lower quadrant.

Which is the most appropriate management?
A. Analgesia, fluids and bowel rest
B. Angioplasty and stenting
C. Antibiotic therapy
D. Anticoagulation
E. Emergency colectomy

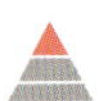 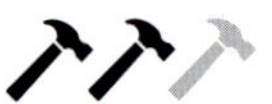 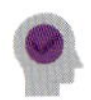

70. A 39-year-old man has sudden onset epigastric pain radiating to the back and vomiting after an alcoholic binge. His temperature is 37.9°C, pulse 107 bpm and BP 108/69 mmHg. Intravenous fluids are started. He subsequently develops chest pain, dyspnoea and diffuse lung field crepitations, with a new oxygen requirement of 4 L to maintain saturations of 96%.

Which is the most likely diagnosis?
A. Acute respiratory distress syndrome
B. Oesophageal rupture
C. Pleural effusion
D. Pneumonia
E. Pulmonary oedema

  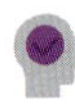

71. A 28-year-old woman has 3 days of perianal discomfort and itch when opening her bowels. She has ulcerative colitis managed with mesalamine. She has a warm, tender subcutaneous mass on the anal margin.

Which is the most appropriate management?
A. Antibiotics
B. Fistulotomy
C. Incision and drainage
D. Laxatives
E. Topical lidocaine

72. A 56-year-old man has 1 month of burning retrosternal pain, worse after meals and at night, with nausea and flatulence. He has type 2 diabetes mellitus and asthma, managed with metformin and salbutamol inhalers.

Investigations:
Figure 11.6 (see Chapter 37).

Which is the most likely diagnosis?
A. Gastroesophageal reflux disease
B. Hiatus hernia
C. Oesophageal adenocarcinoma
D. Oesophagitis
E. Peptic ulcer disease

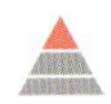 

73. An 82-year-old man has 2 days of abdominal pain and dark, offensive stools. He has atherosclerosis, managed with atorvastatin, and has smoked 40 cigarettes a day for 30 years. His temperature is 37.2°C, pulse 121 bpm and BP 92/64 mmHg. He has left-sided abdominal tenderness and distention, and dark red blood per rectum.

Which is the most likely diagnosis?
A. Angiodysplasia
B. Diverticular bleeding
C. Ischaemic colitis
D. Peptic ulcer disease
E. Ulcerative colitis

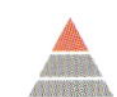 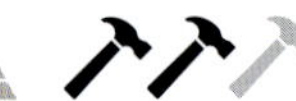

74. A 71-year-old man has 1 month of mild upper abdominal discomfort and 4 kg of weight loss. He has alcoholic liver disease managed with propranolol, ciprofloxacin and spironolactone. He is cachexic, with mild abdominal distention, distended paraumbilical veins and scleral icterus.

Which is the most likely diagnosis?
A. Decompensated cirrhosis
B. End-stage liver disease
C. Hepatocellular carcinoma
D. Liver fibrosis
E. Schistosomiasis

 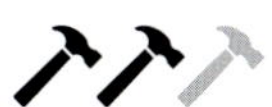 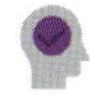

75. A 34-year-old man has 2 weeks of severe pain when opening his bowels and bright red blood when he wipes. He opens his bowels once a day. He has a midline fissure in the posterior anal sphincter.

Which is the most appropriate management?

A. Anal dilatation
B. Botulinum A toxin injection
C. Lateral internal sphincterotomy
D. Laxatives
E. Topical glyceryl trinitrate ointment

 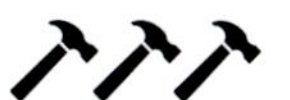 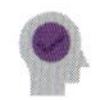

76. A 55-year-old man has 1 week of rectal bleeding and lower abdominal discomfort. He has HIV with undetectable viral load, managed with antiretroviral combination therapy.

Investigations:
Colonoscopy: T3N1M0 tumour of the anal canal.

Which is the most appropriate management?

A. Abdominoperineal resection
B. Anterior resection
C. Neoadjuvant chemotherapy
D. Palliation
E. Radiochemotherapy

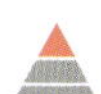 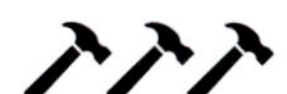 

77. A 43-year-old man has 1 month of intermittent pain and regurgitation when swallowing. He has gastroesophageal reflux disease, managed with omeprazole and over-the-counter antacids.

Investigations:
Barium swallow: narrowing of the gastroesophageal junction.

Which is the most appropriate management?

A. Chemoradiotherapy
B. Endoscopic dilation
C. Endoscopic stent placement
D. Increase omeprazole dose
E. Surgical resection

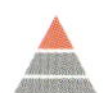  

78. A 64-year-old man has 3 months of swallowing discomfort, with nausea and three stones of weight loss. He has peptic ulcer disease, managed with omeprazole. He is pale, cachexic, with a palpable epigastric mass.

Investigations:
Endoscopy: T3N0M0 lesion in the gastric cardia.

Which is the most appropriate management?

A. Endoscopic mucosal resection
B. Palliation
C. Radiochemotherapy
D. Subtotal gastrectomy
E. Total gastrectomy

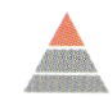 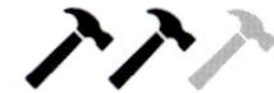 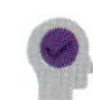

79. A 58-year-old woman has severe abdominal pain, vomiting and constipation, after 6 months of intermittent upper abdominal pain after meals lasting several hours. Her temperature is 36.8°C, pulse 92 bpm and BP 92/67 mmHg. She has dry mucous membranes, a distended abdomen, right-sided abdominal tenderness and hyperactive bowel sounds.

Investigations:
Abdominal X-ray: multiple distended small bowel loops and air in the biliary tree.

Which is the most appropriate management?

A. Cholecystectomy
B. Cholecystostomy
C. Endoscopic retrograde cholangiopancreatography
D. Enterolithotomy
E. Intravenous antibiotics

 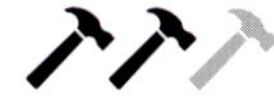

80. A 32-year-old man has 2 weeks of severe pain when opening his bowels, with bright red blood and perianal itch. He typically opens his bowels twice a week. He has Crohn disease, managed with azathioprine. There is a superficial laceration in the posterior anal canal, with no mass, erythema or perianal discharge.

Which is the most likely diagnosis?

A. Anal abscess
B. Anal fissure
C. Anal fistula
D. Haemorrhoids
E. Pruritus ani

Cardiothoracics and vascular

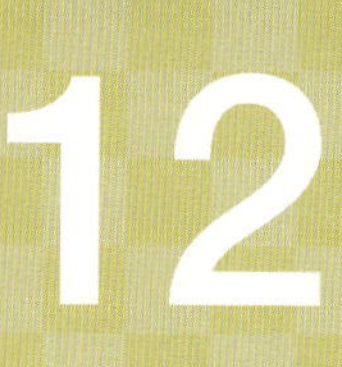

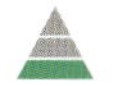  

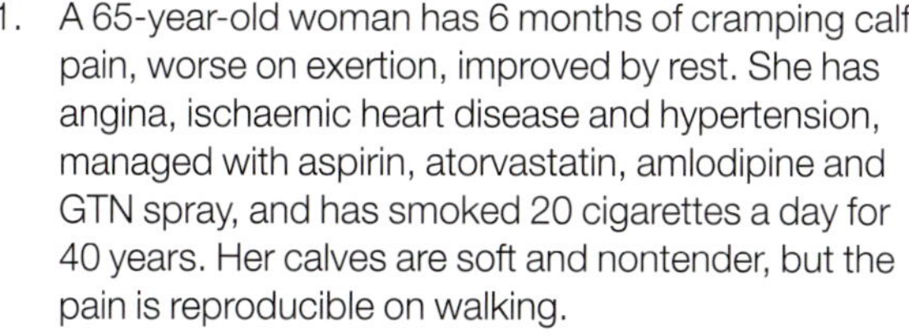

1. A 65-year-old woman has 6 months of cramping calf pain, worse on exertion, improved by rest. She has angina, ischaemic heart disease and hypertension, managed with aspirin, atorvastatin, amlodipine and GTN spray, and has smoked 20 cigarettes a day for 40 years. Her calves are soft and nontender, but the pain is reproducible on walking.

Which is the most appropriate management?

A. Alcohol reduction
B. Dietary modifications
C. Smoking cessation
D. Structured exercise therapy
E. Weight loss

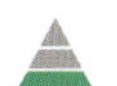 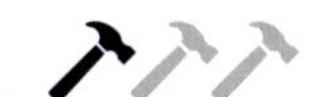 

2. A 73-year-old man has a 1 hour episode of left sided visual loss which has now resolved. He has type 2 diabetes mellitus and hypertension, managed with metformin, dapagliflozin and ramipril, and has smoked 20 cigarettes a day for 40 years. There is an audible carotid bruit on the left.

Which is the most appropriate investigation?

A. Carotid duplex ultrasound
B. CT angiography
C. CT scan of head
D. Digital subtraction angiography
E. MR angiography

3. A 42-year-old man has 1 day of right calf swelling and tenderness. He has ulcerative colitis, managed with mesalamine, and has smoked 20 cigarettes a day for 15 years. His right lower leg is swollen, tender, warm and erythematous.

Which is the most likely diagnosis?

A. Cellulitis
B. Compartment syndrome
C. Deep vein thrombosis
D. Lymphedema
E. Superficial thrombophlebitis

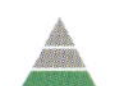 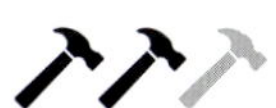 

4. A 54-year-old woman has sudden sharp right-sided chest pain, cough and shortness of breath. She had her gallbladder removed 1 week ago, but is otherwise well. Her temperature is 37.8°C, pulse 131 bpm, BP 117/91 mmHg, respiratory rate 31 breaths per minute and oxygen saturation 91% on breathing air. Her chest is clear to auscultation.

Which is the most appropriate management?

A. Apixaban
B. Clopidogrel
C. Enoxaparin
D. Unfractionated heparin
E. Warfarin

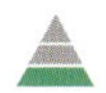 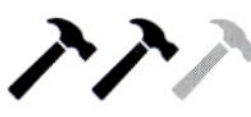 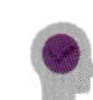

5. A 56-year-old man has 2 months of dull central lower back pain. He has high cholesterol and hypertension, managed with atorvastatin and ramipril, and has smoked 30 cigarettes a day for 30 years. He has an expansile central abdominal mass and audible bruit.

Which is the most appropriate investigation?

A. Abdominal X-ray
B. CT of abdomen
C. MR of lumbar spine
D. Ultrasound of abdomen
E. X-ray lumbar spine

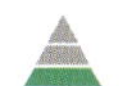 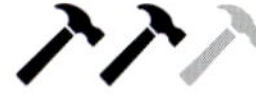 

6. A 63-year-old man has sudden tearing central chest pain radiating to the back, with nausea and lightheadedness. He has hypertension and high cholesterol, managed with ramipril, amlodipine and atorvastatin, and has smoked 30 cigarettes a day for 40 years. His temperature is 36.9°C, pulse 141 bpm and BP 175/95 mmHg. He has a strong right radial pulse, but the left is barely palpable.

Which is the most appropriate investigation?
  A. Chest X-ray
  B. CT angiogram
  C. CT scan of pulmonary arteries
  D. ECG
  E. Echocardiogram

 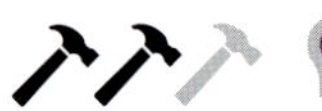

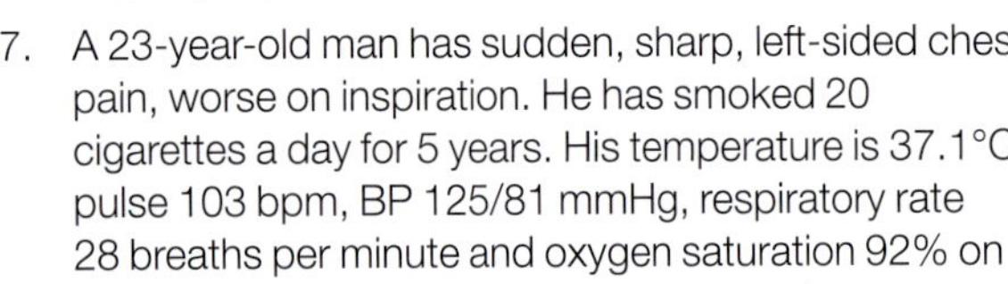

7. A 23-year-old man has sudden, sharp, left-sided chest pain, worse on inspiration. He has smoked 20 cigarettes a day for 5 years. His temperature is 37.1°C, pulse 103 bpm, BP 125/81 mmHg, respiratory rate 28 breaths per minute and oxygen saturation 92% on breathing air. He has reduced air entry and hyperresonant percussion on the left.

Figure 12.1 (see Chapter 37).

Which is the most appropriate management?
  A. Chest drain
  B. Needle decompression in the second intercostal space
  C. Pleurodesis
  D. Repeat chest X-ray in 2 weeks
  E. Treatment dose low-molecular-weight heparin

 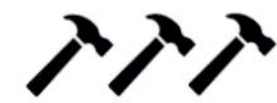

8. A 68-year-old man has 6 months of numbness, tingling and burning in his feet. He has bilateral sensory loss to the mid shin, and a painless, deep ulcer at the base of the first metatarsal, with surrounding callous.

Investigations:
Ankle brachial pressure index: 1.4.

Which is the most likely diagnosis?
  A. Chronic venous insufficiency
  B. Critical limb ischaemia
  C. Diabetic neuropathy
  D. Intermittent claudication
  E. Spinal stenosis

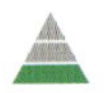 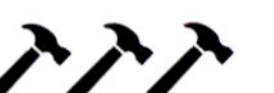 

9. A 61-year-old man has 2 weeks of worsening right foot pain, after 6 months of constant burning pain in his right calf and foot. He has type 1 diabetes mellitus, peripheral arterial disease and CKD 4, managed with insulin, clopidogrel, ramipril and atorvastatin. His temperature is 38.1°C, pulse 96 bpm and BP 116/87 mmHg.

Figure 12.2 (see Chapter 37).

Which is the most appropriate management?
  A. Amputation
  B. Angioplasty and stenting
  C. Optimise glycaemic control
  D. Peripheral artery bypass
  E. Structured exercise therapy

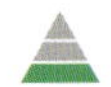 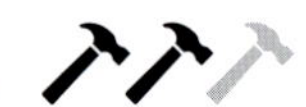 

10. A 67-year-old man has 6 months of cramping lower leg pain, worse on exertion, relieved by rest. He has atrial fibrillation and CKD 3, managed with bisoprolol, apixaban and atorvastatin, and has smoked 20 cigarettes a day for 40 years. His calves are soft, pale and cool. Posterior tibial and dorsalis pedis pulses are diminished on the left, and absent on the right.

Which is the most appropriate investigation?
  A. Ankle brachial pressure index
  B. Digital subtraction angiography
  C. Duplex ultrasound
  D. MR angiography
  E. Transcutaneous oximetry

 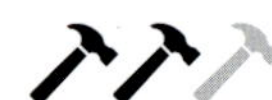

11. A 62-year-old man has sudden onset, severe pain, tingling and weakness in his left lower leg. He has atrial fibrillation and hypertension, managed with bisoprolol and ramipril. His left calf is pale, cool to touch, with absent pedal pulses.

Which is the most likely diagnosis?
  A. Acute limb ischaemia
  B. Deep vein thrombosis
  C. Intermittent claudication
  D. Compartment syndrome
  E. Critical limb ischaemia

 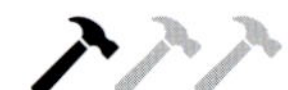 

12. A 62-year-old woman has 6 months of worsening lower leg pain, swelling and itch, worse in the heat or after standing. She has bilateral nonpitting oedema to the knees, with superficial telangiectasia and dilated tortuous lower leg veins.

Which is the most appropriate management?
  A. Compression stockings
  B. Ligation and vein stripping
  C. Radiofrequency ablation
  D. Sclerotherapy
  E. Structured exercise therapy

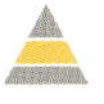 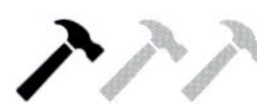 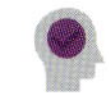

13. A 65-year-old male is diagnosed with a 4.2 cm abdominal aortic aneurysm following screening. He has no back or abdominal pain. He has hypertension, managed with ramipril, and is an ex-smoker of 20 pack years.

Which is the most appropriate management?
  A. CT angiography at 12 months
  B. Endovascular aneurysm repair
  C. Open surgical repair
  D. Repeat ultrasound at 12 months
  E. Repeat ultrasound at 6 months

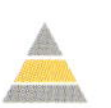 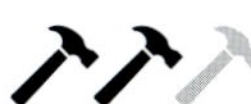 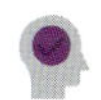

14. A 64-year-old woman has 2 months of exertional breathlessness, palpitations and fatigue. She has hypertension, high cholesterol and coronary artery disease, managed with losartan, amlodipine, atorvastatin and bisoprolol. She has a pansystolic murmur in the mitral area radiating to the axilla.

Which is the most appropriate investigation?
  A. BNP
  B. Chest X-ray
  C. Coronary angiography
  D. ECG
  E. Transthoracic echocardiogram

 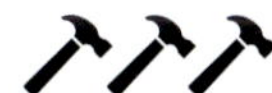 

15. A 64-year-old man has sudden central chest pain radiating to the back, with nausea and dizziness. He has hypertension and high cholesterol, managed with ramipril, amlodipine, indapamide and atorvastatin, and has smoked 40 cigarettes a day for 30 years. His temperature is 37.3°C, pulse 119 bpm and BP 165/61 mmHg.

Investigations:
Chest X-ray: widened mediastinum.
CT aortogram: dilation of the descending aorta with intimal flap and double lumen.

Which is the most appropriate management?
  A. Endovascular stent implantation
  B. Inotropes
  C. Intravenous labetalol
  D. Open graft repair
  E. Sodium nitroprusside

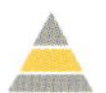 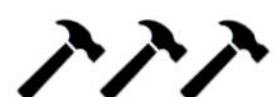

16. A 63-year-old man has 3 weeks of worsening retrosternal chest pain, breathlessness and nausea. He has mesothelioma and is undergoing radiochemotherapy. His temperature is 37.1°C, pulse 123 bpm, BP 85/57 mmHg, respiratory rate 22 breaths per minute and oxygen saturation 91% on breathing air. He is pale, with distended neck veins and a JVP 6 cm above the sternal angle. He has bibasal crepitations in the lung fields and soft heart sounds.

Which is the most likely diagnosis?
  A. Cardiac tamponade
  B. Haemopericardium
  C. Pericardial effusion
  D. Pleural effusion
  E. Pulmonary oedema

 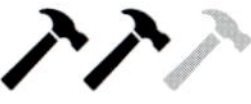 

17. A 64-year-old man has 2 years of bilateral cramping lower leg pain, initially on exertion only but now constant, worse at night. He has peripheral arterial disease and hypertension, managed with atorvastatin, clopidogrel, amlodipine and losartan, and has smoked 20 cigarettes a day for 40 years.

Figure 12.3 (see Chapter 37).

Which is the most appropriate management?
  A. Aspirin
  B. Phosphodiesterase inhibitor
  C. Revascularization
  D. Smoking cessation adverse
  E. Structured exercise therapy

 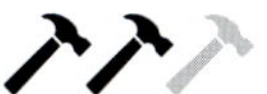 

18. An 82-year-old woman has 1 month of a painless, itchy right ankle ulcer.

Figure 12.4 (see Chapter 37).

Which is the most likely diagnosis?
  A. Arterial ulcer
  B. Diabetic ulcer
  C. Neuropathic ulcer
  D. Pressure ulcer
  E. Venous ulcer

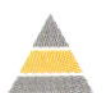 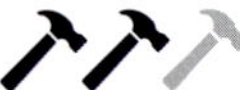 

19. A 32-year-old woman has 3 days of aching central chest discomfort and breathlessness, worse lying flat. She has systemic lupus erythematosus, managed with hydroxychloroquine. Her temperature is 37.2°C, pulse 82 bpm, BP 113/83 mmHg, respiratory rate 22 breaths per minute and oxygen saturation 93% on breathing air. Her chest is clear and heart sounds are present, but the apex beat is not palpable.

Which is the most appropriate investigation?

A. Chest X-ray
B. CT scan of pulmonary arteries
C. CT of thorax
D. ECG
E. Echocardiogram

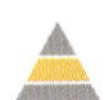 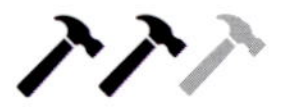 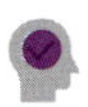

20. A 73-year-old man has 2 months of dull upper back pain, dry cough and pain when swallowing. He has hypertension, managed with ramipril and amlodipine, and has smoked 20 cigarettes a day for 40 years.

Which is the most appropriate investigation?

A. Chest X-ray
B. Coronary angiogram
C. CT angiogram
D. MR angiography
E. Transthoracic echocardiogram

21. A 94-year-old woman has a 1 hour vacant episode with left sided weakness, which has now resolved. She has hypertension and type 2 diabetes mellitus, managed with ramipril, amlodipine and metformin, and is an ex-smoker of 40 pack years.

Investigations:
CT angiogram carotid arteries: 60% stenosis of the right carotid artery.

Which is the most appropriate management?

A. Aspirin
B. Carotid artery bypass grafting
C. Carotid artery stenting
D. Carotid endarterectomy
E. Thrombectomy

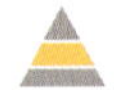 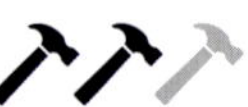

22. A 75-year-old lady has 3 months of exertional central chest pain, breathlessness and lightheadedness. She has hypertension, managed with amlodipine. She has an ejection systolic murmur radiating to the carotids.

Investigations:
ECG: left axis deviation and tall R waves in V5/6.
Echocardiogram: significant calcification and narrowing of the aortic valve and left ventricular concentric hypertrophy.

Which is the most appropriate management?

A. Anticoagulation
B. Echocardiogram monitoring
C. Open aortic valve replacement
D. Percutaneous balloon valvuloplasty
E. Transcatheter aortic valve replacement

 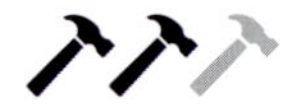 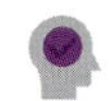

23. A 72-year-old man has sudden severe abdominal pain radiating down his legs, with nausea and lightheadedness. He has hypertension and diabetes, managed with ramipril and metformin, and has smoked 20 cigarettes a day for 40 years. His temperature is 36.8°C, pulse 122 bpm and BP 93/61 mmHg. He has a painful pulsatile abdominal mass.

Which is the most appropriate management?

A. Blood transfusion
B. Emergency open surgical repair
C. Endovascular aneurysm repair
D. Explorative laparotomy
E. Palliation

  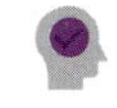

24. A 55-year-old woman has 6 months of bilateral lower leg discomfort, itch and ankle swelling, worse on exertion or after standing, relieved by leg elevation. She is overweight, and has smoked 10 cigarettes a day for 30 years. She has bilateral nonpitting oedema to the mid shins, and tortuous dilated veins on the posterior calves.

Which is the most appropriate investigation?

A. ABPI
B. Echocardiogram
C. MR venography
D. Plethysmography
E. Venous duplex ultrasound

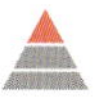  

25. A 24-year-old woman has intermittent pain and discoloration of her fingers in the cold or when distressed. Her fingers go numb, white and blue, then painful and red, before normalizing. She has anxiety, managed with sertraline.

Which is the most appropriate management?
   A. Botox injections
   B. Nifedipine
   C. Sildenafil
   D. Topical GTN
   E. Trigger avoidance

 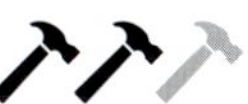

26. A 63-year-old woman has 3 months of cramping pain in her buttocks and thighs on exertion. She has ischaemic heart disease, managed with aspirin, ramipril, bisoprolol and GTN spray. She has wasting of the thighs and buttocks with absent femoral pulses.

Which is the most likely cause?
   A. Aortoiliac occlusive disease
   B. Femoral arteritis
   C. Femoral artery occlusive disease
   D. May-Thurner syndrome
   E. Spinal stenosis

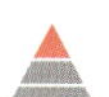 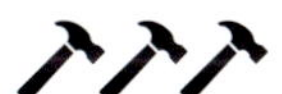 

27. A 72-year-old man has 3 weeks of breathlessness, aching left-sided chest pain and a nonproductive cough, after 3 months of fatigue and 5 kg of weight loss.

Investigations:
Chest X-ray: left sided white out with meniscal level to the mid zone.
Pleural fluid analysis:
Appearance: bloody.
pH: 7.21.
Protein: 0.8 (1–2 g/dL).
Glucose: 103 mg/dL (<60 mg/dL).
LDH: 285 U/L.
Cholesterol: 84 mg/dL.

Which is the most likely diagnosis?
   A. Cirrhosis
   B. Congestive heart failure
   C. Lung cancer
   D. Nephrotic syndrome
   E. Pneumonia

 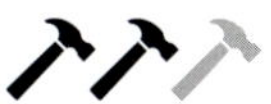

28. A 56-year-old woman has 2 months of bilateral lower leg swelling and discomfort, worse after standing, improved by elevation. She had a total abdominal hysterectomy and bilateral salpingo-oophorectomy with radical regional radiotherapy for ovarian cancer 6 months ago. She has nonpitting oedema of the left leg, with firm, tight skin.

Which is the most likely diagnosis?
   A. Chronic venous insufficiency
   B. Deep vein thrombosis
   C. Right heart failure
   D. Lipoedema
   E. Lymphoedema

 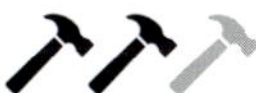 

29. A 62-year-old man has 6 weeks of a nonproductive cough and shortness of breath, with fatigue and 3 kg of weight loss.

Investigations:
Endobronchial ultrasound and biopsy: T2N0M0 adenocarcinoma of the left upper lung lobe.

Which is the most appropriate management?
   A. Chemotherapy
   B. Lobectomy
   C. Pneumonectomy
   D. Radiotherapy
   E. Wedge resection

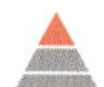  

30. A 73-year-old male has 2 days of worsening breathlessness, cough and pain when swallowing. He has a left lung adenocarcinoma and is an ex-smoker of 60 pack years. His temperature is 36.5°C, pulse 134 bpm, BP 95/64 mmHg, respiratory rate 31 breaths per minute and oxygen saturation 88% on breathing air. He has marked facial plethora, a JVP 5 cm above the sternal angle, with prominent chest wall veins.

Which is the most appropriate management?
   A. Dexamethasone
   B. Endovascular venography and stenting
   C. Intravenous furosemide
   D. Pneumonectomy
   E. Radiotherapy

Orthopaedics

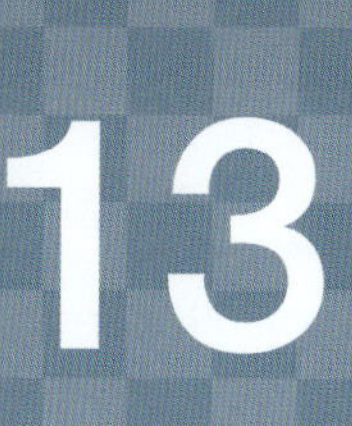

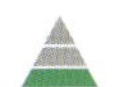  

1. A 50-year-old man has 3 days of worsening left calf pain and malaise. He has type 1 diabetes mellitus, managed with insulin. His temperature is 38.1°C, pulse 98 bpm and BP 133/84 mmHg. He has diffuse erythema, warmth, swelling and tenderness over the left lower calf, with a small graze over the shin.

Which is the most appropriate management?
  A. Apixaban
  B. Intravenous flucloxacillin
  C. Surgical debridement
  D. Topical ibuprofen gel
  E. Unfractionated heparin

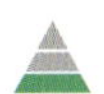 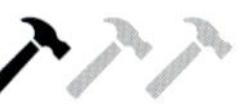 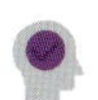

2. A 62-year-old man has 12 hours of worsening right knee pain, swelling and stiffness. He has type 2 diabetes mellitus and high cholesterol, managed with metformin, gliclazide and atorvastatin. His temperature is 38.1°C, pulse 102 bpm and BP 137/84 mmHg. His right knee is erythematous and warm, with boggy swelling around the joint and reduced range of flexion and extension.

Which is the most appropriate investigation?
  A. Aspiration of left knee joint for microscopy and culture
  B. Blood cultures
  C. MR of Knee
  D. Ultrasound of knee
  E. X-ray of knee

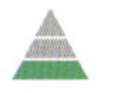  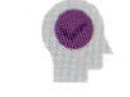

3. A 24-year-old man has sudden left lower leg pain and swelling. He had a left Achilles tendon rupture 1 week ago managed with plaster cast immobilization. He has an exquisitely tender and swollen left lower leg, with sensory loss to mid shin and absent pedal pulses.

Which is the most appropriate immediate management?
  A. Apixaban
  B. Cast removal
  C. Intravenous fluids
  D. Intravenous morphine
  E. Leg elevation

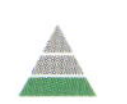 

4. A 72-year-old man has 6 months of bilateral knee pain and stiffness, worse on exertion and relieved by rest. He has hypertension and type 2 diabetes mellitus, managed with ramipril and metformin. He has an antalgic gait, with knee extension and flexion limited by pain, and palpable crepitus on passive joint movement.

Which is the most likely diagnosis?
  A. Gout
  B. Osteoarthritis
  C. Osteoporosis
  D. Reactive arthritis
  E. Rheumatoid arthritis

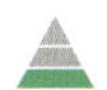 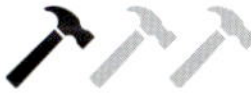 

5. A 74-year-old woman has 3 days of worsening right hip pain and pain when walking. She has hypertension and osteoarthritis, managed with amlodipine and codeine, and had a right hip intraarticular steroid injection 1 week ago. Her temperature is 37.8°C. She has a tender, warm right hip, with boggy joint swelling.

Investigations:
MR hip: cortical destruction and bone marrow oedema.

Which is the most appropriate management?
  A. Intravenous antibiotic therapy
  B. Oral morphine
  C. Physiotherapy
  D. Surgical debridement
  E. Therapeutic arthrocentesis

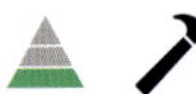 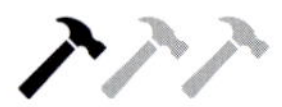 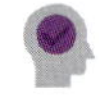

6. A 59-year-old woman has 2 days of worsening right knee pain, stiffness and inability to weight bear. She has rheumatoid arthritis and osteoporosis, managed with methotrexate, alendronic acid, Adcal D3 and lansoprazole. Her temperature is 37.9°C, pulse 102 bpm and BP 128/74 mmHg. Her right knee is swollen, warm and painful, with reduced range of flexion and extension.

Investigations:
Aspiration of knee joint: turbid fluid, WBC >80,000 mm^3, 99% neutrophils.

Which is the most appropriate management?
   A. Colchicine
   B. Empirical antibiotic therapy
   C. Intravenous hydrocortisone
   D. Intraarticular hydrocortisone
   E. Oral morphine

 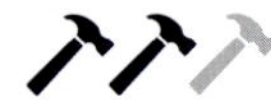 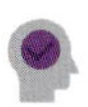

7. A 74-year-old man has severe right hip pain and inability to weight bear after a fall. He has hypertension, managed with ramipril. He has a shortened and externally rotated right hip, with pain on palpation of the greater trochanter.

Pelvic X-ray: nondisplaced intracapsular fracture of the right femoral neck

Which is the most appropriate management?
   A. Dynamic hip screw
   B. Hemiarthroplasty
   C. Intramedullary nail
   D. Open reduction and internal fixation
   E. Total hip replacement

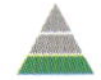 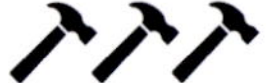 

8. A 38-year-old man has severe left leg pain after a motorcycle accident. He has severe pain and tense swelling in his left calf, worse on passive movement and is unable to weight bear. Pedal pulses are absent.

Which is the most appropriate management?
   A. Apixaban
   B. Fasciotomy
   C. Intravenous fluids
   D. Morphine
   E. Thrombolysis

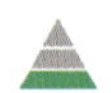 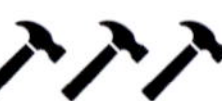 

9. A 68-year-old man has 12 hours of worsening right calf pain, malaise and fevers. He has type 2 diabetes mellitus, managed with metformin and gliclazide, and has recently had antibiotics for cellulitis. His temperature is 38.3°C, pulse 105 bpm and BP 143/94 mmHg. He has extreme pain, diffuse erythema and violaceous discolouration of the right lower leg, with subcutaneous induration and palpable crepitus.

Which is the most appropriate long-term management?
   A. Fasciotomy
   B. Intravenous antibiotics
   C. Intravenous immunoglobulins
   D. Oral morphine
   E. Surgical exploration and debridement

 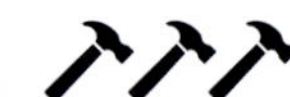 

10. A 23-year-old man has 3 days of worsening right hip pain. He is an intravenous drug user. His temperature is 38.3°C and pulse 132 bpm. He has a tender, warm right hip, with boggy swelling around the joint and reduced range of motion.

Which is the most appropriate management?
   A. Arthroscopy and irrigation
   B. Arthrotomy and debridement
   C. Empirical antibiotic therapy
   D. Intravenous morphine
   E. Therapeutic arthrocentesis

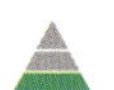 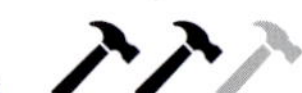 

11. A 65-year-old man has 1 week of left foot pain. He has insulin-dependent type 2 diabetes mellitus, hypertension and gout, managed with insulin, ramipril, amlodipine and allopurinol. His temperature is 38.3°C and pulse 118 bpm. His left foot is tender, swollen and warm, with a deep sloughy ulcer at the base of the first metatarsal, with surrounding callous. There is bilateral lower limb sensory loss to the ankle.

Which is the most appropriate investigation?

A. Aspiration of left knee joint for microscopy and culture
B. Blood cultures
C. Bone biopsy
D. MR of foot
E. X-ray of foot

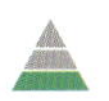 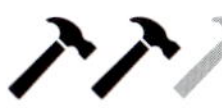

12. A 54-year-old man has 2 days of left knee pain, swelling and stiffness. He had a left knee replacement 6 months ago for osteoarthritis. His temperature is 38.7°C, pulse 121 bpm, BP 117/64 mmHg, respiratory rate 21 breaths per minute and oxygen saturation 98% on breathing air. His left knee is warm, tender and swollen, and he is unable to weight bear.

Investigations:
Synovial fluid analysis:
Appearance: yellow green
WBC >60,000 mm^3
Neutrophils 98%
Glucose 1.3 g/dL
Gram stain: gram-positive cocci in clusters
Crystal microscopy: negative

Which is the most likely diagnosis?

A. Gout
B. Idiopathic arthritis
C. Pseudogout
D. Reactive arthritis
E. Septic arthritis

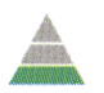 

13. A 52-year-old woman has 2 days of worsening lower back pain and difficulty mobilizing. She has L4 disc protrusion, managed with physiotherapy and codeine. She has severe lumbosacral tenderness, reduced tone and left leg weakness, with loss of sensation in the inner thigh and perineum.

Which is the most likely diagnosis?

A. Cauda equina syndrome
B. L4 disc prolapse
C. L4 radiculopathy
D. Spinal cord compression
E. Spondylosis

 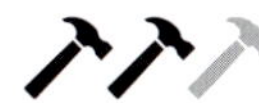 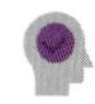

14. A 54-year-old man has worsening left knee pain and stiffness. He has osteoarthritis, managed with morphine, naproxen and multiple intraarticular steroid injections. He has pain and reduced range of motion in the left knee, with crepitus on joint movement.

Which is the most appropriate management?

A. Arthrodesis
B. Arthroplasty
C. Arthroscopy
D. Osteotomy
E. Physiotherapy

 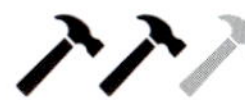

15. A 73-year-old man has worsening left lower leg pain, sensory loss and confusion. He has type 2 diabetes mellitus, CKD 3 and peripheral arterial disease, managed with metformin, gliclazide, atorvastatin and clopidogrel. His temperature is 38.9°C, pulse 131 bpm and BP 105/84 mmHg.

Figure 13.1 (see Chapter 37).

Which is the most likely diagnosis?

A. Cellulitis
B. Compartment syndrome
C. Deep vein thrombosis
D. Erysipelas
E. Necrotizing fasciitis

 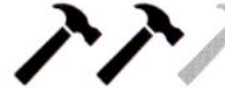 

16. A 38-year-old man has 3 days of worsening right groin pain. He is an intravenous drug user. His temperature is 38.8°C and pulse 129 bpm. He has severe perineal pain, with diffuse purple skin discolouration, tissue induration, bullae and palpable subcutaneous crepitus.

Which test is most likely to confirm the diagnosis?

A. Blood cultures
B. CT pelvis
C. Deep tissue biopsy
D. MRI pelvis
E. Skin scrape

 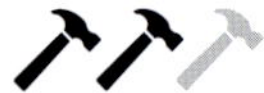 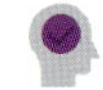

17. A 64-year-old man has 1 day of worsening right lower leg pain. He has chronic venous insufficiency managed with regular compression bandaging of his lower legs. He has severe pain in his right lower leg, worse on passive movement and is unable to weight bear. His right calf is swollen >3 cm more than the right, and there is sensory loss and paraesthesia in the right foot. Pedal pulses are palpable.

Which is the most appropriate investigation?
   A. Compartmental pressures
   B. Creatine kinase levels
   C. Doppler ultrasound
   D. MR angiography
   E. X-ray of right lower leg

  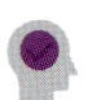

18. A 22-year-old man has an open, displaced fracture of the right femur after a road traffic accident. There is visible profusion of the distal femur and significant overlying tissue loss, but no sensory loss, and palpable lower limb pulses.

Which is the most appropriate management?
   A. Antibiotic therapy and wound dressing
   B. Closed reduction and dressing
   C. Debridement and external fixation
   D. Intramedullary nailing
   E. Open reduction and internal fixation

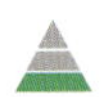 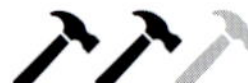 

19. A 72-year-old woman has 2 months of worsening back pain and difficulty mobilizing. She had breast cancer 2 years ago, managed with radical mastectomy and regional lymph node dissection. She has focal L2/L3 tenderness, bilateral weakness to hip flexion and knee extension, with lower limb sensory loss and brisk lower limb reflexes.

Which is the most appropriate investigation?
   A. Bladder scan
   B. CT myelogram
   C. MR of lumbosacral spine
   D. Nerve conduction studies
   E. X-ray of lumbar spine

 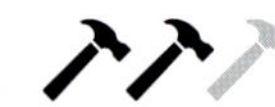

20. A 78-year-old woman has severe right-sided groin pain and inability to weight bear after a fall. She has a shortened and externally rotated right leg, with pain on palpation from the greater trochanter into the groin.

Figure 13.2 (see Chapter 37).

Which is the most likely diagnosis?
   A. Intertrochanteric fracture
   B. Fracture of the femoral head
   C. Neck of femur fracture
   D. Pubic rami fracture
   E. Trochanteric fracture

21. A 52-year-old woman has 3 months of pain and tingling in her left thumb, index and middle fingers, worse at night and after typing at her computer, relieved by shaking the hand. She has type 2 diabetes mellitus and hypothyroidism, managed with metformin and levothyroxine. Her symptoms are reproducible when her wrists are held in full flexion for 1 minute.

Which is the most appropriate management?
   A. Carpal tunnel release
   B. Oral hydrocortisone
   C. Physiotherapy
   D. Steroid injection
   E. Wrist splinting

 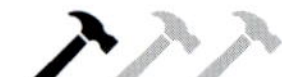 

22. A 67-year-old woman has 2 months of right hip pain, worse on exertion, improved by rest, with morning stiffness. She has an antalgic gait and limited range of movement of the right hip, with tenderness and palpable joint crepitus.

Which is the most appropriate investigation?
   A. Hip joint aspirate
   B. No investigation required
   C. MR of hip
   D. Ultrasound of hip
   E. X-ray of hip

 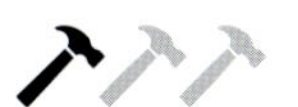 

23. A 54-year-old woman has 2 months of dull lower back pain. She has hypothyroidism and peptic ulcer disease, managed with levothyroxine and omeprazole, and has smoked 20 cigarettes a day for 30 years. She has focal L2 tenderness.

Investigations:
X-ray of spine: increased radiolucency and cortical thinning of the thoracic and lumbar spine, with nondisplaced L1/2 wedge fracture.

Which is the most appropriate management?
A. Adcal D3
B. Alendronic acid
C. Denosumab
D. Oral analgesia
E. Physiotherapy

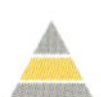 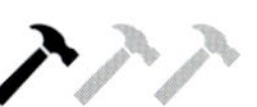 

24. A 71-year-old woman has 1 year of worsening bilateral finger pain, swelling and stiffness, worse in the morning and after use. She has bilateral stiffness and reduced range of movement in the first phalanx, with pain and thickening of the distal and proximal interphalangeal joints.

Figure 13.3 (see Chapter 37).

Which is the most appropriate management?
A. Arthroplasty
B. Ibuprofen gel
C. Intraarticular hydrocortisone
D. Topical capsaicin
E. Tramadol

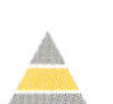  

25. A 35-year-old man has right knee pain and swelling after a direct blow to the knee. He has extensive boggy swelling of the right knee joint, with pain on passive and active extension and flexion of the knee, and a positive anterior drawer test.

Which is the most appropriate investigation?
A. CT of knee
B. Joint aspirate
C. MR of knee
D. Ultrasound of knee
E. X-ray of knee

 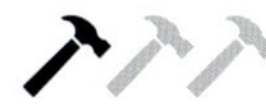

26. A 72-year-old man has 1 month of neck pain, with shooting pain down his left arm and left arm weakness. He has osteoarthritis, managed with naproxen and omeprazole. He has focal C6/C7 tenderness, with weakness to wrist flexion and finger extension, and sensory loss over the medial forearm.

Which is the most appropriate investigation?
A. CT myelogram
B. MR of cervical spine
C. Nerve conduction studies
D. Wrist series
E. X-ray of cervical spine

 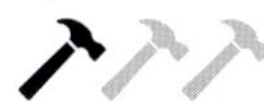

27. A 32-year-old woman who is 33 weeks pregnant has 2 months of burning and tingling in her right thumb, index and middle finger, worse at night, with difficulty buttoning her clothes and holding a pen. She has sensory loss over the right index and middle finger, with weakness in thumb abduction and thenar atrophy. Her symptoms are reproducible with tapping over the volar wrist.

Which is the most likely diagnosis?
A. Carpal tunnel syndrome
B. Cervical radiculopathy
C. De Quervain's tenosynovitis
D. Osteoarthritis
E. Ulnar neuropathy

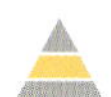 

28. A 72-year-old man has 6 weeks of left foot pain and difficulty walking. He has type 2 diabetes mellitus and high cholesterol, managed with metformin, dapagliflozin, linagliptin and atorvastatin. He has a mildly tender, warm left foot, with a callous ulcer over the first metatarsal and adjacent pus-draining sinus tract.

Investigations:
X-ray of foot: bone destruction and periosteal reaction.

Which is the most likely diagnosis?
A. Avascular necrosis
B. Charcot arthropathy
C. Chronic osteomyelitis
D. Diabetic foot ulcer
E. Septic arthritis

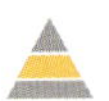 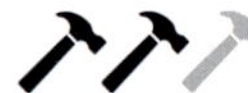 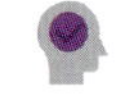

29. An 18-year-old girl has ankle pain after a fall. She has tenderness in the left lateral and medial malleolus and bruising extending to the midfoot, and is unable to weight bear.

Investigations:
X-ray of ankle: displaced bimalleolar fracture.

Which is the most appropriate management?
A. Open reduction and internal fixation
B. Oral analgesia
C. Physiotherapy
D. Rest, ice, compression and elevation
E. Short leg cast

 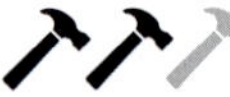 

30. A 24-year-old man has a sudden pop in his left ankle while running, with subsequent severe pain and inability to weight bear. He has calf swelling and tenderness to palpation over the posterior ankle. Plantar flexion on left calf compression is absent.

Which is the most appropriate investigation?
A. CT of ankle
B. MR of ankle
C. No investigations required
D. Ultrasound of ankle
E. X-ray of ankle

 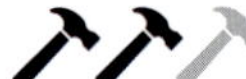 

31. A 44-year-old woman has 1 month of worsening shoulder stiffness and pain following surgical repair of a right rotator cuff tear. She has severe restriction of external rotation and abduction of the right shoulder, with pain on palpation over the glenohumeral joint.

Which is the most appropriate management?
A. Arthroplasty
B. Hydrodilatation
C. Intraarticular joint injection
D. Opiate analgesia
E. Physiotherapy

 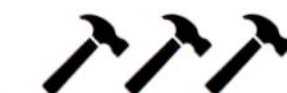 

32. An 86-year-old woman has 1 month of worsening right groin pain radiating to the knee. She has rheumatoid arthritis, managed with methotrexate, alendronic acid and Adcal D3, and recent prednisolone for a flare. She has pain on right groin palpation, with reduced active and passive hip movement.

Investigations:
X-ray pelvis: cystic and sclerotic changes of the femoral head, with flattening and subchondral collapse.

Which is the most appropriate management?
A. Bed rest
B. Hemiarthroplasty
C. Hip resurfacing
D. Morphine
E. Physiotherapy

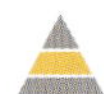 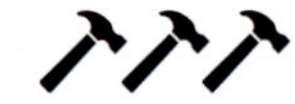 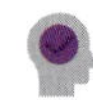

33. An 18-year-old boy has severe left knee pain after a blow to the outer knee. He marked left knee swelling, with diffuse bruising and medial joint line tenderness. There is medial laxity of the knee with valgus force in full extension.

Which is the most appropriate management?
A. Functional brace and physiotherapy
B. Intra Articular steroid injections
C. Rest, ice and elevation
D. Surgical repair
E. Topical ibuprofen

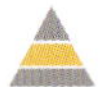 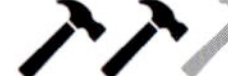

34. An 18-year-old man has sudden sharp left knee pain, locking and difficulty weight bearing while playing football. He has medial joint line tenderness, reduced range of knee extension, suprapatellar effusion and clicking of the knee on passive movement.

Which is the most likely diagnosis?
A. Anterior cruciate ligament tear
B. Medial collateral ligament tear
C. Meniscal tear
D. Patella tendon rupture
E. Prepatellar bursitis

 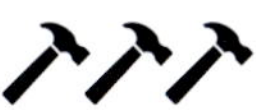 

35. An 85-year-old woman has severe right groin pain and inability to weight bear after a fall. She has a shortened and externally rotated right leg, with swelling and bruising over the greater trochanter.

Investigations:
X-ray pelvis: displaced subtrochanteric fracture of the femoral shaft.

Which is the most appropriate management?
 A. Controlled traction
 B. Dynamic hip screw
 C. Hemiarthroplasty
 D. Intramedullary nail
 E. Total hip replacement

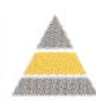  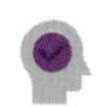

36. A 28-year-old boy has left shoulder pain and inability to weight bear after falling on an outstretched hand. He had a previous rotator cuff tear, managed with surgical repair. He has tenderness over the anterior left shoulder joint, numbness over the lateral shoulder and is unable to abduct the arm.

Figure 13.4 (see Chapter 37).

Which is the most appropriate management?
 A. Analgesia
 B. Closed reduction
 C. Open reduction and internal fixation
 D. Shoulder brace
 E. Sling immobilization

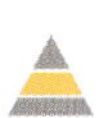 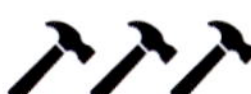

37. A 48-year-old woman has 3 months of right groin pain radiating to the knee. She has systemic lupus erythematosus, managed with hydroxychloroquine, and a recent course of prednisolone for a flare. She has pain and limited active and passive movement of the right hip.

Which is the most likely diagnosis?
 A. Osteoarthritis
 B. Osteonecrosis
 C. Osteoporosis
 D. Reactive arthritis
 E. Synovitis

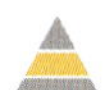  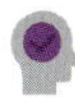

38. A 62-year-old woman has hip pain after a fall. She has chronic obstructive pulmonary disease, managed with prednisolone, salmeterol and tiotropium inhalers, and has smoked 20 cigarettes a day for 40 years. She has groin tenderness and a shortened, externally rotated leg.

Investigations:
X-ray of hip: nondisplaced intracapsular femoral neck fracture.

Which test is most likely to confirm the cause of injury?
 A. Bone profile
 B. DEXA scan
 C. MRI hip
 D. Parathyroid hormone
 E. Vitamin D levels

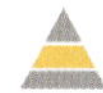 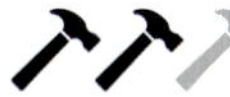

39. A 48-year-old woman has 1 month of worsening dull left shoulder pain and stiffness. She has type 2 diabetes mellitus and hypothyroidism, managed with metformin and levothyroxine. She has severe restriction of active and passive external rotation in the left shoulder, with abduction limited to 60 degrees.

Which is the most likely diagnosis?
 A. Adhesive capsulitis
 B. Osteoarthritis
 C. Subacromial bursitis
 D. Subacromial impingement
 E. Rotator cuff tear

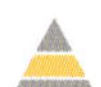 

40. A 23-year-old man has left ankle pain after a fall. He has pain and swelling over the left lateral malleolus, with reduced range of plantar and dorsiflexion, and is unable to weight bear.

Figure 13.5 (see Chapter 37).

Which is the most likely diagnosis?
 A. Bimalleolar fracture
 B. Medial malleolar fracture
 C. Trimalleolar fracture
 D. Weber A fracture
 E. Weber B fracture

 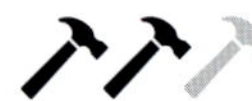 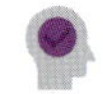

41. An 82-year-old man has left hip pain and difficulty mobilizing following a fall. He has temporal arteritis, managed prednisolone, and has smoked 20 cigarettes a day for 40 years. He has a shortened, externally rotated left hip, with pain on groin palpation.

Investigations:
X-ray of hip: no acute bony injury.

Which is the most appropriate next step?
 A. MR of hip
 B. Oral analgesia
 C. Physiotherapy
 D. Radioisotope bone scan
 E. Reassure and discharge

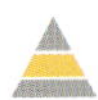 

42. A 59-year-old woman has 2 months of dull central lower back pain and sharp shooting pain down the back of her left leg. She has focal L4 tenderness, sensory loss over the left lateral thigh, knee and dorsum of the foot, with weakness in foot dorsiflexion and foot drop. The posterior tibial reflex is absent.

Which is the most likely diagnosis?
 A. Disc herniation
 B. Spinal cord compression
 C. Spinal stenosis
 D. Spondylolisthesis
 E. Spondylolysis

 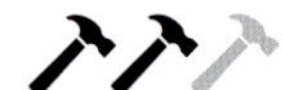 

43. A 24-year-old man has sudden severe right shoulder pain and inability to weight bear after falling on his shoulder while playing rugby. He has severe pain on passive and active shoulder abduction between 60 and 120 degrees and weakness of external rotation. There is tenderness over the acromioclavicular joint and deltoid muscle.

Which is the most appropriate management?
 A. Analgesia
 B. Intraarticular steroid injections
 C. Physiotherapy
 D. Rotator cuff repair
 E. Subacromial decompression

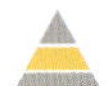 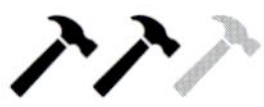 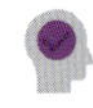

44. A 28-year-old woman has left ankle pain after a fall. She has left ankle swelling and tenderness, with midfoot bruising and reduced range of movement in all planes. She is able to mobilize with assistance in the emergency department.

Which is the most appropriate investigation?
 A. CT of foot
 B. MR of foot
 C. No investigation required
 D. Ultrasound of ankle
 E. X-ray of ankle with lateral and oblique views

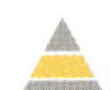  

45. A 56-year-old man has 1 month of neck pain, with bilateral upper arm weakness and difficulty gripping his pen. He has focal C4/5 tenderness, bilateral weakness to shoulder abduction and elbow flexion, sensory loss over the anterior shoulder and reduced biceps reflexes.

Which is the most appropriate management?
 A. Discectomy
 B. Intrathecal steroids
 C. Oral steroids
 D. Physiotherapy
 E. Spinal cord decompression

46. A 35-year-old woman has severe left shoulder pain and inability to weight bear after a seizure. She has epilepsy, managed with lamotrigine. She has left shoulder joint tenderness, and is unable to externally rotate the arm. Her arm is held in adduction and internal rotation.

Figure 13.6 (see Chapter 37).

Which is the most likely diagnosis?
 A. Acromioclavicular joint dislocation
 B. Anterior shoulder dislocation
 C. Inferior shoulder dislocation
 D. Nondisplaced proximal humeral fracture
 E. Posterior shoulder dislocation

47. A 28-year-old man has 2 weeks of left leg pain and difficulty mobilizing following a left tibial fracture 3 months ago managed with closed reduction and backslab immobilization. He has an antalgic gait, with tenderness, swelling and reduced range of motion of the left knee and ankle.

Which is the most likely diagnosis?
- A. Avascular necrosis
- B. Complex regional pain syndrome
- C. Fracture nonunion
- D. Osteomyelitis
- E. Posttraumatic osteoarthritis

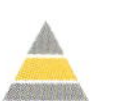  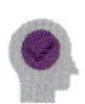

48. A 34-year-old woman has 6 months of bilateral pain and stiffness in her hands and fingers, worse in the morning, improving throughout the day.

Figure 13.7 (see Chapter 37).

Which test is most likely to confirm the diagnosis?
- A. ANA antibodies
- B. Anti-CCP antibodies
- C. CRP and ESR
- D. p-ANCA antibodies
- E. Rheumatoid factor

 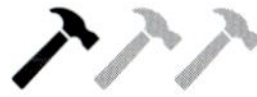

49. A 54-year-old woman has 2 weeks of severe mouth pain and bleeding gums. She had a tooth extraction 1 month ago, but otherwise has good oral hygiene. She has rheumatoid arthritis, managed with methotrexate, folic acid, alendronic acid, Adcal D3 and omeprazole.

Figure 13.8 (see Chapter 37).

Which is the most likely diagnosis?
- A. Gingivitis
- B. Osteonecrosis of the jaw
- C. Periodontitis
- D. Temporomandibular joint dysfunction
- E. Trigeminal neuralgia

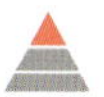 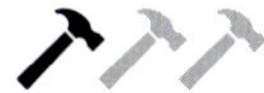

50. A 54-year-old woman has 3 weeks of elbow pain radiating to the back of the forearm, worse on typing and lifting. She has tenderness over the lateral aspect of the elbow and extensor tendon, reduced grip strength and pain on wrist dorsiflexion.

Which is the most likely diagnosis?
- A. Elbow synovitis
- B. Lateral epicondylitis
- C. Medial epicondylitis
- D. Olecranon bursitis
- E. Osteoarthritis

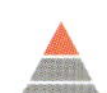  

51. A 46-year-old man has 6 months of worsening back pain and difficulty mobilizing. He has ankylosing spondylitis, managed with infliximab, naproxen and omeprazole. He has severe, dull lower back pain, with a fixed flexion deformity of the lumbar spine and thoracic kyphosis of 40 degrees.

Which is the most appropriate management?
- A. Hydrocortisone
- B. Opiate analgesia
- C. Physiotherapy
- D. Spinal osteotomy
- E. Sulphasalazine

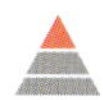 

52. A 34-year-old woman has 2 weeks of aching pain at the base of the thumbs and outer wrists. She gave birth 1 month ago to her first child. She has pain and numbness at the base of the first metacarpal and the thenar muscle, with weakness to thumb and wrist abduction.

Which is the most likely diagnosis?
- A. Carpal tunnel syndrome
- B. Cervical nerve root entrapment
- C. De Quervain tenosynovitis
- D. Morton neuroma
- E. Osteoarthritis

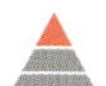  

53. A 28-year-old man has third-degree burns of the chest and lower limbs after a house fire. After initial resuscitation, he develops severe, worsening right lower leg pain, worse on passive movement, with paraesthesia and numbness in the right foot. Pedal pulses are palpable.

Which is the most appropriate management?
A. Escharotomy
B. Fasciotomy
C. Intravenous fluids
D. Revascularization
E. Surgical debridement

 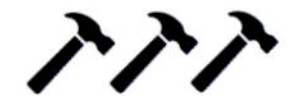

54. A 19-year-old boy has 2 weeks of worsening right shoulder pain and swelling, after 2 months of fatigue, poor appetite and 5 kg of weight loss. He has focal tenderness over the anterior and lateral shoulder, with soft tissue swelling, erythema and warmth.

Figure 13.9 (see Chapter 37).

Which is the most likely diagnosis?
A. Chondrosarcoma
B. Chordoma
C. Ewing sarcoma
D. Osteomyelitis
E. Osteosarcoma

 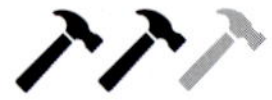

55. A 25-year-old woman has 2 months of dull pain in the outer left knee radiating to the thigh, worse while running and improved by rest. She has pain on passive flexion of the knee when pressure is applied to the lateral femoral epicondyle, and weakness in left hip abduction.

Which is the most likely diagnosis?
A. Achilles tendinitis
B. Iliotibial band syndrome
C. Lateral collateral ligament strain
D. Lateral meniscal bursitis
E. Patellar tendonitis

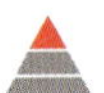 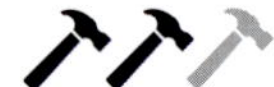

56. A 57-year-old woman has 3 months of worsening left hip pain radiating to the outer thigh, worse on exertion and at night. She takes over-the-counter ibuprofen and paracetamol for her pain. She has an antalgic gait with right hip drop, tenderness over the left greater trochanter and pain on left hip abduction, internal and external rotation.

Which is the most likely diagnosis?
A. Avascular necrosis of the femoral head
B. Gluteal tendon tear
C. Iliotibial band syndrome
D. Neck of femur fracture
E. Trochanteric bursitis

 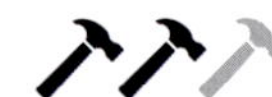 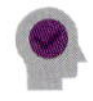

57. A 74-year-old woman has 2 weeks of dull central lower back pain. She has peptic ulcer disease, hypertension and CKD 3, managed with omeprazole, amlodipine and losartan. She has focal lumbar spinal tenderness.

Investigations:
X-ray of lumbar spine: L2 wedge compression fracture.
DEXA scan: T score –2.8 SDs.

Which is the most appropriate management?
A. Alendronic acid
B. Calcitonin
C. Denosumab
D. Teriparatide
E. Raloxifene

  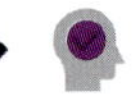

58. A 62-year-old woman has 6 months of burning right hip pain radiating to the thigh, worse at night. She has rheumatoid arthritis, managed with methotrexate, alendronic acid, omeprazole and Adcal D3, and is taking regular over-the-counter ibuprofen and paracetamol for her pain. She has tenderness over the right greater trochanter, with pain on internal and external rotation and reduced range of hip abduction, and left hip droop on mobilizing.

Which is the most appropriate management?
A. Intraarticular steroid injections
B. Infliximab
C. Naproxen
D. Morphine
E. Prednisolone

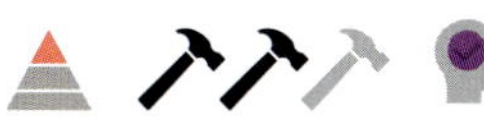

59. A 54-year-old woman has 2 weeks of right shoulder pain, worse on movement and at night. She has tenderness at the superior and medial aspects of the shoulder joint, and pain on shoulder abduction between 60 and 120 degrees and external rotation.

Which is the most appropriate management?
A. Analgesia
B. Intraarticular steroid injections
C. Physiotherapy
D. Rotator cuff repair
E. Subacromial decompression

60. A 28-year-old man has 2 months of right arm pain, numbness and tingling while lifting weights, which resolves within 1 hour of activity stopping.

Which is the most likely diagnosis?
A. Carpal tunnel syndrome
B. Chronic compartment syndrome
C. Repetitive strain injury
D. Stress fracture
E. Tendonitis

Urology

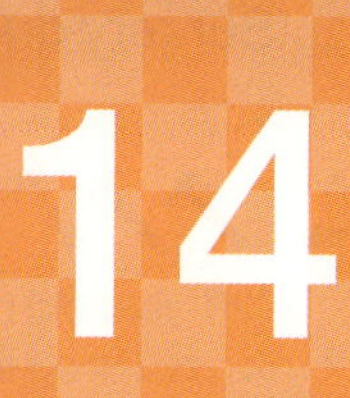

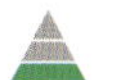  

1. A 28-year-old man has 2 weeks of a left groin lump and dull scrotal discomfort. He has a 2 cm solid mass on the left testis, which does not transilluminate.

Which is the most appropriate investigation?
A. Alpha-fetoprotein
B. CT of testes
C. Fine needle aspiration
D. Human chorionic gonadotropin
E. Ultrasound of testes

2. A 22-year-old woman has 2 days of urinary frequency and pain when passing urine. Her temperature is 37.2°C, pulse 92 bpm and BP 108/81 mmHg. She has suprapubic tenderness.

Investigations:
Urine dipstick: + leucocytes, + nitrites, + blood.

Which is the most appropriate management?
A. Intravenous antibiotics
B. Oral analgesia
C. Oral antibiotics
D. Oral fluids
E. Reassurance and discharge

 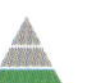  

3. A 73-year-old man has sudden painful inability to pass urine. He has benign prostatic hyperplasia, managed with tamsulosin. He has marked suprapubic distention, a tender, palpable bladder and is restless and agitated.

Which is the most appropriate management?
A. Bladder irrigation
B. Finasteride
C. Oral antibiotics
D. Suprapubic catheterization
E. Transurethral catheterization

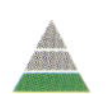 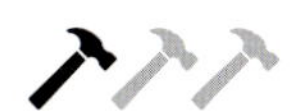 

4. A 62-year-old woman has 3 days of worsening left flank pain, fevers and rigors. She has type 2 diabetes mellitus, managed with metformin. Her temperature is 38.1°C, pulse 112 bpm and BP 117/74 mmHg. She has left costovertebral angle tenderness.

Which is the most appropriate investigation?
A. Blood cultures
B. CT of kidneys, ureters, bladder
C. Ultrasound of abdomen
D. Urinalysis and MC&S
E. Urine dipstick

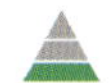 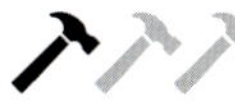

5. A 77-year-old man has 2 months of increased urinary frequency, hesitancy, nocturia and terminal dribbling. His temperature is 36.9°C, pulse 86 bpm and BP 138/82 mmHg. He has a symmetrically enlarged, firm prostate with a rubbery texture.

Which is the most likely diagnosis?
A. Benign prostatic hyperplasia
B. Bladder outlet obstruction
C. Prostate cancer
D. Prostatic abscess
E. Prostatitis

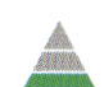 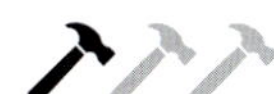 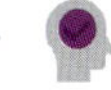

6. An 18-year-old man has sudden severe scrotal pain and vomiting. He has an exquisitely tender right hemiscrotum, with a swollen, high riding testis with a transverse lie. The cremasteric reflex is absent.

Which is the most appropriate management?
A. Intravenous antibiotics
B. Manual detorsion
C. Opiate analgesia
D. Orchiectomy
E. Surgical reduction and orchiopexy

  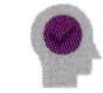

7. A 28-year-old man has 2 days of worsening left scrotal pain radiating to his left flank, with increased urinary frequency and pain when passing urine. He had unprotected sexual intercourse with a new female partner 1 week ago. His temperature is 37.9°C. He has an exquisitely tender, swollen left hemiscrotum with erythema of the overlying skin.

Which is the most appropriate management?
   A. Ceftriaxone and doxycycline
   B. Ice packs
   C. Levofloxacin
   D. Naproxen
   E. Scrotal elevation

  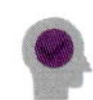

8. A 16-year-old boy has sudden onset severe left scrotal pain and vomiting. He has lower abdominal tenderness, a swollen and tender left hemiscrotum with a high-riding testis with a transverse lie. Elevation of the scrotum does not relieve the pain.

Which is the most appropriate investigation?
   A. Nucleic acid amplification test
   B. MR of testicles
   C. Ultrasound of testicles
   D. Urine dipstick
   E. Urine microscopy, culture and sensitivity

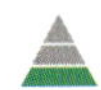  

9. A 65-year-old man has 2 weeks of urinary frequency and urgency. He has smoked 20 cigarettes a day for 30 years.

Investigations:
Urinalysis: 2+ blood.

Which test is most likely to confirm the diagnosis?
   A. CT KUB
   B. CT urogram
   C. Cystoscopy and biopsy
   D. Urea and electrolytes
   E. Urinalysis and MC&S

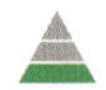 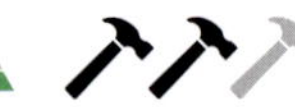 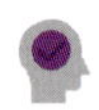

10. A 72-year-old man has 1 month of urinary frequency, urgency, hesitancy, nocturia and terminal dribbling, and the sensation of incomplete bladder emptying. He has benign prostate hyperplasia, managed with finasteride and tamsulosin. He has an enlarged, nontender, smooth prostate, with a rubbery texture.

Which is the most appropriate management?
   A. Prostatectomy
   B. Radiofrequency thermotherapy
   C. Transurethral incision of the prostate
   D. Transurethral resection of the prostate
   E. Watchful waiting

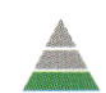 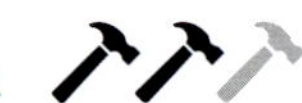 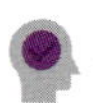

11. A 35-year-old man has 1 day of worsening right testicular pain, with increased urinary frequency and pain when passing urine. His temperature is 37.8°C, pulse 66 bpm and BP 137/85 mmHg. He has a swollen, erythematous right hemiscrotum. The pain is reduced upon elevation of the affected side.

Which test is most likely to confirm the diagnosis?
   A. Full blood count
   B. Nucleic acid amplification test
   C. Ultrasound scrotum
   D. Urine dipstick
   E. Urine MC&S

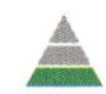 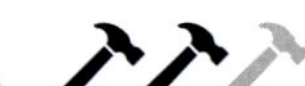

12. A 58-year-old man has 3 weeks of suprapubic discomfort and urinary frequency. He is otherwise well. He has smoked 30 cigarettes a day for 30 years. He has mild suprapubic tenderness.

Urinalysis: 2+ blood.

Which is the most likely diagnosis?
   A. Bladder cancer
   B. Interstitial cystitis
   C. Nephritis syndrome
   D. Renal stones
   E. Urinary tract infection

 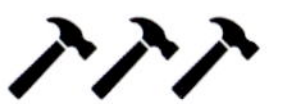 

13. A 68-year-old man has 1 month of urinary hesitancy and terminal dribbling. He has a firm, asymmetrical nodule on the right lobe of the prostate.

Investigations:
Transrectal ultrasound and biopsy: T1N0M0 prostate adenocarcinoma.

Which is the most appropriate management?
A. Active surveillance
B. Androgen deprivation therapy
C. Brachytherapy
D. Radical prostatectomy
E. Watchful waiting

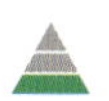 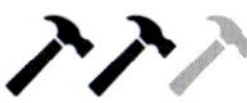 

14. A 62-year-old man has 3 weeks of visible blood in the urine and lower abdominal pain. He has smoked 20 cigarettes a day for 40 years. He has mild suprapubic tenderness and a palpable suprapubic mass.

Investigations:
Urinalysis: 2+ blood.
Cystoscopy: papillary nodular mass extending into the detrusor muscle.
Histology: transitional cell carcinoma.
CT of thorax, abdomen, pelvis: no regional or distant metastatic disease.

Which is the most appropriate management?
A. Immunotherapy
B. Platinum-based chemotherapy
C. Radical cystectomy
D. Targeted radiotherapy
E. Transurethral resection of bladder tumour

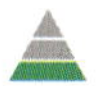  

15. A 62-year-old man 1 day of right flank pain, dysuria and urinary frequency, with nausea, vomiting and fever. His temperature is 38.2°C, pulse 122 bpm and BP 97/62 mmHg. There is pain on percussion of the right flank.

Which is the most appropriate management?
A. Intravenous antibiotics
B. Intravenous fluids
C. Oral antibiotics
D. Percutaneous nephrostomy
E. PR diclofenac

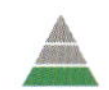 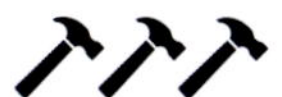 

16. A 78-year-old man has 2 weeks of urinary frequency, urgency, hesitancy and nocturia, after 5 kg of weight loss over 1 month. He has benign prostatic hyperplasia, managed with finasteride. His abdomen is soft and nontender. His prostate is symmetrically enlarged, smooth and firm.

Which is the most appropriate investigation?
A. Multiparametric MR of prostate
B. Prostate biopsy
C. PSA
D. Transrectal ultrasound of prostate
E. Urinalysis and microscopy, culture and sensitivity

17. A 72-year-old man has sudden lower abdominal pain and inability to pass urine. He has Parkinson disease, managed with levodopa and ropinirole. He has suprapubic tenderness and a distended, palpable bladder.

Which is the most appropriate investigation?
A. Bladder scan
B. CT of kidneys, ureters, bladder
C. Transrectal ultrasound of prostate
D. Urodynamic studies
E. Urinalysis and microscopy, culture and sensitivity

 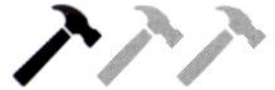

18. A 25-year-old man has 2 days of left testicular pain radiating to the flank, with dysuria and urinary frequency. He has a tender, swollen, erythematous left testicle, with purulent urethral discharge. His pain is reduced upon elevation of the left testicle.

Which is the most likely aetiology?
A. Chlamydia trachomatis
B. *E. coli*
C. Klebsiella
D. Pseudomonas
E. Trichomonas vaginalis

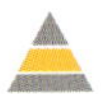 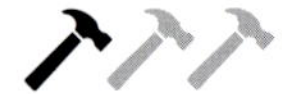 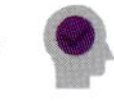

19. A 27-year-old man has 1 month of dull scrotal pain and a left testicular lump. He has a 3 cm, solid, fixed lump on his left testis, which does not transilluminate.

Investigations:
AFP 480 ng/mL (0–40).
Ultrasound of testes: calcified inhomogeneous lesion with variable echogenicity.

Which is the most appropriate management?
A. Active surveillance
B. Bilateral orchiectomy
C. Chemotherapy
D. Radical inguinal orchiectomy
E. Radiotherapy

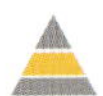 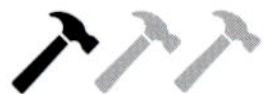 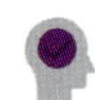

20. A 71-year-old man has 6 months of urinary frequency, nocturia, hesitancy and terminal dribbling. His abdomen is soft and nontender, with no palpable bladder. He has a symmetrically enlarged, smooth, nontender prostate.

Investigations:
Urinalysis: 3+ blood.

Which is the most appropriate management?
A. Bladder retraining
B. Oral antibiotics
C. Reduce fluid intake
D. Tamsulosin
E. Transurethral resection of the prostate

21. A 12-year-old boy has sudden abdominal pain and vomiting. His temperature is 36.8°C, pulse 86 bpm and BP 112/68 mmHg. He has suprapubic tenderness. The left hemiscrotum is empty.

Which is the most likely diagnosis?
A. Appendicitis
B. Epididymo-orchitis
C. Prostatitis
D. Testicular torsion
E. Urinary tract infection

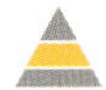 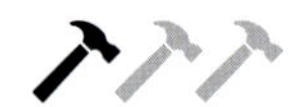

22. A 32-year-old man has 2 days of a painless left groin lump. He has a translucent, fluctuant lump in the left scrotum, isolated from the testis, which is irreducible, and does not transilluminate.

Which is the most likely diagnosis?
A. Epididymal cyst
B. Hydrocele
C. Inguinal hernia
D. Testicular tumour
E. Varicocele

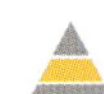  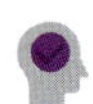

23. A 22-year-old woman has 3 hours of intermittent severe right back pain radiating to the groin, with nausea, vomiting, dysuria and urinary frequency. Her temperature is 37.2°C, pulse 121 bpm and BP 127/92 mmHg. She is agitated and restless, with severe pain on percussion on the right flank.

Which is the most appropriate analgesia?
A. Codeine
B. Ibuprofen
C. Morphine
D. Paracetamol
E. PR diclofenac

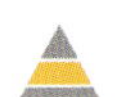 

24. A 49-year-old woman has 2 months of dull right back pain, visible blood in the urine, fatigue and 3 kg of weight loss. She has hypertension and hypothyroidism, managed with ramipril and levothyroxine, and has smoked 20 cigarettes a day for 25 years. She has tenderness in the right flank and a palpable mass.

Which is the most appropriate investigation?
A. Abdominal X-ray
B. CT of abdomen
C. Intravenous urogram
D. Ultrasound of abdomen
E. Urinalysis and microscopy, culture and sensitivity

25. A 24-year-old man has 1 week of a gradually enlarging groin lump. He had oral antibiotics for epididymo-orchitis 2 weeks previously. He has a painless, fluctuant left scrotal swelling, which reduces on lying flat, with red cystic structures evident on transillumination.

Which is the most appropriate management?
   A. Hernioplasty
   B. Hydrocelectomy
   C. Percutaneous aspiration
   D. Sclerotherapy
   E. Watchful waiting

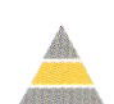 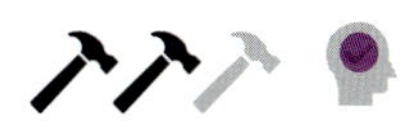

26. A 65-year-old man has severe penile pain following transurethral catheterization for acute urinary retention. He has a firm, oedematous glans penis, with a tight retracted foreskin and band of constricting tissue at the coronal sulcus.

Which is the most appropriate management?
   A. Circumcision
   B. Dorsal slit reduction surgery
   C. Manual foreskin reduction
   D. Reassurance
   E. Vertical foreskin incision

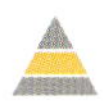 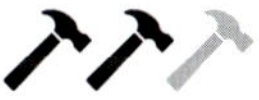 

27. A 32-year-old man has 6 hours of severe right flank pain radiating to the groin, with nausea, vomiting, urinary frequency and pain and visible blood when passing urine. His temperature is 36.7°C, pulse 102 bpm and BP 128/81 mmHg. He has pain on percussion of the right flank.

Which is the most appropriate investigation?
   A. CT of kidneys, ureters, bladder
   B. Intravenous urogram
   C. Ultrasound of abdomen
   D. Urinalysis and microscopy, culture and sensitivity
   E. Urine dipstick

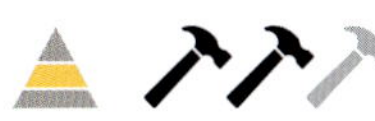

28. A 74-year-old man has 1 month of nocturnal incontinence. He has benign prostatic hyperplasia, managed with tamsulosin. He has mild suprapubic distention and a symmetrically enlarged, smooth, nontender prostate.

Investigations:
Postvoid residual bladder scan: 357 mL.

Which is the most likely diagnosis?
   A. Acute urinary retention
   B. Benign prostatic hyperplasia
   C. Chronic urinary retention
   D. Detrusor muscle underactivity
   E. Neurogenic bladder

 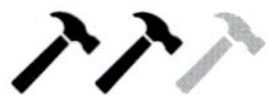 

29. A 54-year-old woman has 3 months of intermittent, involuntary urinary leakage when coughing or sneezing. She has hypertension and asthma, managed with indapamide and a salbutamol inhaler. Her abdomen is soft and nontender.

Which is the most appropriate management?
   A. Bladder retraining
   B. Medication review
   C. Modify fluid intake
   D. Pelvic floor exercises
   E. Weight loss

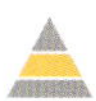  

30. A 28-year-old woman has 2 hours of intermittent, severe pain in the right flank radiating to the groin, with nausea, vomiting and urinary frequency. Her temperature is 37.1°C, pulse 105 bpm and BP 121/81 mmHg. She is agitated and restless, with pain on percussion on the right flank.

Investigations:
Urinalysis: 2+ blood.
CT kidneys, ureters, bladder: 8 mm stone in the right distal ureter.

Which is the most appropriate management?
   A. Extracorporeal shockwave lithotripsy
   B. Oral antibiotics
   C. Percutaneous nephrolithotomy
   D. Tamsulosin
   E. Ureteral stenting

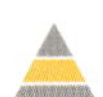 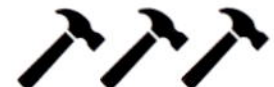 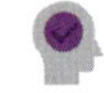

31. An 82-year-old man has 3 months of weak urinary stream, terminal dribbling, hesitancy, urinary frequency and nocturia. His abdomen is soft and nontender. He has a symmetrically enlarged, smooth, nontender prostate.

Which is the most appropriate investigation?

A. Postvoid residual bladder scan
B. PSA
C. Transrectal ultrasound of prostate
D. Urea and electrolytes
E. Urinalysis

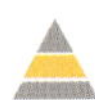 

32. A 72-year-old woman has 1 month of intermittent urinary urgency and urinary incontinence. There is no leakage of urine on coughing or sneezing. She has diverticular disease, managed with laxatives.

Investigations:
Postvoid residual bladder scan: 10 mL.

Which is the most likely diagnosis?

A. Mixed incontinence
B. Overflow incontinence
C. Stress incontinence
D. Total incontinence
E. Urge incontinence

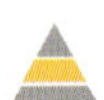 

33. A 25-year-old man has 1 month of painless right scrotal swelling. His right hemiscrotum is mildly swollen compared to the left. There is no transillumination.

Investigations:
Ultrasound of testes: hypoechoic mass on the right testis.

Which is the most likely diagnosis?

A. Testicular hydrocele
B. Testicular microlithiasis
C. Testicular nonseminoma
D. Testicular seminoma
E. Testicular varicocele

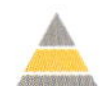 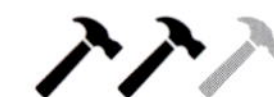 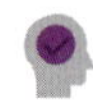

34. A 62-year-old man has 12 hours of worsening abdominal pain and inability to pass urine. He has benign prostatic hyperplasia, managed with tamsulosin, and had a stent for a urethral stricture 1 month ago. He has marked suprapubic tenderness and a palpable bladder.

Investigations:
Postvoid residual bladder scan: 758 mL.

Which is the most appropriate management?

A. Bladder irrigation
B. Radical cystectomy
C. Suprapubic catheterization
D. Transurethral catheterization
E. Urethral stenting

35. A 26-year-old man has 2 days of pain and swelling of the glans penis, with white discharge and pain when passing urine. He has a swollen and erythematous glans penis and foreskin, with thick white discharge and ulcerated lesions on foreskin retraction.

Which is the most likely diagnosis?

A. Balanitis
B. Balanoposthitis
C. Penile cancer
D. Phimosis
E. Urinary tract infection

 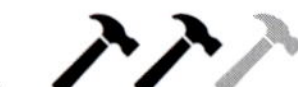

36. A 68-year-old man has 3 weeks of urinary urgency, frequency and difficulty initiating the urine stream. He has benign prostatic hyperplasia, managed with tamsulosin. He has mild suprapubic tenderness and a symmetrically enlarged, smooth, nontender prostate.

Investigations:
Figure 14.1 (see Chapter 37).

Which is the most likely diagnosis?

A. Benign prostatic hyperplasia
B. Bladder cancer
C. Cystolith
D. Urinary retention
E. Urinary tract infection

37. A 64-year-old woman has sudden severe back radiating down the left leg and inability to pass urine. She has osteoarthritis and degenerative disc disease, managed with ibuprofen and tramadol. She has gross lower abdominal swelling and tenderness, with bilateral lower limb weakness and saddle anaesthesia.

Investigations:
Postvoid residual bladder scan: 789 mL.

Which is the most likely aetiology?
   A. Autonomic neuropathy
   B. Detrusor sphincter dyssynergia
   C. Mechanical obstruction
   D. Medication side effect
   E. Neurogenic bladder

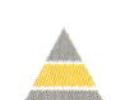 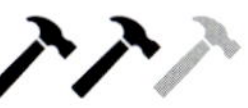 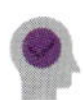

38. A 68-year-old man has 2 months of dull lower back and hip pain, with fatigue and 5 kg of weight loss. He has an antalgic gait and tenderness of the lumbar spinal and greater trochanters bilaterally.

Investigations:
Figure 14.2 (see Chapter 37).

Which is the most appropriate investigation?
   A. Chest X-ray
   B. DEXA scan
   C. Full blood count
   D. PSA
   E. Serum-free light chains

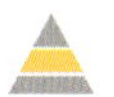 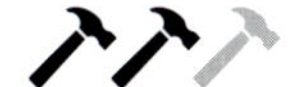 

39. A 75-year-old male has sudden severe right flank pain radiating to the groin, with nausea, vomiting, dysuria and visible blood in the urine. This is his third episode of these symptoms in the past 3 months.

Investigations:
CT of kidneys, ureters, bladder: 5 mm stone in the right ureter.

Which is the most appropriate long-term management?
   A. Allopurinol
   B. Increase daily fluid intake
   C. Indapamide
   D. Low calcium diet
   E. Urine alkalinization

 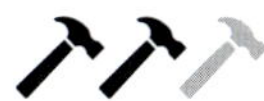 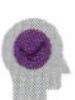

40. A 46-year-old man has 3 days of penile swelling and tenderness, with itching and thick white penile discharge. He has a swollen, erythematous glans penis, with pain and ulcerated lesions evident on foreskin retraction.

Which is the most appropriate management?
   A. Emollients
   B. Foreskin reaction and bathing
   C. Oral antibiotics
   D. Topical clotrimazole
   E. Topical corticosteroid

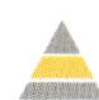  

41. A 54-year-old man requests screening for prostate cancer. He has no urinary symptoms, abdominal pain, fatigue or weight loss. He has benign prostatic hyperplasia managed with finasteride. His abdomen is soft and nontender. His prostate is symmetrical, enlarged, firm and smooth.

Which is the most appropriate management?
   A. Multiparametric MRI
   B. PSA level
   C. Reassurance and discharge
   D. Transrectal ultrasound of the prostate
   E. Urinalysis and MC&S

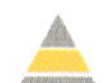 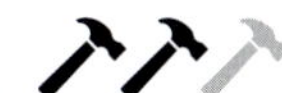

42. A 75-year-old man has 6 hours of severe left back pain radiating to his groin, nausea, vomiting and pain when passing urine. He has myelodysplastic syndrome and gout, managed with colchicine. He has tenderness on percussion of the left flank.

Investigations:
Urine dipstick: 2+ blood.
CT of kidneys, ureters, bladder: left hydronephrosis and peripancreatic fat stranding.
A diagnosis of renal stones is suspected.

Which is the most likely composition of his stone?

A. Calcium oxalate
B. Cystine
C. Struvite
D. Uric acid
E. Xanthine

43. A 65-year-old man has 2 days of increased urinary frequency, pain and visible blood when passing urine. He has type 2 diabetes mellitus and chronic kidney disease, managed with metformin, ramipril, atorvastatin and clopidogrel. His temperature is 37.1°C, pulse 86 bpm and BP 147/92 mmHg. He has suprapubic tenderness.

Which is the most appropriate investigation?

A. CT of kidneys, ureters, bladder
B. No investigation required
C. Ultrasound of kidneys, ureters, bladder
D. Urinalysis and MC&S
E. Urine dipstick

 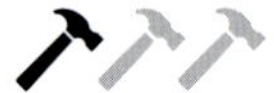 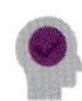

44. A 59-year-old man has 1 month of dull left flank pain and visible blood in the urine, with fatigue and 4 kg of weight loss. He has hypertension, managed with ramipril, and has smoked 20 cigarettes a day for 30 years. There is left flank pain and a palpable mass.

Investigations:
CT of abdomen: 7 mm mass confined to the left renal pole.

Which is the most appropriate management?

A. Cryoablation
B. Immunotherapy
C. Partial nephrectomy
D. Radical nephrectomy
E. Radiochemotherapy

45. A 62-year-old man has 2 days of urinary frequency, dysuria and lower back pain. His temperature is 38.1°C, pulse 108 bpm and BP 129/71 mmHg. He has suprapubic tenderness and a tender, enlarged, boggy prostate.

Which is the most likely diagnosis?

A. Epididymo-orchitis
B. Prostatic abscess
C. Prostatitis
D. Pyelonephritis
E. Urinary tract infection

 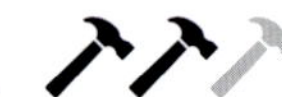

46. A 22-year-old man has 2 weeks of a painless left groin lump. He has a 2 cm, firm mass on the left testis, which is irreducible and does not transilluminate, and bilateral, tender subareolar breast swelling.

Which is the most likely diagnosis?

A. Leydig cell tumour
B. Testicular lymphoma
C. Testicular seminoma
D. Testicular teratoma
E. Yolk sac tumour

47. A 64-year-old man has 3 months of urinary frequency, urgency and nocturia, with intermittent pain on ejaculation and blood in his semen. He has erectile dysfunction, managed with sildenafil. He has mild prostatic tenderness on digital rectal examination.

Investigations:
PSA 107 ng/mL (<3).

Which is the most appropriate management?

A. Degarelix
B. Finasteride
C. Naproxen
D. Oral antibiotics
E. Tamsulosin

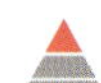 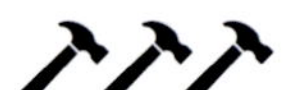 

48. A 65-year-old man has 2 days of crampy abdominal pain, vomiting and diarrhoea, and an itchy rash on the hands and feet. He had a renal transplant 2 months ago for end-stage renal disease and takes cyclosporin. He has generalized abdominal tenderness, hepatosplenomegaly, scleral icterus and a diffuse maculopapular rash on the hands and feet.

Which is the most appropriate management?
A. Cyclosporin
B. Graft removal
C. Intravenous hydrocortisone
D. Intravenous immunoglobulins
E. Plasmapheresis

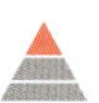  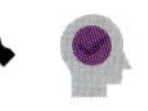

49. A 65-year-old man 1 day posttransurethral resection of the prostate loses consciousness and has continuous rhythmic tonic–clonic movements of the limbs.

Which is the most likely cause of his seizures?
A. Hypercalcaemia
B. Hyperkalaemia
C. Hypokalaemia
D. Hypomagnesaemia
E. Hyponatraemia

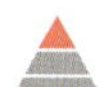  

50. A 28-year-old woman has 3 days of worsening right flank pain, fever and dysuria, following 1 week of analgesia for a right kidney stone. Her temperature is 37.9°C, pulse 102 bpm and BP 106/80 mmHg. She has pain on percussion of the right flank and a palpable mass.

Which is the most appropriate management?
A. Intravenous antibiotics
B. Nephrectomy
C. Percutaneous drainage
D. Percutaneous nephrolithotomy
E. PR diclofenac

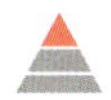 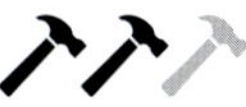 

51. A 55-year-old woman has 1 week of worsening left flank pain, fever, rigors and pain when passing urine. She has type 2 diabetes mellitus, managed with metformin and dapagliflozin. Her temperature is 38.3°C, pulse 109 bpm and BP 96/78 mmHg. She has left costovertebral angle tenderness and a palpable mass.

Which is the most appropriate investigation?
A. Blood cultures
B. CT of abdomen
C. CT of kidneys, ureters, bladder
D. Urinalysis and microscopy, culture and sensitivity
E. Ultrasound of abdomen

 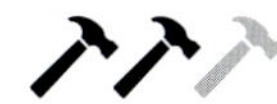

52. A 41-year-old man has 1 week of urinary frequency, urgency and pain when passing urine. He has epilepsy, managed with sodium valproate, and is taking over-the-counter ibuprofen for knee pain. He has bilateral flank and suprapubic tenderness.

Investigations:
Urinalysis: 2+ blood, 2+ leucocytes.
Urine microscopy, culture and sensitivity: no growth.

Which is the most likely diagnosis?
A. Epididymo-orchitis
B. Interstitial cystitis
C. Prostatitis
D. Pyelonephritis
E. Urinary tract infection

 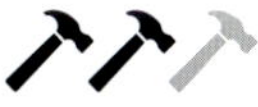 

53. A 28-year-old woman has 6 months of urinary urgency, frequency and nocturia. There is no urinary incontinence. She has anxiety, managed with sertraline. Her temperature is 36.7°C, pulse 54 bpm and BP 126/81 mmHg. Her abdomen is soft and nontender.

Which is the most appropriate management?
A. Bladder retraining
B. Duloxetine
C. Oxybutynin
D. Pelvic floor exercises
E. Vaginal pessary

 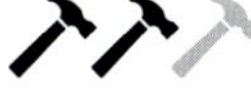

54. A 32-year-old man has 6 weeks of dull right scrotal pain and swelling after three episodes of severe scrotal pain, swelling and fever in the past year. He has mild tenderness and swelling of the right hemiscrotum, with a thick, palpable epididymis.

Which is the most likely diagnosis?
A. Chronic epididymitis
B. Epididymo-orchitis
C. Hydrocele
D. Inguinal hernia
E. Varicocele

 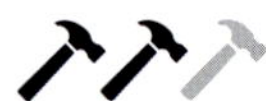

55. A 69-year-old man has 1 month of urinary hesitancy, weak urinary stream and a feeling of incomplete bladder emptying. He has benign prostatic hyperplasia, recurrent urinary tract infections and three episodes of acute urinary retention in the past year. His abdomen is soft and nontender. He has a symmetrically enlarged, smooth, nontender prostate.

Which is the most likely diagnosis?
A. Bladder stone
B. Urethral carcinoma
C. Ureteral stenosis
D. Urethritis
E. Urethral stricture

 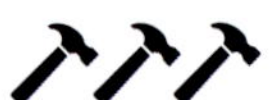

56. A 28-year-old man suddenly collapses with rhythmic controlled jerking of the arms and limbs, which spontaneously resolves. He has 2 months of worsening fatigue and poor appetite, with 5 kg of weight loss.

Investigations:
Figure 14.3 (see Chapter 37).

Which is the most likely diagnosis?
A. Lung cancer
B. Prostate cancer
C. Renal cell carcinoma
D. Testicular cancer
E. Tuberculosis

57. A 52-year-old woman has 6 months of intermittent involuntary leakage of urine. There is no urgency, or worsening of symptoms when coughing or sneezing. She has multiple sclerosis, managed with ocrelizumab.

Investigations:
Postvoid residual bladder scan: 30 mL.

Which is the most appropriate management?
A. Bethanechol
B. Intermittent self-catheterization
C. Long-term catheter
D. Mirabegron
E. Oxybutynin

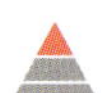 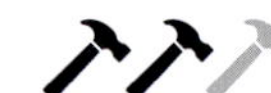 

58. A 73-year-old man has 3 days of dysuria, urinary frequency, fevers and perineal pain. He has benign prostatic hyperplasia, managed with finasteride. His temperature is 38.6°C, pulse 121 bpm and BP 119/84 mmHg. He has suprapubic tenderness and a tender, fluctuant prostate.

Which is the most appropriate investigation?
A. Postvoid residual bladder scan
B. PSA
C. Transrectal ultrasound of prostate
D. Urethral swab and culture
E. Urinalysis

 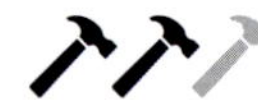 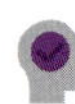

59. A 50-year-old man has 1 month of dull right scrotal pain and a heavy, 'dragging' sensation. He has a mass along the right spermatic cord with palpable soft bands, which is irreducible, and does not transilluminate.

Which is the most appropriate investigation?
A. Abdominal X-ray
B. CT of abdomen
C. PSA
D. Ultrasound of scrotum
E. Urinalysis

60. A 22-year-old man has difficulty retracting the foreskin, after 1 week of pain, swelling and redness of the glans penis. He has a tight ring of foreskin around the tip of the penis that is difficult to retract fully.

Which is the most appropriate management?
A. Circumcision
B. Oral analgesia
C. Reassurance and safety netting
D. Topical corticosteroids
E. Vertical foreskin incision

Breast surgery

1. A 78-year-old woman suddenly loses consciousness with rhythmic, controlled jerking of the upper limbs and incontinence, which spontaneously resolves after 2 minutes. There is no history of seizures. She had breast-conserving surgery for medullary breast cancer 3 months ago, and drinks a bottle of wine a week. Her temperature is 36.7°C, pulse 86 bpm and BP 122/82 mmHg. There are no focal neurological symptoms.

Which is the most likely diagnosis?
   A. Alcohol withdrawal
   B. Cerebral metastasis
   C. Epilepsy
   D. Ischaemic stroke
   E. Meningitis

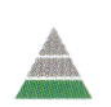  

2. A 35-year-old woman 2 weeks postpartum has 2 days of right breast swelling and tenderness, with increasing pain and difficulty breastfeeding. Both she and her baby are otherwise well. Her temperature is 38.2°C, pulse 83 bpm and BP 121/82 mmHg. The right breast is tender, firm and erythematous.

Which is the most appropriate investigation?
   A. Breast milk culture
   B. Core needle biopsy
   C. Mammogram
   D. No investigations required
   E. Ultrasound of breast

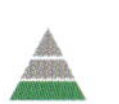  

3. A 28-year-old woman 6 weeks postpartum has 1 week of left breast swelling, pain and difficulty with breastfeeding. Both she and her baby are otherwise well. There is a firm, tender swelling in the left subareolar areas with overlying skin erythema.

Which is the most appropriate management?
   A. Cessation of breastfeeding
   B. Fine needle aspiration
   C. Oral antibiotics
   D. NSAIDs
   E. Warm and cold compresses

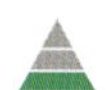 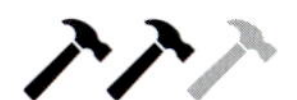 

4. A 45-year-old woman wants to discuss her breast cancer risk. She has a positive BRCA1 mutation and two first-degree relatives with breast cancer. She is asymptomatic and a routine mammogram is normal. She wants to discuss surgery to reduce her future cancer risk.

Which is the most appropriate management?
   A. Breast-conserving surgery
   B. Double mastectomy
   C. Modified radical mastectomy
   D. Radical chest wall radiotherapy
   E. Skin sparing mastectomy

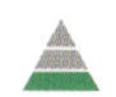 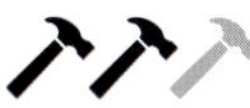 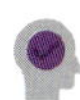

5. A 29-year-old woman has 1 week of a painless right breast lump. There is a firm nodule in the upper outer aspect of the right breast, which is fixed to the underlying breast tissue, with overlying skin dimpling and retraction.

Which is the most appropriate investigation?
   A. Core needle biopsy
   B. Fine needle aspiration
   C. Mammogram
   D. MR of breast
   E. Ultrasound of breast

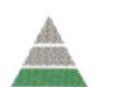 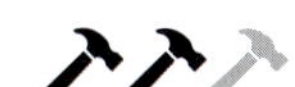 

6. A 56-year-old woman has 1 month of a painless firm lump in her right breast. There is a 3 cm fixed mass in the superolateral aspect of the right breast, with tethering to the underlying tissue, skin retraction and dimpling, with axillary lymphadenopathy.

Investigations:
Core needle biopsy and histology: T3N0M0 HER2+ve, ER/PR-ve invasive ductal carcinoma.

Which is the most appropriate adjuvant management following surgery?

A. Aromatase inhibitors
B. Herceptin
C. Raloxifene
D. Radiotherapy
E. Tamoxifen

  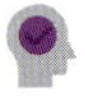

7. A 50-year-old woman wants to discuss breast cancer screening. She feels well, with no breast pain, lump, skin or nipple changes. There is no personal or family history of breast, ovarian or endometrial cancer. She has two children and takes the combined hormonal replacement pill.

Which is the most appropriate management?

A. Annual mammography
B. Annual MRI
C. Mammography every 3 years
D. Mammography every 2 years
E. No screening required

 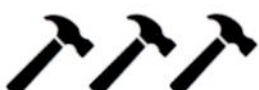 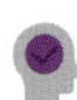

8. A 27-year-old woman 4 weeks postpartum has 2 days of worsening left breast pain, swelling, redness and difficulty when breastfeeding. Her temperature is 38.1°C, pulse 131 bpm and BP 105/75 mmHg. There is a fluctuant, tender mass in the left breast, with oedema, erythema and violaceous discolouration of the overlying skin.

Investigations:
Ultrasound of breast: irregular hypoechoic lesions in the left areolar region with inflammatory axillary lymphadenopathy.

Which is the most appropriate management?

A. Excisional biopsy
B. Fine needle aspiration
C. Incision and drainage
D. Mastectomy with axillary dissection
E. Percutaneous drainage

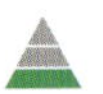  

9. A 69-year-old woman has 1 week of a painless left breast lump. She has smoked 20 cigarettes a day for 40 years. There is a nontender, 3 cm firm nodule in the inferior outer aspect of the left breast, with poorly defined margins, tethering to the underlying tissue, nipple inversion and blood-stained nipple discharge.

Which is the most appropriate investigation?

A. Breast fluid MC&S
B. Mammogram
C. MR breast
D. Ultrasound breast
E. X-ray of breast

10. A 69-year-old woman has a painless right breast lump. There is a firm, 2 cm nodule in the upper outer aspect of the left breast, with puckering and retraction of the overlying skin, and nipple inversion.

Investigations:
Breast biopsy and histology: T2N1M0 invasive ductal carcinoma of the left breast.

Which is the most appropriate management?

A. Breast-conserving surgery
B. Double mastectomy
C. Excisional biopsy
D. Radical mastectomy
E. Total mastectomy with axillary dissection

11. A 14-year-old boy has 3 months of breast swelling and tenderness. There is bilateral firm, tender subareolar swelling.

Which is the most appropriate management?

A. Lipectomy
B. Reassurance
C. Subcutaneous mastectomy
D. Tamoxifen
E. Testosterone replacement therapy

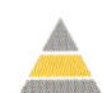 

12. A 31-year-old woman has 2 weeks of a painless left breast lump. There is a 2 cm rubbery lump in the inferior outer quadrant of the left breast that is mobile, with no tethering or skin changes.

Which is the most likely diagnosis?
A. Breast cancer
B. Breast cyst
C. Duct ectasia
D. Fat necrosis
E. Fibroadenoma

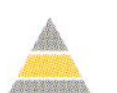  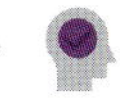

13. A 48-year-old woman has 2 weeks of profuse, milky discharge from both nipples. She has schizophrenia, managed with risperidone. Milky discharge is expressible from both breasts.

Which is the most appropriate investigation?
A. Breast milk culture
B. Mammogram
C. Prolactin level
D. Thyroid function tests
E. Ultrasound of breast

  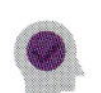

14. A 32-year-old woman has 1 week of a right breast lump. There is a tense, mildly tender mobile lump in the upper outer quadrant of the right breast, with no skin or nipple changes.

Investigations:
Ultrasound of breast: well-defined solid and cystic lesion within the left breast, with internal septations and mural thickening.

Which is the most appropriate management?
A. Excisional biopsy
B. Fine needle aspiration
C. Incision and drainage
D. Mastectomy
E. Oral antibiotics

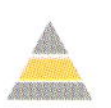  

15. A 32-year-old woman has a painless right breast lump. There is a small, firm, nontender, mobile mass in the upper outer quadrant of the right breast, with no skin or nipple changes.

Investigations:
Ultrasound of breast: 2 cm well-defined anechoic thin-walled cystic lesion in the right breast.

Which is the most appropriate management?
A. Core needle biopsy
B. Excisional biopsy
C. Fine needle aspiration
D. Incision and drainage
E. Reassurance

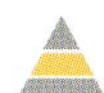 

16. A 45-year-old woman has 3 days of left breast tenderness, swelling, fevers and chills. She has type 2 diabetes mellitus, managed with metformin, and has smoked 20 cigarettes a day for 20 years. Her temperature is 38.6°C, pulse 102 bpm and BP 118/92 mmHg. There is left subareolar tenderness, swelling and erythema, with palpable axillary lymph nodes.

Figure 15.1 (see Chapter 37).

Which is the most likely diagnosis?
A. Breast abscess
B. Inflammatory breast cancer
C. Paget disease of the nipple
D. Periductal mastitis
E. Puerperal mastitis

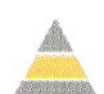 

17. A 72-year-old woman has 2 weeks of a painless left breast lump. She takes hormone replacement therapy for menopausal symptoms but is otherwise well. There is a firm 4 cm mass in the upper outer aspect of the left breast, with poorly defined margins, and tethering to the underlying tissues.

Investigations:
Mammogram: grouped microcalcifications in the left breast, with no stromal invasion.

Which is the most likely diagnosis?
A. Ductal carcinoma in situ
B. Fibroadenoma
C. Inflammatory breast cancer
D. Invasive ductal carcinoma
E. Lobular carcinoma in situ

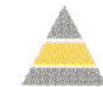 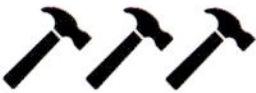

18. A 64-year-old woman has 2 weeks of right breast tenderness, warmth and redness, with occasional blood-stained nipple discharge.

Figure 15.2 (see Chapter 37).

Which is the most likely diagnosis?
A. Breast abscess
B. Breast eczema
C. Inflammatory breast cancer
D. Mastitis
E. Paget disease of the breast

 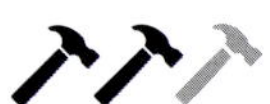 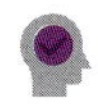

19. A 72-year-old woman has 2 weeks of worsening swelling, discomfort and difficulty lifting the right arm. She had a right total mastectomy with axillary node clearance for invasive ductal carcinoma 3 months previously. There is nonpitting oedema to the mid shaft of the humerus, with hardening and tightening of the overlying skin.

Which is the most appropriate management?
A. Elevation of the affected limb
B. Manual lymphatic drainage
C. Oral analgesia
D. Lymphatic vessel resection
E. Lymph node transfer

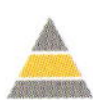 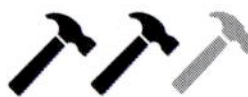

20. A 65-year-old has 2 weeks of an itchy rash on the left breast, with blood-stained nipple discharge. There is an erythematous, scaly rash in the left areolar area, with nipple retraction and ulceration.

Which is the most likely diagnosis?
A. Inflammatory breast cancer
B. Mammillary eczema
C. Mastitis
D. Nipple thrush
E. Paget disease of the nipple

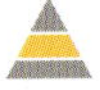 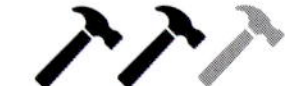 

21. A 23-year-old woman 2 weeks postpartum has 3 days of left breast redness, swelling and pain and difficulty with breastfeeding. Both she and her baby are otherwise well. She has type 1 diabetes mellitus, managed with insulin. Her temperature is 38.3°C, pulse 103 bpm and BP 113/84 mmHg. There is a fluctuant, left subareolar mass, with erythema, oedema and purulent nipple discharge.

Which is the most appropriate investigation?
A. Breast milk culture
B. Fine needle aspiration
C. Mammogram
D. Nipple swabs
E. Ultrasound of breast

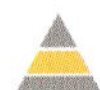 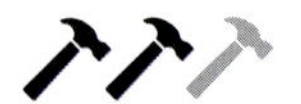 

22. A 30-year-old woman has 3 months of bilateral breast pain and multiple breast lumps, worse in the week before her menstrual cycle. She takes the combined oral contraceptive pill. There is bilateral tender nodularity of the breasts, with clear nipple discharge.

Which is the most appropriate investigation?
A. Core needle biopsy
B. Fine needle aspiration
C. Mammogram
D. MR of breast
E. Ultrasound of breast

 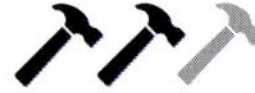 

23. A 74-year-old woman has 2 weeks of a painful, itchy left breast rash with blood-stained nipple discharge. She takes oestradiol and norethisterone hormone replacement therapy.

Figure 15.3 (see Chapter 37).

Which is the most appropriate management?
A. Breast-conserving surgery
B. Chemotherapy
C. Double mastectomy
D. Radical mastectomy
E. Topical emollients

 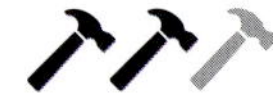

24. A 32-year-old woman 3 weeks postpartum has 1 week of worsening right breast pain, swelling and poor milk supply. Her temperature is 38.9°C, pulse 121 bpm and BP 108/64 mmHg. The right breast is swollen, with diffuse erythema, purulent nipple discharge and a fluctuant mass in the inferior outer quadrant.

Which is the most likely diagnosis?
A. Breast abscess
B. Fat necrosis
C. Inflammatory breast cancer
D. Mammary duct ectasia
E. Mastitis

 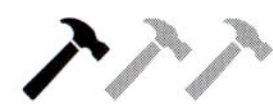 

25. A 38-year-old woman 2 weeks postpartum has breast pain, which starts after breastfeeding and lasts up to an hour, with itching and flaking of the areolar skin. She has type 2 diabetes mellitus, managed with metformin. There is bilateral flaking and patchy discolouration of the areolar area bilaterally.

Which is the most appropriate investigation?
- A. Core needle biopsy
- B. Mammogram
- C. Nipple swabs
- D. No investigations required
- E. Punch biopsy

 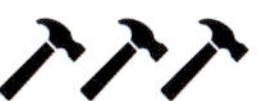 

26. A 52-year-old woman has 1 week of painless blood-stained right nipple discharge. There is a 1 cm right retroareolar mass, with bloody discharge expressible from the nipple.

Investigations:
Mammogram: well-defined mass in the right breast with lactiferous duct calcification.

Which is the most appropriate management?
- A. Core needle biopsy
- B. Fine needle aspiration
- C. Mastectomy
- D. Surgical duct excision
- E. Surveillance

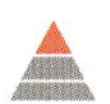  

27. A 23-year-old woman has recurrent bilateral, breast pain the week before her menstrual cycle, which resolves upon menstruation. She takes the combined oral contraceptive pill. There is bilateral breast tenderness worse in the upper outer quadrant.

Which is the most appropriate management?
- A. Combined oral contraceptive pill
- B. Oral antibiotics
- C. Oral NSAIDs
- D. Reassurance
- E. Topical NSAIDs

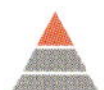 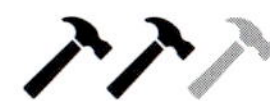

28. A 67-year-old woman has 1 month of a left breast lump following breast-conserving surgery for invasive ductal carcinoma. She has a nontender, firm, well-defined lump in the left upper outer quadrant deep to the surgical incision, which is clean, soft and nontender, with no erythema.

Which is the most likely diagnosis?
- A. Breast cyst
- B. Breast abscess
- C. Fat necrosis
- D. Fibroadenoma
- E. Invasive ductal carcinoma

29. A 44-year-old woman has intermittent bilateral breast pain and green nipple discharge. She has type 2 diabetes mellitus and polycystic ovarian syndrome, managed with metformin and the combined oral contraceptive pill, and has smoked 20 cigarettes a day for 20 years. There is bilateral nipple inversion.

Which is the most likely diagnosis?
- A. Breast cyst
- B. Duct ectasia
- C. Galactocele
- D. Intraductal papilloma
- E. Periductal mastitis

 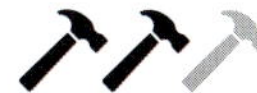

30. A 52-year-old woman has 1 month of a painless left breast lump. There is a 7 cm firm lump in the left breast, with no skin or nipple changes.

Investigations:
Mammogram: hyperintense cystic mass.
Core needle biopsy: leaf-like architecture with stromal cellularity.

Which is the most likely diagnosis?
- A. Breast abscess
- B. Breast cyst
- C. Fibroadenoma
- D. Invasive breast cancer
- E. Phyllodes tumour

Section 3
MEDICINE ANSWERS

Cardiology 16

EXPLANATIONS

Question 1

D. (Lateral STEMI) Sudden, severe chest pain radiating to the left jaw, on the background of hyperlipidaemia combined with being clammy to touch, and ST elevation in leads I, V5 and V6 on ECG suggests a lateral STEMI.

Type of STEMI	Coronary Artery Affected	Leads Affected
Inferior	Right Coronary Artery	II, III and aVF
Lateral	Left Circumflex Artery	I, V5 and V6
Anterior	Left Anterior Descending Artery	V1-V4

Question 2

E. (Right coronary artery) Sudden crushing chest pain radiating up to the left jaw, with an elevated troponin and ST elevation suggests a STEMI. ST elevation in leads II, III and aVF (inferior leads), points to the right coronary artery is the vessel affected.

Question 3

D. (Echocardiogram) Dyspnoea, fatigue, bilateral knee-level pitting oedema, and an S3 heart sound indicate heart failure. The S3 sound results from blood oscillating within the ventricular walls in systolic heart failure. An echocardiogram is optimal for assessing ejection fraction to direct management.

Question 4

A. (Acute pericarditis) Pleuritic chest pain on the background of a recent upper respiratory tract infection with a pericardial rub suggests acute pericarditis. Acute pericarditis causes widespread, concave ST elevation due to abnormal repolarisation secondary to pericardial inflammation.

Question 5

C. (Furosemide) Reduced exercise capacity and orthopnoea following a STEMI three years prior, along with elevated JVP, displaced apex beat, and a low ejection fraction (<0.40), suggest heart failure with reduced ejection fraction (HFrEF). Furosemide is the most suitable next step to alleviate pulmonary oedema.

Question 6

B. (NSAID + colchicine) Nonproductive cough and pleuritic chest pain following a recent Coxsackie B virus infection, along with widespread concave ST elevation and PR depression on ECG, indicate acute pericarditis. Management involves NSAIDs and colchicine for symptom relief and to prevent recurrence.

Question 7

E. (Unstable angina) Sudden chest pain at rest, on the background of hyperlipidaemia combined with an unremarkable cardiovascular examination and normal troponin levels but ST depression in the lateral leads suggests unstable angina.

Question 8

E. (Ramipril) She has a BP >150/80 mmHg and, therefore needs pharmacological management for her hypertension. If >55 years old, the first line is usually a calcium channel blocker i.e. amlodipine. However, in type 2 diabetics, ACE inhibitors such as ramipril are preferred as it has been shown to reduce ischaemic events in diabetics.

Question 9

C. (Pericardiocentesis) Dyspnoea after trauma with symptoms of Beck's triad on examination (raised JVP, dampened heart sounds and hypotension) suggests cardiac tamponade. Electrical alternans (QRS complexes of alternative heights) are indicative of cardiac tamponade. Pericardiocentesis is indicated to aspirate fluid from the pericardium and correct hypotension.

Question 10

A. (Immediate DC Cardioversion) Palpitations and dizziness with tachycardia and hypotension suggest an arrhythmia with haemodynamic instability. A monomorphic, broad complex tachycardia on ECG suggests ventricular tachycardia. Immediate DC cardioversion is indicated to correct arrhythmias in the context of haemodynamic instability.

Question 11

C. (Ventricular Fibrillation) Sudden chest pain combined with pallor and clammy to touch on examination before becoming unresponsive. After becoming unresponsive, his ECG shows irregular deflections of varying amplitude, with no discernable p waves and QRS complexes, suggesting ventricular fibrillation. Myocardial infarction progressing into cardiac arrest suggests ventricular fibrillation.

Question 12

E. (Spironolactone) Heart failure symptoms (paroxysmal nocturnal dyspnoea, bilateral pitting oedema) and a reduced ejection fraction despite medical management necessitate further management. Aldosterone antagonists i.e. spironolactone should be added to reduce morbidity and mortality in HFrEF.

Question 13

A. (Candesartan) For blood pressure >150/95 mmHg in the clinic or 140/80 mmHg at home unresponsive to amlodipine, add an aldosterone antagonist for gout, avoiding thiazides which can raise uric acid and worsen gout.

Question 14

E. (Percutaneous coronary intervention) Sudden dyspnoea with a W-shaped wave in lead V1 and an M-shaped wave in V6 suggests a new-onset left bundle branch block. This combined with ST elevation in leads V1-V4 suggests an anterior STEMI. Percutaneous coronary intervention is the management of choice because the presentation is within 12 hours of symptom onset.

Question 15

B. (CT pulmonary angiogram) Sudden pleuritic chest pain, on the background of an elective left knee replacement three weeks ago combined with left chest crepitations and leg swelling bilaterally, with dilated, swollen, tender lower leg veins. A Wells score of 4.5 (3 - an alternative diagnosis is less likely than PE, 1.5 - surgery in past four weeks), suggests pulmonary embolism. The investigation for a PE if the Wells score is >4, is a CT pulmonary angiogram (provided there are no contraindications such as renal impairment)

Question 16

B. (Kerley B lines) Gradually worsening dyspnoea on the background of hyperlipidaemia combined with raised JVP, hepatomegaly, bibasal crepitations and tachycardia on examination suggests heart failure. ABCDE can summarise the signs of heart failure on the CXR:
A = Alveolar oedema, B = Kerley B lines,
C = Cardiomegaly, D = Upper lobe diversion, E = Pleural effusions - blunted costophrenic angles; hence the correct sign on CXR out of the possible options is Kerley B lines.

Question 17

A. (Amlodipine) For stable angina not managed with a beta-blocker, add on a long-acting dihydropyridine calcium channel blocker such as amlodipine.

Question 18

E. (Ramipril) Dry cough on the background of heart failure suggests the causative drug is ramipril. Ramipril is an ACE inhibitor and is thought to induce the cough reflex by accumulation of bradykinin in the upper and lower respiratory tracts.

Question 19

B. (One shock followed by two minutes of CPR) Cardiac arrest caused by ventricular fibrillation (irregular deflections and lack of p waves and QRS complexes) indicates management for a shockable rhythm. The correct management is one shock by defibrillator followed by two minutes of CPR with a 30:2 ratio between chest compressions and breaths respectively.

Question 20

D. (NYHA Class IV) The inability to carry out any physical activity without discomfort with symptoms such as bilateral leg swelling suggests very severe symptoms of HF. This would be classed as NYHA Class IV, the highest severity of HF.

Question 21

D. (Amiodarone 300 mg and adrenaline 1 mg) Cardiac arrest after an anterior STEMI combined with ventricular fibrillation on ECG, indicates three shocks via the defibrillator have been given. Amiodarone 300 mg and adrenaline 1 mg are the correct doses and drugs used to treat a shockable rhythm after three shocks with the defibrillator.

Question 22

B. (First-degree heart block) Unremarkable cardiovascular examination and a prolonged PR interval on ECG (normal range: 120-200ms) suggest a first-degree heart block.

Question 23

D. (Intraosseous route) Unresponsive and pulselessness after a car accident combined with a regular broad complex tachycardia on ECG suggests pulseless ventricular tachycardia. Pulseless VT should be managed with adrenaline and amiodarone intravenously; however, medical team is unable to gain IV access; hence the ALS guidelines suggest the intraosseous route.

Question 24

C. (Carotid sinus massage) Intermittent palpitations for two months, on the background of recreational cocaine usage combined with a narrow complex tachycardia with absent p waves on ECG suggests supraventricular tachycardia (SVT). The management of choice for SVT is vagal manoeuvres such as a carotid sinus massage.

Question 25

B. (Atrial flutter) Dyspnoea and palpitations combined with a narrow complex tachycardia with rapid, undulating waves in the inferior leads on ECG suggest atrial flutter.

Question 26

E. (Widened Mediastinum) Sudden chest pain and dyspnoea in a hypertensive patient with recreational cocaine usage suggest aortic dissection. The CXR finding associated with aortic dissection is a widened mediastinum due to the formation of a false lumen.

Question 27

E. (Posterior STEMI) Sudden chest pain in a patient with stable angina combined with a raised troponin suggests myocardial infarction. ST depression and tall R waves in leads V1-V3 on ECG suggest a posterior STEMI.

Question 28

E. (Wolff-Parkinson-White Syndrome) Intermittent palpitations, on the background of thyrotoxicosis combined with a short PR interval (<0.12 seconds) and broad QRS complexes on ECG suggest Wolff-Parkinson-White syndrome. Wolff-Parkinson-White is an accessory pathway disorder, caused by the presence of the Bundle of Kent (accessory conduction pathway) and the ECG findings seen are caused by the lack of impulse slowing properties of the AV node.

Question 29

B. (Aortic Dissection) Sudden chest pain in a Marfan's patient with a weak brachial pulse and an aortic regurgitation murmur suggests an aortic dissection. This is confirmed by the presence of a false lumen in the ascending aorta.

Question 30

A. (<2%) The Pulmonary Embolism Rule-out Criteria (PERC) criteria consists of eight criteria and is used to exclude PE in patients known to have a low pretest PE probability (<15%). If all eight of the PERC criteria are absent, then there is less than a <2% chance of a PE.

Question 31

A. (Autosomal Dominant) Syncope during physical exertion combined with a jerky carotid pulse and an aortic stenosis murmur suggests Hypertrophic Obstructive Cardiomyopathy (HOCM). HOCM's characteristic ECG findings are deep Q waves in the lateral/inferior leads caused by septal hypertrophy. HOCM is an autosomal dominant condition.

Question 32

A. (IV alteplase) Sudden pleuritic chest pain on the background of recent surgery suggest a pulmonary embolism. This is confirmed by dilated, swollen, tender lower leg veins and tachycardia on examination, giving a Wells score above 4. The haemodynamic instability suggested by an SBP <90mmHg indicates thrombolysis through IV alteplase as the management of choice.

Question 33

D. (IV magnesium sulphate) Dyspnoea for 48 hours, on the background of mycoplasma pneumoniae infection managed with erythromycin combined with dizziness and ventricular tachycardia with a prolonged QT interval on ECG suggests Torsades de Pointes. The management of choice is IV magnesium sulphate, to stabilise the cardiac membrane.

Question 34

B. (Anterolateral NSTEMI) Sudden chest pain radiating to the left shoulder, on the background of hyperlipidaemia combined with a raised troponin and T wave inversion in leads I, aVL and V3-V6 on ECG suggests an anterolateral NSTEMI.

Question 35

D. (Immediate synchronised DC cardioversion) Acute palpitations with haemodynamic instability (SBP<90mmHg) and an irregularly irregular rhythm on ECG suggests atrial fibrillation, The haemodynamic instability indicates immediate synchronised DC cardioversion, as it classically requires less energy than defibrillation.

Question 36

D. (IV calcium gluconate) Hyperkalaemia with significant ECG changes (tall, tented T waves and broad QRS complexes) suggest the next appropriate step to be IV calcium gluconate, to stabilise the cardiac membrane.

Question 37

E. (Radiofrequency ablation of the accessory pathway) Palpitations noticeable after exertion, on the background of a family history of sudden cardiac death combined with short PR intervals, delta waves and widened QRS complexes on ECG suggests Wolff-Parkinson-White syndrome. The definitive management for this is radiofrequency ablation of the accessory pathway.

Question 38

E. (Right coronary artery) Sudden central crushing chest pain on the background of hypercholesterolaemia combined with ST elevation leading to a STEMI diagnosis. 12 hours after PCI, the patient is pale and clammy to touch and is bradycardic, with ECG showing complete P: QRS dissociation suggesting complete heart block, hence the right coronary artery is most likely affected (as this supplies the atrioventricular node).

Question 39

C. (Transoesophageal echocardiogram) Sudden, tearing chest pain radiating to the back, on the background of Ehlers-Danlos syndrome combined with absent femoral pulses and an aortic regurgitation murmur on examination with tachycardia, tachypnoea and hypotension suggests aortic dissection with haemodynamic instability. The most suitable investigation for aortic dissection is CT angiography chest/abdomen/pelvis, however in haemodynamically instability, the use of contrast is contraindicated, and therefore, a transoesophageal echocardiogram is the suitable investigation.

Question 40

E. (Transcatheter aortic valve replacement) A loud ejection systolic murmur with a soft S2 suggests aortic stenosis. This patient is symptomatic (pleuritic chest pain, dizziness) with multiple comorbidities suggesting the need for transcatheter aortic valve replacement (TAVR). TAVR is preferred to open heart surgery, due to reduced surgical complication risk.

Question 41

E. (Tricuspid regurgitation) Dyspnoea on the background of IV drug use combined with petechial lesions on the palms and soles and a pansystolic murmur on examination with vegetation on the valvular leaflet on echocardiogram suggests infective endocarditis. Given the history of IV drug use, the tricuspid valve is the most likely to be affected as it is the first valve venous blood encounters in the heart.

Question 42

C. (Electrocardiogram) Syncope after collapsing in football training combined with dizziness before the collapse suggests cardiomyopathy like hypertrophic obstructive cardiomyopathy; hence an ECG is the most suitable initial investigation. An ECG would show prominent Q waves and QRS complexes tallest in the mid-precordial leads.

Question 43

C. (Hypertrophic obstructive cardiomyopathy) Chest pain and dyspnoea on the background of a family history of sudden cardiac death combined with a jerky carotid pulse suggests Hypertrophic Obstructive Cardiomyopathy (HOCM). This is confirmed by marked left ventricular hypertrophy and systolic anterior motion of the mitral valve on echocardiogram.

Question 44

D. (Right bundle branch block) Palpitations on the background of myocarditis combined with an M-shaped wave in lead V1 and a W-shaped wave in lead V6 on examination suggest a right bundle branch block.

Question 45

D. (Stage IV hypertensive retinopathy) Visual disturbances with an enlarged blind spot, on the background of poorly controlled hypertension suggest hypertensive retinopathy. Optic margin blurring and venous engorgement on fundoscopy are indicative of papilloedema, which is stage IV hypertensive retinopathy.

Question 46

D. (Torsades de pointes) Dizziness and palpitations causing syncope on the background of CAP managed with erythromycin combined with restlessness, ventricular tachycardia and a prolonged QT interval (350-450ms) on ECG suggests Torsades de Pointes.

Question 47

B. (IV labetalol) Sudden chest pain in a hypertensive patient with weak femoral pulses bilaterally indicates aortic dissection, classified by Stanford as Type A (ascending aorta) and Type B (distal to right brachiocephalic trunk). CT findings show a Type B dissection (false lumen in descending aorta), which is less risky than Type A. Management starts with BP control using IV labetalol, followed by surgical intervention with TEVAR for Type B dissection.

Question 48

D. (Roth spots) Dyspnoea and fever combined with splinter haemorrhages and Osler nodes in the hands, and a mitral regurgitation murmur on examination and a mitral valve vegetation on the echocardiogram suggest infective endocarditis. On fundoscopy, Roth spots (white central retinal haemorrhages) can be seen, with the appearance caused by coagulated fibrin.

Question 49

C. (Rivaroxaban for three months) Sudden pleuritic chest pain and haemoptysis on the background of an elective left hip replacement around three weeks ago combined with bibasilar crepitations, leg swelling bilaterally with dilated, swollen, tender lower leg veins and tachycardia on examination suggests pulmonary embolism. As this is a provoked PE (by surgery), the management of choice is rivaroxaban for three months.

Question 50

C. (Modified Duke criteria) Dyspnoea and chest pain on the background of mitral valve replacement combined with a mitral regurgitation murmur and Janeway lesions on the hands-on examination with mitral valve vegetation on echocardiogram suggests infective endocarditis. The diagnostic tool for infective endocarditis is the modified Duke's criteria, with definitive endocarditis diagnosed if 2 major criteria or 5 minor criteria or 1 major w/ 3 minor criteria are present.

Question 51

A. (Aortic regurgitation) Sudden tearing chest pain and dyspnoea, on the background of hypertension combined with weak brachial pulses and an early diastolic murmur best heard on expiration on examination with a false lumen in the ascending aorta on echocardiogram suggests aortic dissection. Aortic dissection causes dilation of the aortic root, which prevents the aortic valve from closing completely during diastole and thereby causes aortic regurgitation.

Question 52

A. (Implantable cardioverter-defibrillator) Palpitations, on the background of a family history of sudden cardiac death combined with T wave inversion in leads V1-3 and a terminal notch in the QRS complex on ECG and an enlarged, hypokinetic right ventricle with a thin free wall on cardiac MRI suggests arrhythmogenic right ventricular cardiomyopathy (ARVC). An implantable cardioverter-defibrillator is the definitive management of choice for ARVC.

Question 53

C. (Left ventricular free wall rupture) Dyspnoea on the background of a lateral STEMI a week ago combined with raised JVP and muffled heart sounds on examination with hypotension and tachycardia and electrical alternans on ECG suggests a left ventricular free wall rupture, which is a rare complication of MI. One of the potential mechanisms of this complication is the infarcted area undergoing a process of remodelling characterized by thinning of the myocardium which weakens the heart wall and increases the risk of rupture.

Question 54

A. (Percutaneous mitral balloon valvotomy) Haemoptysis and dyspnoea on the background of rheumatic fever combined with malar flush and a mitral stenosis murmur on examination suggest mitral stenosis. Symptomatic mitral stenosis should be treated with percutaneous mitral balloon valvotomy.

Question 55

A. (Dressler syndrome) Signs of acute pericarditis (pleuritic chest pain, widespread concave ST elevation) four weeks after a STEMI suggests Dressler's syndrome. Dressler's syndrome is thought to occur as an autoimmune reaction to myocardial neo-antigens post-MI.

Question 56

D. (Transoesophageal echocardiography) Chest pain and shortness of breath for two weeks, on the background of prior heart valve replacement surgery combined with splinter haemorrhages, mitral regurgitation and a low-grade fever suggests infective endocarditis. The most suitable investigation for infective endocarditis is transthoracic echocardiography, however, the previous history of valve replacement contraindicates this, therefore, transoesophageal echocardiography is the most suitable investigation

Question 57

E. (V/Q scan) Sudden pleuritic chest pain and dyspnoea with basal crepitations in the left lung and bilateral leg swelling suggest pulmonary embolism. An EGFR of 51 mL/min/1.73 m^2, classifies her as having CKD stage 3a, hence a V/Q scan is preferred due to the risk of contrast-induced nephropathy with CTPA.

Question 58

D. (Severe valvular incompetence) Fever, chills and fatigue for a week and new onset dyspnoea and chest pain combined with a mitral regurgitation murmur on examination with positive strep viridans blood cultures and vegetation on the anterior mitral leaflet on echocardiogram suggests infective endocarditis. Whilst infective endocarditis is usually managed with antibiotics, there are a few indications for surgery, such as severe valvular incompetence, aortic abscess and recurrent emboli after antibiotic therapy.

Question 59

D. (Hypokalaemia) Palpitations and light-headedness for a week combined with tachycardia on examination and a prolonged QT interval (350-450ms) on examination, and out of the options, hypokalaemia is the only option that prolongs the QT interval.

Question 60

D. (Rheumatic Fever) Dyspnoea and haemoptysis combined with mid-late diastolic murmur with a loud S1 and malar flush on examination suggests mitral stenosis. The most likely cause of mitral stenosis is rheumatic fever, which can be diagnosed using the Jones criteria.

Question 61

C. (Dilated cardiomyopathy) Chest pain, dyspnoea and fatigue on the background of a recent respiratory tract infection combined with bilateral crepitations and muffled heart sounds on examination and a raised CRP, suggests myocarditis. Dilated cardiomyopathy is a recognised late complication of myocarditis.

Question 62

B. (Brugada Syndrome) Syncope on the background of a family history of arrhythmia combined with partial right bundle branch block and convex ST elevation of 3 mm in leads V1-V2 followed by a negative T wave on ECG suggests Brugada Syndrome. Brugada syndrome is a autosomal dominant channelopathy, most commonly caused by a mutation in SCN5A, which encodes a cardiac sodium channel, which predisposes the heart to arrythmias.

Question 63

D. (Pericardiectomy) Signs of RHF (oedema, elevated JVP, loud S3 heart sound) with pericardial calcifications on CXR suggest constrictive pericarditis. The management is a pericardiectomy, which removes the stiffened part of the pericardium, which causes the symptoms.

Question 64

C. (Eisenmenger's syndrome) Worsening breathlessness and haemoptysis for six weeks, on the background of a ventricular septal defect combined with a fixed, widely split S2 on examination and gross dilatation of the main, left and right pulmonary arteries on CXR suggests Eisenmenger's syndrome. Eisenmenger's syndrome is a reversal of the usual left-to-right shunt due to pulmonary hypertension.

Question 65

B. (Cholesterol embolism) Severe pain at rest in both her feet, on the background of unstable angina combined with toes are cold and purple, but present major arterial pulses in the lower limbs and intravascular cholesterol clefts on renal biopsy suggests cholesterol embolism. Procedures such as cardiac catheterisation can dislodge plaques in the arteries causing cholesterol embolism.

Question 66

C. (Myocarditis) Dyspnoea on the background of a recently recovered viral illness combined with bibasilar crepitations, a low-grade fever, tachycardia and tachypnoea on examination and bilateral pulmonary infiltrates and cardiomegaly on CXR suggests myocarditis.

Question 67

A. (Alcoholism) Exertional dyspnoea gradually worsening for two months combined with orthopnoea and pitting ankle oedema on examination and dilation of all four chambers and thinning of both ventricular walls on echocardiogram suggests dilated cardiomyopathy. Of the provided options, alcoholism is the most associated with dilated cardiomyopathy, which points to this being the most likely cause of his diagnosis.

Question 68

C. (Atrial myxoma) Dyspnoea and unintentional weight loss for three months combined with finger clubbing bilaterally and a mitral stenosis murmur on examination with a pedunculated heterogenous mass attached to the fossa ovalis on examination suggests atrial myxoma. Atrial myxoma's are the most common primary cardiac tumour and whilst the majority occur sporadically, it can be associated with inherited conditions like Carney syndrome (skin pigmentation + benign tumours).

Question 69

D. (Mitral valve prolapse) Chest pain and exertional dyspnoea on the background of Marfan syndrome (upwards lens dislocation, pectus excavatum), with a mitral regurgitation murmur suggests a mitral valve prolapse, is a common complication of Marfan's syndrome.

Question 70

B. (Labetalol) Blurred vision and limb swelling, on the background of being 30 weeks pregnant combined with pitting oedema in her limbs and a raised BP on examination suggests gestational hypertension. The management for gestational hypertension is oral labetalol, unless if asthmatic in which case nifedipine is usually preferred.

Question 71

B. (Coarctation of the aorta) Radio femoral delay and a mid-systolic murmur best heard over the back in a child with positive Roesler sign (notching of inferior borders of posterior ribs on CXR) suggests coarctation of the aorta. Coarctation of the aorta is a congenital narrowing of descending aorta, leading to increased pressure proximal to the narrowing and decreased blood flow distal to the narrowing (radio-femoral delay).

Question 72

E. (Takotsubo cardiomyopathy) Severe chest pain and dyspnoea for a month associated with severe hypokinesis of the mid and apical segment of the left ventricle on echo suggests Takotsubo cardiomyopathy. Takotsubo is a stress-related cardiomyopathy, with the name meaning “octopus trap” referring to the shape seen on echo.

Question 73

B. (Left ventricular aneurysm) Dyspnoea after a recent inferolateral STEMI with signs of left ventricular failure (S3 heart sound and pitting oedema) and persistent ST elevation suggests left ventricular aneurysm. This complication of an MI is caused by a weakened myocardium.

Question 74

E. (Ventricular septal defect) A baby with a harsh pansystolic murmur best heard at the lower left sternal border combined with a left-to-right shunt on echocardiogram suggests a ventricular septal defect, which is the most common type of congenital heart disease. It classically presents with features of volume overload and pulmonary hypertension.

Question 75

D. (PKP2) Exertional palpitations and dizziness, on the background of sudden cardiac depth, combined with enlarged, hypokinetic right ventricle and a terminal notch in the QRS complex suggest arrhythmogenic right ventricular cardiomyopathy (ARVC). The terminal notch is caused by delayed right ventricular conduction causing a delayed action potential at the terminal phase of the QRS complex. Plakophilin-2 (PKP2) is found in cardiac desmosomes and is the most common gene mutation seen in ARVC.

Question 76

A. (Anti-beta2 glycoprotein I antibody) Sudden pleuritic chest pain on the background of systemic lupus erythematosus and two miscarriages for four years combined with a prolonged aPTT and raised d-dimer suggests antiphospholipid syndrome. Antiphospholipid syndrome predisposes patients to arterial and venous thrombosis and the antibodies involved are anti-cardiolipin antibodies, anti-beta2 glycoprotein I (anti-beta2GPI) antibodies and lupus anticoagulant.

Question 77

B. (Ajmaline) Syncope, on the background of sudden cardiac death in the family, with saddleback ST elevation in leads V1-V3 suggests a type II Brugada pattern. After the challenge, the ECG shows convex ST elevation in leads V1-V3 followed by a negative T wave, a type I Brugada pattern; hence Brugada syndrome can be diagnosed. Ajmaline is a sodium channel blocker given in the challenge as Brugada syndrome is caused by sodium channel mutations such as SCN5A.

Question 78

B. (Benzylpenicillin and Colonoscopy) Fever and myalgia with bilateral lower leg oedema and bibasilar crackles on examination. Growth of streptococcus with these symptoms suggests infective endocarditis with severe valvular involvement, mimicking a heart failure presentation. Streptococcus gallolyticus, a member of the streptococcus bovis group indicates the need for benzylpenicillin, the preferred antibiotic for a streptococcal infection. Furthermore, the association between streptococcus bovis and colorectal cancer necessitates a colonoscopy in this man.

Gastroenterology 17

EXPLANATIONS

Question 1

B. (Acute pancreatitis) Sudden, severe epigastric pain radiating to the back, with sweating, epigastric tenderness and abdominal guarding, suggests acute pancreatitis, confirmed by the significant elevation in amylase. Acute pancreatitis is caused by autodigestion of pancreatic tissue by the pancreatic enzymes, leading to necrosis and is most commonly by gallstones or alcohol use (other causes can be summarised by the acronym GET SMASHED).

Question 2

A. (Acute cholecystitis) Sudden RUQ pain radiating to the right shoulder, with RUQ tenderness and guarding without fever or signs of jaundice suggests acute cholecystitis. Acute cholecystitis is the inflammation of the gall bladder, which is caused in 90% of cases by gallstones (calculous cholecystitis). The impacted gallstone causes bile to become trapped in the gallbladder, causing irritation and increased pressure in the gallbladder.

Question 3

A. (Acute appendicitis) Generalized lower abdominal pain, associated with nonbloody vomiting a low-grade fever tenderness and neutrophilia suggests acute appendicitis. The Alvarado score is a 10-point score that can help in the diagnosis of acute appendicitis, with a score of 5 or 6 compatible with acute appendicitis. Both ovarian torsion and ectopic pregnancy are important differentials to exclude in a woman with lower abdominal pain; however, these don't present with a fever.

Question 4

C. (Laparoscopic cholecystectomy) Severe, intermittent right upper quadrant pain radiating to the right shoulder, tenderness and guarding in the right upper quadrant without jaundice suggests acute cholecystitis, confirmed by gallstones on US. Laparoscopic cholecystectomy is the management of acute cholecystitis to remove the gallstones, with the guidelines changing to early laparoscopic cholecystectomy (within a week) from cholecystectomy after the inflammation has subsided (usually after weeks).

Question 5

E. (Ulcerative colitis) Diarrhoea and rectal bleeding for 3 weeks, on the background of his mother having inflammatory bowel disease combined with severe LLQ abdominal pain, suggests ulcerative colitis. Ulcerative colitis' inflammation starts at the rectum and typically presents with bloody diarrhoea and has extra-intestinal manifestations like uveitis through a combination of immune dysregulation, genetic predisposition and microbial factors, whilst Crohn's typically presents with nonbloody diarrhoea and are less likely to present with extra-intestinal manifestations.

Question 6

E. (Biliary colic) Severe right upper quadrant pain radiating to the right shoulder after having a fatty meal combined with RUQ tenderness and Murphy's sign negative on examination suggests biliary colic over acute cholecystitis. Whilst biliary colic and acute cholecystitis both involve gallstone-related pathology, the absence of inflammation in biliary colic typically precludes the presence of Murphy's sign.

Question 7

B. (GORD) Recurrent heartburn and regurgitation, leaving an unpleasant taste, with these symptoms occurring after meals and improved by antacids, with 20 pack-year smoking history suggesting gastro-oesophageal reflux disease (GORD). GORD refers to oesophagitis secondary to refluxed gastric contents, with obesity and smoking being major risk factors.

Question 8

C. (Elevated neutrophils) Lower abdominal pain, with a low-grade fever and positive Rovsing's sign and tenderness and guarding over McBurney's point on examination, suggest acute appendicitis. Acute appendicitis is inflammatory, so it would be associated with elevated C-reactive protein (CRP), as well as leucocytosis and neutrophilia (both components of the Alvarado score for appendicitis). Neutrophils and other granulocytes are often increased first which then release cytokines such as TNF-α, IL-1β and IFN-γ, which causes an increase in acute phase proteins such as CRP. Furthermore, a fever would also be induced by the release of cytokines such as IL-1 and IL-6.

Question 9

A. (Acute fatty liver of pregnancy) Severe abdominal pain for a week, on the background of being 30 weeks pregnant combined with scleral icterus and RUQ pain on examination and and ALT > 500 U/L suggest an acute fatty liver of pregnancy. Obstetric cholestasis would present with a raised bilirubin causing an itch and HELLP syndrome would present with Haemolysis, Elevated Liver enzymes and Low Platelets.

Question 10

E. (Mesenteric adenitis) Right iliac fossa pain on the background of an upper respiratory tract infection combined with an unremarkable examination and bloods suggests mesenteric adenitis. Mesenteric adenitis is caused by inflammation of lymph nodes in the mesentery, and whilst it presents similarly to appendicitis, bloods (raised inflammatory markers and WCC) can differentiate between the two.

Question 11

A. (Acetylcysteine) Unconsciousness after excess paracetmol ingestion, with jaundice (scleral icterus) and coagulopathy (raised prothrombin time), suggests acute liver failure secondary to paracetamol overdose. Paracetamol overdose causes liver failure by increased metabolism of paracetamol via the cytochrome P450 enzyme system, particularly the CYP2E1 isoenzyme, resulting in a larger amount of N-acetyl-p-benzoquinone imine (NAPQI), a highly reactive and toxic metabolite. Acetylcysteine is indicated in the management of a paracetamol overdose, if the paracetamol concentration is above the treatment line on the treatment nonogram or if there are signs of acute liver injury such as raised prothrombin time. Activated charcoal is only indicated if patients present within 1 hour of ingestion to reduce absorption of paracetamol.

Question 12

C. (ERCP) Severe epigastric pain radiating through the back combined with Grey-Turner's sign (flank discolouration) and epigastric tenderness on examination suggests acute pancreatitis. Flank discolouration is caused in severe pancreatitis, where inflammation and enzymatic digestion of pancreatic tissue can lead to the erosion of blood vessels within the pancreas and adjacent retroperitoneal space. The abdominal US shows gallstones with evidence of cholangitis or bile duct obstruction so an ERCP is preferred.

Question 13

B. (Prothrombin time) Confusion and asterixis three days after a paracetamol overdose, when she presented with jaundice and right upper quadrant pain, suggests the development of encepahlopahty as a result of acute liver failure. Prothrombin time is the investigation of choice to investigate coagulopathy in acute liver failure, and it is considered better than LFTs because unlike some LFTs, which can be influenced by factors unrelated to liver function (e.g., muscle injury, bone disease), PT is a more specific indicator of hepatic synthetic function.

Question 14

A. (Gluten-free diet) Malaise, stomach cramps and pale diarrhoea for 3 months, on the background of type 1 diabetes mellitus combined with abdominal bloating and duodenal biopsy showing intraepithelial lymphocytes suggests coeliac disease (although villous atrophy and crypt hyperplasia are more classic). A gluten-free diet is the management of choice for coeliac disease because it is caused by an inflammatory reaction to gliadins and glutenins.

Question 15

B. (ALT high, ALP normal) Confusion after ingesting a paracetamol excess combined with scleral icterus, and coagulopathy (due to increased PT) suggests acute liver failure. In paracetamol overdose, LFTs showing hepatocyte damage (in this case ALT and AST) are high, and LFTs that show cholestasis (in this case ALP and GGT) are normal.

Question 16

B. (Acute diverticulitis) Sudden left lower quadrant pain and change in bowel habit combined with LLQ tenderness and guarding and reduced bowel sounds on examination with a raised white cell count suggest acute diverticulitis. Acute diverticulitis occurs when diverticula, which are caused by increased intra-colonic pressure and usually occur along the weaker areas of the wall, become infected. The sigmoid colon is the most affected area of the colon because of high intraluminal pressure, reduced colon wall thickness, anatomic factors, reduced perfusion, and delayed transit time compared to other parts of the colon.

Question 17

E. (Malnutrition Universal Screening Tool) Unintentional weight loss and myalgia for 5 months due to a poor appetite and decreased food intake combined with an underweight BMI, muscular atrophy and generalized weakness on examination suggest malnutrition. Malnutrition Universal Screening Tool (MUST) should be used to categorize the severity of the woman's malnutrition and is composed of 3 parameters: BMI, unplanned weight loss in the past 3-6 months and the patient is acutely ill and there has been or is likely to be no nutritional intake for >5 days.

Question 18

B. (Colonoscopy and biopsy) Bloody diarrhoea, faecal urgency and left lower quadrant pain for 6 months combined with erythema nodosum and left lower quadrant tenderness on examination suggests ulcerative colitis. Colonoscopy and biopsy is the investigation of choice for ulcerative colitis (UC) to look for features such as mucosal inflammation.

Question 19

E. (Prednisolone) Nonbloody diarrhoea and weight loss combined with lower right quadrant tenderness and perianal skin tags on examination with noncaseating granuloma and serosal inflammation on a biopsy suggests Crohn's disease. Glucocorticoids such as prednisolone manage to induce remission in Crohn's disease, by suppressing inflammation, reducing vascular permeability and promoting apoptosis of activated immune cells.

Question 20

B. (Omeprazole) Recurrent heartburn and regurgitation exacerbated by meals and when lying down despite weight loss and avoiding triggers suggests gastro-oesophageal reflux disease (GORD). The management for GORD that is not managed by lifestyle changes is a month trial of a proton pump inhibitor like omeprazole. Surgery is indicated for patients who have a good response to PPIs, but who are nonadherent to therapy or do not wish to take long-term medical treatment.

Question 21

D. (Loperamide) Recurrent abdominal pain and bowel habit alternating between diarrhoea and constipation, associated with bloating suggests irritable bowel syndrome (IBS) (triad of abdominal pain, bloating and changes in bowel habit - **ABC**). The main concern is diarrhoea affecting daily activities; hence, the appropriate management is loperamide. Loperamide acts on μ-opioid receptors in the myenteric plexus of the large intestine thereby it decreases the tone of the longitudinal and circular smooth muscles of the intestinal wall, causing decreased gastric motility.

Question 22

E. (Primary sclerosing cholangitis) Fatigue and pruritus combined with scleral icterus and hepatomegaly on examination, with multiple biliary strictures on ERCP, suggest primary sclerosing cholangitis. Primary sclerosing cholangitis is the fibrosis of the intra- and extrahepatic ducts, with 80% of patients with PSC having UC, classically would present with a raised ALP and a "beaded" appearance on ERCP.

Question 23

A. (Dermatitis herpetiformis) Fatigue and diarrhoea for 4 months, on the background of Hashimoto's thyroiditis, combined with a pruritic, vesicular skin lesion on the extensor surfaces on examination, despite a false negative coeliac result (due to IgA deficiency) suggests coeliac disease. Dermatitis herpetiformis is the dermatological manifestation associated with coeliac disease, which presents with an intense itch and a symmetrical blistering rash.

Question 24

C. (Ascending cholangitis) RUQ pain, fever and jaundice (scleral icterus) is known as Charcot's triad and is associated with ascending cholangitis, which is an infection of the biliary tree. The bile duct stones are a predisposing factor to ascending cholangitis.

Question 25

D. (Liver cirrhosis) RUQ pain and abdominal swelling combined with peripheral stigmata of chronic liver disease (scleral icterus, leukonychia and spider naevi) with an AST: ALT ratio > 2 suggests alcoholic liver cirrhosis. Although the patient has features consistent with advanced liver disease, such as jaundice, the absence of overt signs of hepatic encephalopathy, severe coagulopathy, or altered mental status suggests that she may not yet have progressed to the stage of liver failure.

Question 26

D. (Infectious mononucleosis) The triad of sore throat, low-grade fever and lymphadenopathy is seen in close to all patients with infectious mononucleosis. Infectious mononucleosis is caused by Epstein-Barr virus (EBV) is the causative organism (also known as human herpesvirus-4), with one important complication to be aware of being a morbilliform rash if amoxicillin is given (as it can often be mistaken for bacterial throat infections).

Question 27

A. (Bed rest and oral rehydration solution) Abdominal pain, watery diarrhoea and persistent vomiting for a day, despite no recent travel or exposure to sick contacts combined with diffuse abdominal tenderness and hyperactive bowel sounds on examination, suggest gastroenteritis. There are no signs of systemic upset or severe disease; hence, bed rest and oral rehydration solution are the management of choice.

Question 28

C. (Hepatitis C) Fatigue, nausea and abdominal discomfort for 3 weeks, on the background of IV drug use and unprotected sexual activity combined with jaundice and hepatomegaly on examination suggests hepatitis B or C (IV drug use and unprotected sexual activity are the main risk factors for Hepatitis **C** (C for RFs associated with **C**irculation), whilst Hepatitis A and E route of transmission is faecal oral – vowels come from the bowel). However, low C4 levels are associated with cryoglobulinaemia, which is a complication of hepatitis C exclusively, whilst extra-hepatic complications of hepatitis B include polyarteritis nodosa.

Question 29

D. (Omeprazole, clarithromycin + metronidazole) Severe epigastric pain relieved by eating combined with a positive urea breath test (*H. pylori* infection) suggests a duodenal ulcer secondary to *H. pylori* infection. *H pylori* infection causes gastric mucin degradation and increased mucosal permeability that are directly cytotoxic to the gastric epithelium. Omeprazole, metronidazole + clarithromycin, commonly called triple therapy, is the management of choice in penicillin-allergic patients for peptic ulcer disease caused by *H. pylori*. Triple therapy allows for high eradication rates, minimizes the risk of antibiotic resistance,

Question 30

E. (Typhoid Fever) A dull, frontal headache and diarrhoea after having street food after a recent trip to South Asia, combined with rose spots (blanching, erythematous maculopapular lesion) and diffuse abdominal tenderness which suggests typhoid fever. Typhoid fever is caused by *Salmonella typhi*, which invades and adheres to the gut wall first, causing diarrhoea and abdominal pain. The management of typhoid fever involves azithromycin and a third-generation cephalosporin like ceftriaxone.

Question 31

C. (Gastric cancer) Persistent epigastric pain and systemic signs of malignancy (unintentional weight loss and pallor) and epigastric tenderness on examination with a large, ulcerated mass in the pyloric antrum on OGD suggest gastric cancer. The cancer seen is a type III gastric cancer as per the Japanese Endoscopic Society classification

Question 32

E. (*Escherichia coli*) RUQ pain, fever and jaundice (scleral icterus) is known as Charcot's triad and is associated with ascending cholangitis. *Escherichia coli* is the most common causative organism of ascending cholangitis, often ascending retrogradely from the duodenum into the bile ducts through the papilla of Vater, leading to infection.

Question 33

A. (Chest X-ray) Sudden severe epigastric pain on the background of recurrent peptic ulcers combined with guarding and rebound tenderness in the epigastric region and hypotension on examination suggests a peptic ulcer perforation. Chest X-ray is the investigation of choice for the perforation of peptic ulcer to look for pneumoperitoneum.

Question 34

E. (Vitamin B12 deficiency) Fatigue and peripheral neuropathy for 2 months, on the background of type 1 diabetes mellitus and macrocytic anaemia on a blood film, suggests pernicious anaemia (autoimmune history), which causes a vitamin B12 deficiency. Whilst anaemia of chronic disease is an important differential given the autoimmune history, it would present with microcytic anaemia not macrocytic.

Question 35

C. (Serum caeruloplasmin) Difficulty writing and slurred speech for 4 months combined with a bilateral resting tremor and aggressiveness on examination with elevated AST and ALT suggest Wilson disease. Serum caeruloplasmin is the investigation of choice for Wilson's disease, where there would be a reduction observed as Wilson's disease is an autosomal recessive disorder characterised by excessive copper deposition in the tissues.

Question 36

D. (Subtotal gastrectomy) Persistent epigastric pain and unintentional weight loss combined with epigastric tenderness and a palpable Virchow's node (left supraclavicular lymph node) on examination with a large, ulcerated pyloric antrum mass on OGD suggests gastric cancer. Subtotal gastrectomy is the management of choice for gastric cancer for localised, distal gastric cancer, whilst proximal tumours can be treated with total gastrectomy. This allows for the preservation of a significant portion of the stomach and allows for better preservation of gastric function, including gastric reservoir capacity and food transit.

Question 37

A. (Achalasia) Dysphagia to solids and liquids and regurgitation for 5 months combined with a grossly expanded oesophagus with a bird's beak appearance on a barium swallow suggests achalasia. Achalasia is caused by a defect in the Auerbach's plexus therefore causing a failure of oesophageal peristalsis and of relaxation of the lower oesophageal sphincter (**A**chalasia = **A**uerbach's plexus).

Question 38

B. (CT pancreas) Back pain and unintentional weight loss, on the background of a 10-pack-year smoking history combined with scleral icterus, and palpable gall bladder on examination suggest pancreatic cancer (Courvoisier's law = palpable gall bladder not down to gallstones). CT pancreas is the investigation of choice for pancreatic cancer, which would demonstrate a mass in the pancreas and the extent of local or distant spread.

Question 39

B. (Haemochromatosis) Arthralgia and RUQ pain combined with skin hyperpigmentation and hepatomegaly on examination suggests haemochromatosis. Haemochromatosis is an autosomal recessive condition caused by a mutation in the HFE gene, which is responsible for hepcidin production, causing iron accumulation (4H's: HFE, Hepatomegaly, High iron and Hepatocellular Carcinoma).

Question 40

C. (CT abdomen) Severe abdominal pain, absolute constipation and bilious vomiting on the background of laparoscopic appendectomy combined with abdominal distension and tinkling bowel sounds on examination suggest small bowel obstruction. CT abdomen is the definitive investigation of choice for small bowel obstruction, because they have the highest sensitivity for detecting both the cause of the obstruction and extent of ischaemia thereby informing the need for urgent surgery.

Question 41

A. (Acute hepatitis B infection) Myalgia, arthralgia and mild abdominal discomfort for a week, on the background of IV drug use and excessive alcohol intake combined with scleral icterus and hepatomegaly on examination with being HBsAg and IgM anti-Hbc positive and anti-Hbs negative on serology suggest acute hepatitis B infection (IgM anti-Hbc positive is diagnostic).

Question 42

E. (Surgical resection) Steatorrhoea and unintentional weight loss for 3 months. On examination, he has scleral icterus and a palpable gall bladder with pancreatic malignancy with no invasion of local structures on CT pancreas, staged as T2N0M0 (stage I tumour), for which surgical resection is the management of choice. Pylorus-preserving pancreaticoduodenectomy (Whipple procedure) is preferred for tumours located in the head of the pancreas due to its advantages in preserving gastrointestinal function, reducing postoperative complications, and improving quality of life for patients undergoing surgery.

Question 43

D. (Anti-smooth muscle (SMA) antibodies) Amenorrhoea and fatigue, on the background of type 1 diabetes mellitus combined with spider naevi and hepatomegaly on examination, suggests autoimmune hepatitis. The specific antibodies are associated with type 1 autoimmune hepatitis, which has a peak incidence between the 4th and 6th decades of life whilst type 2 autoimmune hepatitis presents in children and young adults. Hence this woman likely has type 1 autoimmune hepatitis, which is associated with anti-smooth muscle antibodies.

Question 44

B. (Ivor-Lewis oesophagectomy) Progressively worsening dysphagia to solids and liquids, unintentional weight loss and episodic haematemesis for 4 months combined with mild cervical lymphadenopathy on examination and a T1N0M0 lesion in the lower third of the oesophagus on biopsy suggest oesophageal adenocarcinoma. Ivor-Lewis oesophagectomy is the management of choice for a T1N0M0 oesophageal adenocarcinoma and is the preferred oncological resection due to preservation of stomach function, reduction of anastomotic complications, and prevention of lymphatic spread.

Question 45

B. (Creon) Constant, dull epigastric pain radiating to the back, on the background of excess alcohol combined with malnourishment and a palpable, tender epigastric mass on examination pancreatic calcifications on AXR, suggests chronic pancreatitis. Creon (pancrealipase) is the management of choice for chronic pancreatitis to replace pancreatic enzymes and aid digestion. A coeliac plexus block would be indicated if there is a persistent pain that is refractory to other treatments and endoscopic decompression indicated if there is a pancreatic pseudocyst.

Question 46

D. (Pneumatic dilatation) Progressive odynophagia to solids and liquids for 6 months combined with an unremarkable examination and a dilated oesophagus with a bird's beak appearance on barium swallow suggests achalasia. Pneumatic dilation (which uses air-inflated balloons to apply mechanical stretch to the lower oesophageal sphincter to tear its muscle fibres) is the first-line management for achalasia and is preferred to surgical options such as Heller cardiomyotomy.

Question 47

B. (Liver CT) RUQ pain and unintentional weight loss on the background of chronic hepatitis B infection combined with scleral icterus and hepatomegaly on examination, with an elevated AFP level, suggests hepatocellular carcinoma. Chronic hepatitis B infection leads to continuous viral replication within hepatocytes, resulting in the production of viral proteins, particularly the HBV X protein (HBx). HBx has been shown to play a crucial role in hepatocarcinogenesis by promoting cellular proliferation, inhibiting apoptosis, and disrupting cell cycle regulation Liver CT is the diagnostic investigation of choice for hepatocellular carcinoma and is indicated if there is elevated alpha-fetoprotein and/or abnormal ultrasound with a focal liver lesion.

Question 48

B. (Enhanced liver fibrosis blood test) Fatigue and RUQ discomfort on the background of T2DM, with hepatomegaly and a "bright liver" on liver US suggests non-alcoholic fatty liver disease (NAFLD) or non-alcoholic steatohepatitis (NASH). The guidelines suggest the use of an enhanced liver fibrosis blood test to check for advanced fibrosis, which is a combination of hyaluronic acid + procollagen III + tissue inhibitor of metalloproteinase 1 to calculate an ELF score (a score above 10.51) suggests advanced fibrosis).

Question 49

D. (Macrogol and senna) Abdominal bloating with constipation for 2 weeks, postsurgery where she has been managing her pain with oxycodone suggests opioid-induced constipation. The management of opioid-induced constipation is with an osmotic laxative such as macrogol and a stimulant laxative such as senna, with bulk-forming laxatives contraindicated because opioids prevent peristalsis of the increased bulk potentially leading to bowel obstruction.

Question 50

D. (Every 6 months) Frequent heartburn and regurgitation for 8 months, not helped by antacids, with metaplastic change (squamous epithelium of the oesophagus is replaced by columnar epithelium) and dysplasia (irregular mucosal pits), suggests Barrett's oesophagus. The evidence of low-grade dysplasia indicated radiofrequency ablation as the management for complete eradication, as well as endoscopic surveillance at 6-monthly intervals for 1 year and then annually unless there is a reversion to nondysplastic Barrett oesophagus.

Question 51

D. (Prednisolone) Right upper quadrant pain (RUQ) for 3 months on the background of excessive alcohol consumption combined with RUQ abdominal tenderness on examination and increased GGT and an AST: ALT ratio >2 suggests alcoholic hepatitis. Prednisolone is used to treat acute alcoholic hepatitis as it has been shown to risk death within 28 days; although it should be started with caution because it is contraindicated in patients with GI bleeding, active infection or hepatorenal syndrome.

Question 52

E. (Venesection) Arthralgia and erectile dysfunction, on the background of both parents having family liver issues (autosomal recessive) combined with skin hyperpigmentation and tender hepatomegaly on examination and an abnormally low liver signal on MRI (iron accumulation reduces parenchymal signal intensity), suggests haemochromatosis. Venesection (therapeutic phlebotomy) is the management of choice for haemochromatosis, with the therapeutic intention of the patient's bone marrow being stimulated to make new red cells using the iron they have in storage.

Question 53

D. (Paracentesis) The triad of fever, abdominal pain and increasing ascites suggests spontaneous bacterial peritonitis, on the background of cirrhosis. The diagnostic investigation for SBP is paracentesis, which looks for a raised neutrophil count (>250 cells/uL), because in SBP the bacteria cannot be phagocytosed by neutrophils, as a lack of opsonisation caused by low complement levels in advanced cirrhosis. This means more neutrophils are realised to compensate.

Question 54

E. (Oral vancomycin + IV metronidazole) Nonbloody diarrhoea on the background of cefaclor usage combined with the positive stool finding of *Clostridium difficile* toxin suggests a *C. difficile* infection. This woman has a life-threatening infection as she is hypotensive (Public Health England Severity Scale), for which oral vancomycin and IV metronidazole are the first-line management. Other factors that are classified as severe are partial or complete ileus, toxic megacolon, or CT evidence of severe disease.

Question 55

A. (Endoscopic dilation) Globus and dysphagia, especially with dry foods, on the background of atopy with white mucosal plaques (eosinophilic infiltration) and oesophageal stenosis on OGD (likely to be the cause of his chest discomfort) suggests eosinophilic oesophagitis. Whilst it is often managed with a high-dose PPI or corticosteroid, the presence of oesophageal narrowing or stricture indicates endoscopic oesophageal dilation,

Question 56

E. (Oral ciprofloxacin) Abdominal distension and right upper quadrant pain on the background of advanced cirrhosis combined with shifting dullness on examination and a protein concentration of 14 g/L on ascitic tap suggest a risk of spontaneous bacterial peritonitis (SBP). NICE recommends offering prophylactic oral ciprofloxacin or norfloxacin for people with cirrhosis and ascites with an ascitic protein of <15 g/L until the ascites have resolved due to the risk of SBP.

Question 57

E. (Transient elastography) Ascites, abdominal pain and a fine tremor in the hands, which, combined with chronic alcohol usage, suggest cirrhosis. NICE suggests transient elastography screening for cirrhosis in certain situations, such as in hepatitis C infection and in women who drink over 35 units of alcohol per week for a sustained period of time. Transient elastrography is a noninvasive, rapid, and reproducible method allowing evaluation of liver fibrosis by measurement of liver stiffness, and is preferred over liver biopsy if both are available.

Question 58

C. (Oral fidaxomicin) Nonbloody diarrhoea and colicky pain after recent hospitalisation on the background of a similar episode 6 weeks ago managed with vancomycin suggests another episode of *C.difficile* colitis. Oral fidaxomicin treats *C. difficile* infections if there is a recurrent episode within 12 weeks of symptom resolution. Fidaxomicin is preferred for recurrence due to it being a narrower spectrum antibiotic, lower recurrence rates, reduced impact on the gut microbiota and a favourable safety profile. Metronidazole is used as either third-line therapy for a first episode of *C.difficile* colitis or along with oral vancomycin for life-threatening infection. IV vancomycin is not indicated however as it is not excreted into the GI lumen, thereby not having therapeutic value.

Question 59

A. (Glucuronosyl transferase) A young man with episodes of jaundice after exertion, on the background of no FH of liver disease, with elevated unconjugated bilirubin suggests Gilbert syndrome. Gilbert syndrome is caused by a deficiency in glucoronosyl transferase, the key enzyme in bilirubin glucuronidation (the conjugation of indirect bilirubin), which is why there are high levels of unconjugated bilirubin in Gilbert's.

Question 60

E. (Negative, Positive, Negative) HbsAg implies active infection, with 1-6 months associated with acute hepatitis B infection and >6 months suggesting chronic hepatitis B infection, anti-HBs is a marker of immunity, either after exposure or immunisation and anti-HBc implies that they have had infection either previously or currently. Therefore, previous hepatitis B immunisation would suggest that only anti-HBs is positive but the other two would be negative because they have not had an infection in the past.

Question 61

E. (Pharyngeal pouch) Dysphagia to solids, Globus and halitosis for 3 months combined with a palpable mass at the level of the cricoid cartilage suggest a pharyngeal pouch. A pharyngeal pouch is defined as a posteromedial diverticulum through Killian's dehiscence (the area of muscular weakness is a triangular region formed between the inferior pharyngeal constrictor and the cricopharyngeus).

Question 62

D. (Primary biliary cirrhosis) Fatigue and pruritus, with xanthelasma and hepatomegaly on examination, positive AMA M2 and IgM antibodies and small bile duct destruction and lymphocytic infiltration on liver biopsy suggest primary biliary cirrhosis. Primary biliary cirrhosis is an autoimmune slow, progressive destruction of the small bile ducts in the liver causing cholestasis. The specific AMA in PBC is against the pyruvate-dehydrogenase complex.

Question 63

B. (Vitamin B3 deficiency) Confusion and diarrhoea for a week combined with a scaly, erythematous rash and confusion on examination suggest vitamin B3 deficiency, also known as pellagra (dermatitis, dementia and diarrhoea triad).

Question 64

D. (Laxative abuse) Colonoscopy showing abnormal colon pigmentation, with PAS staining showing pigment-laden macrophages within the mucosa, suggesting melanosis coli. Melanosis coli is an abnormal pigmentation of the colon, commonly associated with laxative abuse, especially anthraquinone laxatives such as senna. The abnormal pigmentation is caused by apoptotic cells taken up by macrophages.

Question 65

E. (Jejunal biopsy) Episodic diarrhoea, epigastric pain, unintentional weight loss for 3 months combined with ankle swelling, tender hepatomegaly and skin hyperpigmentation on examination suggests Whipple's disease, which is caused by *Tropheryma whipplei*. A jejunal biopsy is the investigation of choice for Whipple disease to look for deposition of macrophages containing periodic acid-Schiff granules, caused by *Tropheryma whipplei* replicating within macrophages.

Question 66

C. (Gallstone ileus) Severe RUQ pain, bilious vomiting and absolute constipation for 48 hours combined with abdominal distension on examination and small bowel dilation, pneumobilia and a calcified gallstone outside the gall bladder (Rigler's triad) on imaging suggest gallstone ileus. Gallstone ileus is a small bowel obstruction caused by an impaction of a gallstone.

Question 67

A. (Abdominal US) Severe, cramping abdominal pain, intermittent vomiting and jelly-like blood in the stool combined with a tender abdomen with guarding on examination and a RUQ mass on imaging suggests intussusception. Intussusception is caused by the invagination of one portion of the bowel into the lumen of the adjacent bowel. The investigation for intussusception is an abdominal US to look for a target-like mass, caused by concentric alternating echogenic and hypoechoic bands caused by the invagination of the bowel.

Question 68

A. (Cholestyramine) Chronic diarrhoea associated with steatorrhoea on the background of laparoscopic cholecystectomy combined with a 12% retention on the SeHCAT scan (>15% is normal) suggests bile acid malabsorption. The management for bile acid malabsorption is bile acid sequestrants like cholestyramine, which lower LDL cholesterol and thereby reduce bile acid production.

Question 69

E. (Hypophosphataemia) Severe muscle weakness and shortness of breath, after aggressive nutritional rehabilitation for anorexia nervosa suggests refeeding syndrome. The most likely electrolyte abnormality would be hypophosphataemia, which is caused by the shift from fat to carbohydrate metabolism which utilises phosphate in patients with chronic malnutrition causing further depletion.

Question 70

A. (Endoscopic diverticulectomy) Dysphagia, especially solid food and globus for 5 months combined with halitosis and outpouching of the posterior hypopharyngeal wall on barium swallow suggests a pharyngeal pouch. Endoscopic diverticulectomy is the management of choice for a pharyngeal pouch, because of its minimally invasive nature, reduced risk of complications, and shorter recovery times.

Question 71

C. (Boerhaave's syndrome) Sudden central, tearing chest pain after suffering from food poisoning 24 hours ago and vomiting every 2 hours since, combined with chest crepitations, with a distal rupture on the left side of the oesophagus on CT contrast swallow suggest Boerhaave syndrome. Boerhaave syndrome is the sudden rupture of the oesophagus due to vomiting causing the cricopharyngeus muscle to not relax, building up intra-oesophageal pressure.

Question 72

A. (Enterolithotomy) Severe, sudden RUQ pain and abdominal swelling combined with a palpable RUQ mass and generalized abdominal tenderness on examination, with small bowel dilation, pneumobilia and a calcified gallstone outside the gall bladder (Rigler's triad) on imaging suggest gallstone ileus. Enterolithotomy is the management of choice for gallstone ileus to extract the gallstone, especially when the gallstone is too large or impacted to be safely retrieved endoscopically or fragmented using lithotripsy techniques.

Question 73

A. (Hepatic vein angioplasty) The triad of sudden-onset abdominal pain, ascites (causing abdominal distension) and tender hepatomegaly suggest Budd-Chiari syndrome. The oral contraceptive pill is thought to cause Budd-Chiari syndrome, by increasing antithrombin III levels, which can predispose individuals to thrombus formation within the hepatic veins. This can lead to venous obstruction and subsequent Budd-Chiari syndrome. Hepatic vein angioplasty is the management for Budd-Chiari syndrome to restore hepatic blood flow.

Question 74

D. (Primary oesophageal repair) Severe chest pain radiating to the back after forceful vomiting, after having 20 units of alcohol preceding the vomiting episode combined with neck and chest crepitations on palpation and a distal rupture of the left side of the oesophagus on imaging suggests Boerhaave syndrome. Thoracotomy and primary oesophageal repair using a two-layer closure is the management of choice with a stent placement being preferred in inoperable patients (e.g. high-performance status).

Question 75

E. (Plummer-Vinson syndrome) The triad of glossitis, iron-deficiency anaemia and dysphagia suggests Plummer-Vinson syndrome, which is thought to occur due to chronic iron deficiency leading to mucosal atrophy and formation of thin, membranous webs in the proximal oesophagus. These webs can cause mechanical obstruction, resulting in dysphagia. Patients typically present with difficulty swallowing solid foods, which is often accompanied by fatigue and pallor due to chronic iron deficiency anaemia.

Question 76

C. (Fasting gastrin level) Persistent epigastric pain and diarrhoea for 2 months, on the background of peptic ulcers not improved by PPIs combined with scleral icterus and epigastric tenderness on examination, suggests Zollinger-Ellison syndrome. Zollinger-Ellison is characterised by the presence of gastrinomas leading to increased gastric acid secretions which leads to treatment-resistant peptic ulcers. Fasting gastrin level is the investigation for Zollinger-Ellison syndrome as a gastrin-secreting tumour of the duodenum/pancreas causes it.

Question 77

C. (Salmonella typhi) RUQ pain, jaundice, on the background of recurrent episodes of pyogenic cholangitis combined with tender hepatomegaly and a double target sign on liver CT suggests a pyogenic liver abscess. *Salmonella typhi* is a rare cause of pyogenic liver abscess (the most common cause is *Escherichia coli*) but in the context of recurrent pyogenic cholangitis, it is the most likely cause.

Question 78

D. (Rifaximin) Chronic diarrhoea and abdominal discomfort on the background of recurrent UTIs treated with broad-spectrum antibiotics, combined with abdominal bloating and a positive hydrogen breath test, suggest small bowel bacterial overgrowth syndrome (SBBOS). The management of choice for SBBOS is rifaximin (a rifamycin antibiotic) due to its unlikelihood for bacteria to form antibiotic resistance

Question 79

B. (Absence of ganglion cells in the myenteric and submucosal plexus) Failure to pass meconium, with an empty rectal vault on examination is highly suggestive of Hirschprung's disease. It is caused by parasympathetic neuroblasts failing to migrate from the neural crest to the distal colon, leading to an absence of ganglion cells in the myenteric and submucosal plexuses causing uncoordinated peristalsis. Whilst cystic fibrosis can also cause meconium ileus, the presence of an empty rectal vault on DRE suggests Hirschsprung's disease.

Question 80

C. (Oral co-trimoxazole) Confusion and malodorous diarrhoea on the background of asthma combined with ophthalmoplegia and skin hyperpigmentation on examination and macrophage deposition containing PAS granules on a jejunal biopsy suggests Whipple disease. Guidelines suggest the management for Whipple disease with CNS involvement (i.e., signs of confusion, ophthalmoplegia) is oral co-trimoxazole because it has the lowest relapse rates.

Respiratory 18

EXPLANATIONS

Question 1

B. (Bronchiectasis) Productive cough with purulent sputum and occasional haemoptysis, on the background of recurrent chest infections combined with bilateral clubbing and coarse crepitations suggests bronchiectasis. Bronchiectasis has dilated, thickened bronchial walls with tramline markings on CXR suggesting cylindrical bronchiectasis, which is the most common type.

Question 2

E. (Pneumothorax) Pleuritic chest pain and dyspnoea on the background of a seven-pack-year smoking history combined with decreased breath sounds and hyperresonance to percussion suggests a pneumothorax. Pneumothorax is caused by lung collapse and hence would present with an absence of lung markings on CXR.

Question 3

A. (Asthma) Sudden dyspnoea and an expiratory wheeze with an atopic history and triggers like cold weather suggest asthma. This is further suggested by a positive fractional nitric oxide (FeNO) test, where >40 parts per billion is positive for adults. The FeNO test measures inflammation of the airways as nitric oxide production is linked to increased inflammation.

Question 4

C. (Chronic obstructive pulmonary disease) Worsening dyspnoea and a productive cough, with a chronic smoking history (40 pack years) combined with expiratory bilateral wheeze, suggests chronic obstructive pulmonary disease (COPD).

Question 5

E. (Salbutamol) Dyspnoea and cough, exacerbated by night, on the background of atopy (eczema) combined with bilateral expiratory wheeze on examination and diurnal variability on PEFR suggest asthma. The first-line management for asthma is short-acting beta2 agonists (SABA) such as salbutamol, which inhibit bronchial smooth muscle contraction thereby making it easier to breathe.

Question 6

C. (Oseltamivir) Guidelines suggest the use of oral oseltamivir for influenza A (confirmed by rapid antigen testing in this scenario) if it can be started within 48 hours of symptom onset or if the patient is from an "at risk" group.

Question 7

D. (COVID-19) Fever and progressive dyspnoea on the background of no recent travel combined with bilateral crepitations and positive SARS-CoV-2 confirms COVID-19.

Question 8

E. (Signet ring sign) Persistent cough, producing yellow-green sputum, on the background of recurrent respiratory infections combined with finger clubbing, coarse crepitations and a bilateral expiratory wheeze on examination suggests bronchiectasis. Signet ring sign is when the dilated bronchus and accompanying pulmonary artery branch are seen in bronchiectasis cross-sections.

Question 9

D. (Postbronchodilator spirometry) Progressive dyspnoea and a chronic, productive cough on the background of a 40-pack-year smoking history combined with a bilateral expiratory wheeze suggest COPD. Postbronchodilator spirometry is the diagnostic investigation in COPD to differentiate it from asthma (which has bronchodilator reversibility).

Question 10

C. (33%–50%) An inability to complete full sentences with subcutaneous emphysema on imaging on the background of asthma suggests acute severe asthma. The PEFR associated with acute severe asthma is 33%–50%.

Question 11

C. (Inspiratory muscle training) Persistent, productive cough and dyspnoea for 9 months, on the background of recurrent respiratory infections combined with bilateral coarse crepitations on examination and enlarged bronchi with a signet ring sign on imaging, suggests bronchiectasis. Inspiratory muscle training is the management of choice for noncystic fibrosis-related bronchiectasis, to enhance muscle strength and endurance and thereby alleviate dyspnoea.

Question 12

A. (Chest X-ray) Sudden pleuritic chest pain and dyspnoea on the background of Marfan syndrome combined with decreased breath sounds and right-sided hyperresonant percussion on examination suggest a secondary pneumothorax. A chest X-ray is the diagnostic investigation for pneumothorax, to look for absent lung markings caused by the collapsed lung.

Question 13

C. (Respiratory acidosis) Acute dyspnoea and chest tightness, on the background of asthma, combined with tachypnoea, a bilateral expiratory wheeze and accessory muscle usage suggest an acute asthma exacerbation. Her ABG shows acidosis (pH <7.35) and an elevated PCO_2 with normoxaemia suggesting respiratory acidosis without compensation as the bicarbonate is normal.

Question 14

E. (Tension pneumothorax) Chest pain after a stab wound combined with right-sided hyperresonance and absent breath sounds on examination, left-sided tracheal deviation and an absence of lung markings on the right on imaging suggests a tension pneumothorax.

Question 15

A. (Atelectasis) Dyspnoea and chest pain postoperatively, with dullness to percussion and decreased breath sounds over the right lung base and right basilar opacification and right-sided tracheal deviation on imaging suggests atelectasis. Atelectasis can occur in surgery as anaesthesia can cause mucus plug formation because you are unable to cough and clear mucus.

Question 16

D. (pH 7.51, PO_2 11.6 kPa, PCO_2 4.4 kPa and bicarbonate 25 mmol/L) Dizziness and dyspnoea secondary to stress, on the background of GAD combined with tachycardia, tachypnoea but no signs of hypoxia suggests hyperventilation. Hyperventilation is associated with respiratory alkalosis; hence, we would see reduced PCO_2 and increased pH.

Question 17

C. (Ipratropium) Chronic cough and exertional dyspnoea on the background of a 25-pack-year history combined with decreased breath sounds bilaterally and prolonged expiration, with an FEV1/FVC ratio of 0.62 (obstructive pattern) suggesting COPD. The first-line management for COPD is a short-acting beta2-agonist (SABA) or short-acting muscarinic antagonist (SAMA), with ipratropium being a SAMA.

Question 18

A. (*Haemophilus influenzae*) Productive cough and dyspnoea combined with bilateral finger clubbing and coarse crepitations on examination with thick-walled dilated bronchi on CXR suggest bronchiectasis. *Haemophilus influenzae* is the most common organism isolated from sputum samples of patients with bronchiectasis.

Question 19

E. (Video-assisted thoracoscopic surgery) Sudden dyspnoea and pleuritic chest pain on the background of recurrent pneumothoraces combined with decreased breath sounds and hyperresonant percussion on examination with pneumothorax on imaging. The management for recurrent pneumothoraces is video-assisted thoracoscopic surgery (VATS), which has shown to reduce recurrent pneumothorax rates from 25% to less than 5%.

Question 20

B. (Continuous positive airway pressure [CPAP]) Exertional dyspnoea combined with bilateral ankle pitting oedema and bibasilar, fine crepitations on examination combined with cardiomegaly and Kerley B lines on imaging suggest acute heart failure. He is unresponsive to treatment, which suggests accompanying respiratory failure, and hence, the management of choice is CPAP. CPAP improves V/Q matching and changes the cardiac output in patients with respiratory failure secondary to heart failure.

Question 21

A. (Acute bronchitis) Productive cough and sore throat for a week, with no fever, chest pain or dyspnoea combined with bilateral scattered wheezes and coarse crepitations on examination suggests acute bronchitis.

Question 22

E. (Tuberculosis) Persistent cough and unintentional weight loss for 2 months, on the background of HIV combined with bilateral lymphadenopathy and crepitations in the right upper lobe of the lung on examination with right upper lobe consolidation and right-sided hilar enlargement suggests tuberculosis.

Question 23

E. (Pneumonia) Worsening productive cough and pleuritic chest pain on the background of hypertension combined with decreased breath sounds and bronchial breathing on the left side and lobar consolidation in the left lower lung lobe on imaging suggests pneumonia.

Question 24

C. (*Mycobacterium tuberculosis*) Productive cough and haemoptysis for 2 months combined with supraclavicular lymphadenopathy and bilateral crepitations with bilateral hilar lymphadenopathy on examination suggest tuberculosis. The causative organism for tuberculosis is *Mycobacterium tuberculosis*.

Question 25

D. (Sarcoidosis) Unintentional weight loss and a dry cough on the background of rheumatoid arthritis combined with erythema nodosum and lupus pernio on examination with hypercalcaemia and bilateral hilar lymphadenopathy on imaging suggests sarcoidosis.

Question 26

A. (Cystic fibrosis) Productive cough on the background of recurrent chest infection combined with lungs that are hyperresonant to percussion, and a bilateral wheeze on examination with multiple dilated bronchi on imaging suggests cystic fibrosis. Her sweat test is >60 mmol/L which is diagnostic for cystic fibrosis.

Question 27

C. (Extrinsic allergic alveolitis) Recurrent productive cough and dyspnoea, exacerbated by cleaning hay in the stables and improved when away from work combined with bibasilar inspiratory crepitations on examination and lymphocytosis on bronchoalveolar lavage suggest extrinsic allergic alveolitis.

Question 28

E. (*Staphylococcus aureus*) Dyspnoea and a productive cough, on the background of IV drug use combined with decreased breath sounds and bronchial breathing on the right side on examination, suggests pneumonia. Given the history of IV drug use, *Staphylococcus aureus* is the most likely causative organism.

Question 29

C. (Lymph node biopsy) Dyspnoea, dry cough and unintentional weight loss combined with lupus pernio and erythema nodosum on examination suggest sarcoidosis. There is no one diagnostic investigation for sarcoidosis but a lymph node biopsy can be used to look for noncaseating granulomas.

Question 30

B. (Lung abscess) Persistent cough with foul-smelling sputum and unintentional weight loss over 3 months, on the background of alcohol misuse combined with decreased breath sounds over the left lower lung lobe and a cavitary lesion with an air-fluid level in the left lower lobe on imaging suggest a lung abscess.

Question 31

D. (Lower zone fibrosis) Gradually worsened exercise tolerance and a dry cough for 2 years, on the background of an occupational history of shipbuilding and insulation installation (asbestos exposure red flag) for 30 years combined with bilateral finger clubbing and bibasal inspiratory crepitations on examination suggests asbestosis. Asbestosis is associated with lower zone fibrosis on imaging.

Question 32

C. (Polysomnography) Daytime somnolence, morning headaches, loud snoring combined with an enlarged neck circumference, tonsils and hypertension on examination suggest obstructive sleep apnoea (OSA). Polysomnography is the investigation of choice for OSA to identify and characterise nature of apnoeic episodes.

Question 33

A. (CFTR) Persistent, productive cough and steatorrhoea on the background of recurrent respiratory infections combined with bilateral crepitations and a barrel-shaped chest on examination with a sweat chloride level >60 mmol/L suggest cystic fibrosis. Cystic fibrosis is caused by a defect in the CFTR gene, which codes a cAMP-regulated chloride channel, that maintains salt and water balance, with the defect causing dehydration of secretions such as mucus.

Question 34

A. (Acute respiratory distress syndrome [ARDS]) Cyanosis and diaphoresis after admission for severe pneumonia with bilateral coarse crepitations and decreased breath sounds on examination with a decreased PaO_2/FiO_2 and diffuse bilateral infiltrates on imaging (meeting the Berlin Criteria) suggest ARDS.

Question 35

E. (Rifampicin, isoniazid, pyrazinamide and ethambutol) Chronic cough and night sweats, on the background of recent Asian travel combined with decreased right lung base breath sounds on examination with right upper lobe consolidation on imaging and acid-fast bacilli on sputum culture suggests tuberculosis. The management for tuberculosis is the RIPE regimen (rifampicin, isoniazid, pyrazinamide and ethambutol), with pyrazinamide and ethambutol for 2 months and rifampicin and isoniazid for an extra 4 months.

Question 36

E. (FEV1 = reduced, FEV1/FVC = increased) Exertional dyspnoea and a dry cough, on the background of being a dockyard worker (asbestos exposure red flag) combined with bibasilar end-inspiratory crepitations on examination and basal opacities obscuring the cardiac borders on imaging, suggest asbestosis. As asbestosis is a restrictive lung disease, we would expect a reduced FEV1 and a significantly decreased FVC, which would cause a normal/increased FEV1/FVC.

Question 37

C. (Right inferior bronchus) Dyspnoea and coughing fits after playing with Lego combined with stridor and reduced air entry on the right and continued right-sided lung expansion on an expiratory chest X-ray suggest an inhaled foreign body on the right side. The foreign body is more likely to end up in the inferior bronchus than the superior bronchus, as it is the most direct path for the object with the least resistance.

Question 38

E. (Urgent admission to hospital) Dyspnoea, confusion and a productive cough combined with dullness when percussing the right lower lobe with confusion and right lower lobe consolidation on imaging suggests pneumonia. Management for pneumonia is dictated by the CURB/CRB-65 score, of which this woman has a score of 3 (respiratory rate >30, AMTS less than 9 and is aged over 65); therefore, the management is urgent admission to the hospital.

Question 39

A. (Bronchoscopy and EBUS-TBNA) Haemoptysis and unintentional weight loss combined with bilateral finger clubbing and a fixed, monophonic wheeze on examination with a solitary pulmonary nodule in the right middle lobe on imaging suggests lung cancer. Bronchoscopy and EBUS-TBNA are the investigation methods of choice for lung cancer, as this allows a biopsy to be taken to obtain a histological diagnosis.

Question 40

B. (*Klebsiella pneumoniae*) Fever and a cough producing red-currant jelly sputum on the background of liver cirrhosis due to chronic alcohol misuse combined with dullness to percussion in the right upper lobe and a cavitary lesion in the right upper lobe on imaging suggests pneumonia caused by *Klebsiella pneumoniae*.

Question 41

D. (Obstructive sleep apnoea) Excessive daytime somnolence and snoring combined with a very obese BMI (47 kg/m^2) and hypertension on examination suggests obstructive sleep apnoea (OSA), confirmed by an apnoea-hypopnoea index of 7 episodes per hour (>5 being diagnostic for OSA).

Question 42

B. (Atorvastatin) Productive cough and pleuritic chest pain, on the background of hypertension, type 2 diabetes mellitus and hypercholesterolemia, and a penicillin allergy combined with reduced breath sounds and bronchial breathing on examination suggests typical community-acquired pneumonia. Given the penicillin allergy, a macrolide antibiotic such as clarithromycin would be started. When combined with macrolides, atorvastatin can increase the risk of myopathy and rhabdomyolysis because it inhibits cytochrome P450 isoenzyme that metabolizes the statin; hence, it is contraindicated with clarithromycin.

Question 43

D. (Pirfenidone) Dry cough and progressive exertional dyspnoea for a year combined with bibasilar inspiratory crepitations on examination and bibasilar reticular opacities on imaging suggest idiopathic pulmonary fibrosis (IPF). Of the options provided, pirfenidone is the most appropriate management for IPF because it has been shown to reduce fibrosis, by decreasing fibroblast proliferation and influences transforming growth factor-beta (TGF-β)-mediated differentiation of fibroblasts into myofibroblasts.

Question 44

E. (Uveitis) Dry cough and dyspnoea for 6 months combined with painful red eyes (anterior uveitis), lupus pernio on examination and bilateral hilar lymphadenopathy on imaging suggest sarcoidosis. Steroids are indicated in sarcoidosis, in cases with hypercalcaemia, eye/heart/neurological involvement and patients with stage 2 or 3 sarcoidosis; hence, as uveitis is one of the ocular features associated with sarcoidosis, this is the correct answer.

Question 45

E. (Protein levels) Progressive dyspnoea and a dry cough on the background of congestive heart failure combined with decreased breath sounds and dull percussion on the right suggest pleural effusion, confirmed by his chest X-ray. The Light's criteria distinguish between a transudate and an exudate, with exudates having a protein level above 30 g/L and transudates having a protein level below 30 g/L.

Question 46

A. (Ethambutol) Pain with eye movement and vision loss, secondary to tuberculosis treatment combined with decreased visual acuity, suggests optic neuritis. Ethambutol is known to cause optic neuritis, which is thought to be through the chelation of copper disrupting oxidative phosphorylation, and causing a neurotoxic effect on the optic nerve.

Question 47

B. (Lofgren syndrome) Dry cough and dyspnoea for 4 days combined with erythema nodosum, polyarthralgia and a low-grade fever on examination and bilateral hilar lymphadenopathy on imaging suggests Lofgren syndrome (very acute presentation of sarcoidosis suggests Lofgren syndrome).

Question 48

C. (Renal cell carcinoma) Haemoptysis and unintentional weight loss on the background of a 30-pack-year smoking history combined with flank pain on examination and cannonball lesions on imaging, consistent with cannonball metastases, suggest renal cell carcinoma. Other less common causes of cannonball metastases are prostate and endometrial cancer.

Question 49

A. (Berlin criteria) Dyspnoea after severe acute pancreatitis combined with cyanosis and tachypnoea, with bilateral coarse crepitations on examination, a reduced PaO_2/FiO_2 ratio and diffuse bilateral infiltrates on imaging suggest acute respiratory distress syndrome (ARDS). ARDS' diagnostic criteria are Berlin criteria, which consist of the following:

- Acute onset within 1 week
- Bilateral infiltrates on chest X-ray
- Noncardiogenic
- PaO_2/FiO_2 <300 mmHg

Question 50

D. (Isocyanates) Recurrent coughing and dyspnoea after work while working in a car painting shop for 15 years, combined with bilateral expiratory wheezes and bronchodilator reversibility on spirometry, suggests occupational asthma. Isocyanates are the most common cause of occupational asthma, and occupations associated with isocyanates are spray painting and foam moulding.

Question 51

B. (Bronchiolitis) Worsening dry cough and dyspnoea after a recent upper respiratory tract infection in a child combined with nasal flaring and diffuse bilateral wheeze on examination with positive RSV pathogens on immunofluorescence suggests bronchiolitis.

Question 52

E. (Thoracoscopy and histology) Productive cough with haemoptysis and unintentional weight loss, on the background of being an insulation factory worker (asbestos exposure red flag) combined with dull percussion on the left side, and a large left-sided opacity causing irregular margins on imaging suggests mesothelioma. The diagnostic investigation for mesothelioma is thoracoscopy and histology, because it has the highest diagnostic yield (around 95%).

Question 53

C. (Prednisolone) Dyspnoea and a productive cough, on the background of asthma combined with a wheeze and multiple dilated bronchi on imaging (bronchiectasis); eosinophilia combined with bronchiectasis, suggests allergic bronchopulmonary aspergillosis. The first-line management for allergic bronchopulmonary aspergillosis is oral glucocorticoids like prednisolone to reduce inflammation.

Question 54

A. (Bilevel-positive airway pressure [BiPAP]) Difficulty breathing on the background of COPD combined with a barrel-shaped chest and a wheeze on examination. A poor response to treatment resulting in an ABG shows acidosis, hypercapnia and hypoxaemia. In COPD patients, there is an indication for noninvasive ventilation if a patient has a pH of between 7.25 and 7.35, and as this woman has hypercapnia and hypoxemia (Type 2 Respiratory Failure), BiPAP is the better choice than CPAP. This is because BiPAP would help the patient both inhale and exhale rather than just inhale (which is what CPAP does).

Question 55

A. (Alpha-1 antitrypsin deficiency) Chronic dyspnoea on the background of hepatocellular carcinoma combined with decreased breath sounds and a bilateral wheeze on examination and an FEV1/FVC of 0.63 (obstructive pattern) on spirometry suggests alpha-1 antitrypsin deficiency (COPD symptoms + lack of smoking).

Question 56

B. (Pancoast tumour) Unintentional weight loss and hoarseness of voice, on the background of 38 pack-year smoking history combined with bilateral finger clubbing and a fixed, monophonic wheeze on examination and a right apical opacification on imaging suggest a Pancoast tumour. The hoarseness of the voice is caused by the tumour compressing the recurrent laryngeal nerve.

Question 57

D. (Doxycycline) Headache and dry cough after recent bird exposure and myalgia and right-sided basilar crepitations with right lower lobe consolidation on imaging suggest psittacosis. The management of choice for psittacosis is tetracyclines such as doxycycline.

Question 58

C. (Egg-shell calcification of the hilar lymph nodes) Persistent cough and progressive dyspnoea, on the background of being a miner (silica exposure red flag) for 28 years combined with blueish discolouration of the lips and bibasal end-inspiratory fine crepitations on examination suggests silicosis. Egg-shell calcification of the hilar lymph nodes is seen in patients with silicosis and describes the peripheral calcification in these patients.

Question 59

B. (Asthma-COPD overlap syndrome) Progressively worsening dyspnoea and cough on the background of a 30-pack-year smoking history combined with bilateral expiratory wheezes on chest auscultation with an obstructive spirometry pattern with postbronchodilator reversibility suggests asthma-COPD overlap syndrome; due to the coexistence of asthma and COPD symptoms.

Question 60

A. (No follow-up needed) Excessive coughing not associated with worsening dyspnoea on the background of being a plumber combined with multiple nodular lesions in the upper lobes bilaterally on imaging suggests pleural plaques. Pleural plaques are the most benign form of asbestos-related lung disease and do not require any follow-up due to no chance of it progressing to malignancy.

Question 61

E. (Pulmonary hypertension) Progressive dyspnoea combined with normal observations, a loud S2 and an ejection systolic murmur on examination with right axis deviation and right ventricular suggests pulmonary hypertension. Although pulmonary hypertension can increase SBP, it will only affect the pulmonary artery pressures in milder cases and thereby keep SBP within the normal range.

Question 62

B. (Kartagener syndrome) Progressively worsening chronic cough, with occasional haemoptysis on the background of recurrent chest infections and infertility, with widespread coarse crepitations suggests Kartagener syndrome. The quiet heart sounds in this woman are likely down to dextrocardia, which is another feature associated with Kartagener syndrome. Kartagener syndrome, also known as primary ciliary dyskinesia, is characterised by a triad of sinus inversus, bronchiectasis and chronic sinusitis.

Question 63

B. (Co-trimoxazole) Dyspnoea and dry cough with scattered crepitations on examination, bilateral interstitial pulmonary infiltrates on imaging and ping-pong ball cysts on bronchoalveolar lavage suggest *pneumocystis jirovecii* pneumonia. Co-trimoxazole combines trimethoprim and sulfamethoxazole and is indicated first line in *P. jirovecii* pneumonia.

Question 64

D. (cANCA) Episodic haemoptysis and epistaxis for a week, combined with a saddle-shaped nose deformity and proptosis on examination, multiple cavitating, ill-defined lesions on imaging and epithelial crescents in the Bowman's capsule on biopsy suggest granulomatosis with polyangiitis. Granulomatosis with polyangiitis is associated with cANCA in 90% of patients which targets Proteinase 3 (PRTN3), a serine protease enzyme in neutrophil granulocytes.

Renal 19

EXPLANATIONS

Question 1

B. (Hypertension) Fatigue, loss of appetite and leg swelling on the background of type 2 diabetes mellitus combined with elevated blood pressure and mild pallor on examination, renal failure (elevated urea and creatinine) and reduced eGFR suggest chronic kidney disease. Hypertension is the most common cause of chronic kidney disease.

Question 2

A. (Acute interstitial nephritis) Maculopapular rash for a week after starting RIPE regimen for TB. The rash combined with renal failure (elevated urea and creatinine) and eosinophilia, suggests acute interstitial nephritis, a type of AKI characterised by interstitial infiltrate and oedema in connective tissue between the tubules. AIN is most commonly caused by drugs in particular antibiotics, so rifampicin is the most likely cause here.

Question 3

E. (Stop ibuprofen) Dyspnoea, reduced urine output and renal failure (elevated urea and creatinine) after post-operative pain relief suggests an AKI. As the symptoms came about after starting ibuprofen (NSAIDs are known to be nephrotoxic due to their inhibition of renal prostaglandins), the management should be to stop the ibuprofen.

Question 4

D. (Ramipril) A raised blood pressure, confirmed to be hypertension by ambulatory monitoring combined with elevated urea and creatinine, reduced eGFR and increased albumin:creatinine ratio (ACR) suggests chronic kidney disease. His ACR is >30 mg/mmol, so he should be started on an ACE inhibitor such as ramipril.

Question 5

B. (Acute tubular necrosis) Bilateral pitting oedema of the legs and dyspnoea after a recent inferior STEMI treated with PCI with contrast dye combined with renal failure (elevated urea and creatinine) suggests acute tubular necrosis. This is an AKI caused by necrosis of the renal tubular epithelial cells, for which the two main causes are ischaemia and nephrotoxins such as radiocontrast dye.

Question 6

B. (Stage 2) An eGFR of between 60 and 90 mL/min/1.73 m^2 suggests some kidney damage and is classified as stage 2 chronic kidney disease if there are abnormal U+Es or proteinuria, and this woman has elevated urea and creatinine; hence she has stage 2 CKD.

Question 7

E. (White cell casts) A large diffuse maculopapular rash and generalized back aches on the background of penicillin use combined with lower back tenderness associated with renal failure (elevated urea and creatinine) and eosinophilia suggest acute interstitial nephritis. White cell casts are the urinary casts associated with acute interstitial nephritis, as they are indicative of inflammation within the kidney parenchyma.

Question 8

C. (Metabolic acidosis) Confusion, nausea and vomiting combined with tachycardia after being admitted with AKI combined with Kussmaul respiration on examination suggest metabolic acidosis as heavy breathing is a compensatory mechanism to excrete carbon dioxide.

Question 9

E. (Furosemide + restrict dietary intake of potassium) Fluid overload on the background of alcohol excess with renal failure (elevated creatinine) and hyperkalaemia suggests an AKI. The hyperkalaemia is mild (<6.0 mmol/L with no ECG changes), and as he has a hypervolaemic AKI (pitting and pulmonary oedema), the management is furosemide and restriction of dietary intake of potassium.

Question 10

C. (Stage 2) Fatigue and decreased urine output, on the background of hypertension, with a creatinine raised >2 times above baseline and a urine output <0.5 mL/kg/h for >12 hours suggests stage 2 AKI as per the KDIGO criteria.

Question 11

B. (Serum creatine kinase) Severe muscular pain and dark red urine (myoglobinuria) on the background of a recent powerlifting competition combined with decreased limb ROM and brown granular casts on urinalysis suggest an ATN secondary to rhabdomyolysis. The investigation for rhabdomyolysis is creatine kinase (CK), with a significant elevation of CK (>5 times the upper limit of normal), suggesting rhabdomyolysis.

Question 12

E. (Raised serum urea:creatinine ratio) Dizziness and decreased urine output on the background of congestive heart failure, with ascites and hypotension suggests a prerenal uraemia, which is caused by hypoperfusion to the kidneys. Prerenal uraemia is associated with increased serum urea: creatinine ratio, due to increased reabsorption of urea in the proximal tubules but increased secretion of creatinine.

Question 13

A. (Haemodialysis) Gradually worsening dyspnoea, whilst recovering from an AKI secondary to rhabdomyolysis, has bilateral basal crepitations and pitting oedema of the ankles on examination and peri-hilar opacities on peri-hilar opacities suggests pulmonary oedema secondary to an AKI. Pulmonary oedema is an indication for haemodialysis treatment for an AKI, along with other complications of AKI such as acidosis, electrolyte disturbances, ingestion of toxins, overload and uraemia (AEIOU).

Question 14

D. (Polycystic kidney disease) Dull abdominal pain for 2 months, on the background of multiple urinary tract infections, combined with elevated blood pressure, bilateral flank masses and hepatomegaly on examination, haematuria on urinalysis and multiple liver cysts on abdominal US suggest polycystic kidney disease. Liver cysts are the most common extra-renal complication of PKD seen in up to 70% of patients.

Question 15

B. (Fatty casts) Periorbital oedema, pitting oedema of the lower limbs and dysuria for 3 days combined with hepatomegaly and proteinuria and hypoalbuminemia on urinalysis suggests nephrotic syndrome. As urinary casts are seen on urinalysis, fatty casts are associated with nephrotic syndrome, due to excess protein in the urine.

Question 16

B. (Renal US) Abdominal pain and haematuria, on the background of polycystic kidney disease, associated with bloating and dysuria combined with hypertension and mild tenderness and palpable kidneys, suggests polycystic kidney disease. Renal US is the investigation of choice for polycystic kidney disease, with the diagnostic criteria being as follows: two cysts, bilateral or unilateral, if aged <30 years, two cysts in both kidneys if aged between 30–59 years or four cysts in both kidneys if > 60 years.

Question 17

D. (Minimal change disease) Facial and leg oedema in a young boy with proteinuria and hypoalbuminaemia on urinalysis suggests nephrotic syndrome. Renal biopsy under electron microscopy shows podocyte fusion and effacement of foot processes, which, combined with him being young and nephrotic syndrome presentation, suggests minimal change disease.

Question 18

B. (Partial nephrectomy) Persistent right-sided flank pain, haematuria and unintentional weight loss combined with a right flank mass on examination and a heterogenous mass on the right kidney on CT abdomen suggest renal cell carcinoma. This is staged as T1N0M0, which should be treated with a partial nephrectomy as there are no contraindications.

Question 19

E. (Poststreptococcal glomerulonephritis) Periorbital oedema and dark urine, on the background of sore throat and fever 2 weeks ago combined with urinalysis showing proteinuria and haematuria suggests nephritic syndrome. His renal biopsy showing endothelial proliferation with neutrophils combined with presentation 2 weeks after sore throat suggests post-streptococcal glomerulonephritis. A similar presentation of nephritic syndrome after 2 days rather than 2 weeks, would suggest IgA nephropathy.

Question 20

E. (Renal artery stenosis) Sudden dyspnoea with no chest pain, on the background of poorly controlled hypertension combined with pulmonary oedema on CXR and a renal artery bruit, suggests renal artery stenosis as the underlying cause of her pulmonary oedema.

Question 21

B. (IgA nephropathy) Haematuria and intermittent flank pain for 24 hours, on the background of a recent upper respiratory tract infection that resolved 2 days ago combined with pitting oedema in the legs and urinalysis reveals proteinuria and haematuria, suggests nephritic syndrome. His renal biopsy shows mesangial hypercellularity, which, combined with his presentation after 2 days of infection, suggests IgA nephropathy.

Question 22

B. (Amlodipine + aspirin + statin) Headaches, on the background of hyperlipidaemia with hypertension and a left flank bruit on examination, raised total and LDL cholesterol and stenosis of the left renal artery >50%, suggest renal artery stenosis secondary to atherosclerosis. The man requires amlodipine to treat hypertension with aspirin and a statin to treat hypercholesterolaemia/atherosclerosis.

Question 23

A. (Antiglomerular basement membrane disease) Dyspnoea and a cough with occasional haemoptysis combined with a low-grade fever and bilateral crepitations on examination and proteinuria and haematuria on urinalysis and renal failure (elevated urea and creatinine) suggest anti-glomerular basement membrane disease. Signs of pulmonary haemorrhage occur in anti-GBM disease because circulating anti-GBM antibodies affect the kidneys and lungs primarily.

Question 24

B. (Fibromuscular dysplasia)cPoorly controlled hypertension, combined with nontender, nonpalpable kidneys and bruit on the left of the umbilicus and multiple outpouchings in both renal arteries (a string of beads) appearance on duplex US, suggest fibromuscular dysplasia causing renal artery stenosis.

Question 25

B. (Anti-GBM) Haemoptysis and haematuria for a week with a fever combined with protein and blood on urinalysis, renal failure (raised urea and creatinine) and linear IgG deposits along the basement membrane suggest antiglomerular basement membrane disease. Anti-GBM antibodies are the primary antibody associated with antiglomerular basement membrane disease and they primarily affect type IV collagen in the kidneys and lungs hence the presentation of glomerulonephritis with pulmonary haemorrhage.

Question 26

D. (Red cell casts) Facial and leg swelling and dark urine on the background of a self-resolved sore throat combined with a decreased urine output on examination and haematuria and proteinuria suggest nephritic syndrome. Red cell casts are associated with nephritic syndrome, due to the blood in the urine.

Question 27

E. (Tolvaptan) Lower back pain and fatigue, on the background of hypertension and a family history of kidney disease combined with palpable kidneys with tenderness and three fluid-filled sacs in the left kidney, suggests polycystic kidney disease (PKD). An eGFR of 51 mL/min/1.73 m^2 suggests stage 3 chronic kidney disease (eGFR between 30-59); hence, tolvaptan would be indicated for PKD.

Question 28

D. (Normal glomeruli) Facial and leg swelling for 4 days, on the background of gout, combined with normotension and hypoalbuminemia and proteinuria on urinalysis, suggests minimal change disease. Minimal change disease is associated with normal glomeruli on light microscopy, with a spike and dome appearance associated with membranous glomerulonephritis and Kimmelstiel-Wilson nodules associated with diabetic nephropathy.

Question 29

C. (Kimmelstiel-Wilson nodules) Severe facial oedema and pitting oedema to the of the thighs on the background of poorly controlled type 1 diabetes mellitus combined with an elevated HbA1c and proteinuria and hypoalbuminaemia suggest diabetic nephropathy. The build-up of collagen, lipid and immune cell deposits that eventually form Kimmelstiel-Wilson nodules in diabetic nephropathy.

Question 30

D. (Membranous glomerulonephritis) Intermittent facial and leg oedema and weight gain, on the background of vitiligo combined with hypoalbuminaemia and proteinuria on urinalysis and basement membrane thickening with spike and dome appearance, suggest membranous glomerulonephritis. Membranous glomerulonephritis is associated with autoimmune diseases like vitiligo but in most cases are idiopathic (associated with anti-phospholipase A2 antibodies in 70% of cases).

Question 31

D. (Plasmapheresis) Haemoptysis and haematuria for a week combined with proteinuria and haematuria on urinalysis and linear IgG deposits along the basement membrane on a renal biopsy suggest antiglomerular basement membrane (anti-GBM) disease. Plasmapheresis is the management of choice for anti-GBM disease, with the aim to reduce the amount of circulating antibodies.

Question 32

D. (Syndrome of inappropriate antidiuretic hormone secretion) Headache and myalgia, whilst recovering from a subarachnoid haemorrhage (SAH) combined with an elevated urinary Na^+ and urinary osmolality suggests syndrome of inappropriate antidiuretic hormone secretion (SIADH).

Question 33

B. (Eosinophilic granulomatosis with polyangiitis) Lower limb petechiae and haematuria, on the background of atopy combined with urinalysis showing nephritic syndrome (proteinuria and haematuria), suggests eosinophilic granulomatosis with polyangiitis. Whilst HSP is a differential to consider given the lack of a purpuric rash and the demographics of the patient (HSP is classically a paediatric presentation), we can exclude this.

Question 34

C. (Prednisolone) Facial and leg oedema associated with dyspnoea for a month, on the background of hepatitis C combined with subendothelial and mesangial immune deposits on a renal biopsy suggests membranoproliferative glomerulonephritis. Steroids like prednisolone are beneficial in membranoproliferative glomerulonephritis.

Question 35

C. (Henoch-Schonlein purpura) A palpable, purpuric rash over the buttocks and legs, lower limb joint pain and haematuria in a young child combined with tenderness and swelling over the knees and ankles suggests Henoch-Schonlein purpura. HSP, also known as IgA vasculitis, causes these symptoms by deposition of immune complexes containing IgA.

Question 36

A. (Amyloidosis) Fatigue and ankle swelling associated with systemic malignancy symptoms combined with ankle oedema and hepatomegaly on examination, proteinuria on urinalysis and apple-green birefringence of abdominal fat on Congo red staining suggests amyloidosis causing nephrotic syndrome. This is done by amyloid buildup in the kidney causing loss of protein in the urine and hypoalbuminaemia.

Question 37

B. (Focal segmental glomerulosclerosis) Fatigue and pitting oedema for a week, on the background of IgA nephropathy, with an elevated blood pressure on examination with areas of mesangial collapse on renal biopsy suggests focal segmental glomerulosclerosis.

Question 38

D. (*Staphylococcus epidermis*) Signs of peritonitis (tenderness and guarding) and a cloudy dialysis effluent suggest peritonitis secondary peritoneal dialysis. Coagulase-negative staphylococci are often indicated with *Staphylococcus epidermis* the most common cause of this.

Question 39

D. (cANCA) Recurrent nosebleeds and nasal stuffiness combined with a low-grade fever and signs of renal failure (elevated urea and creatinine) suggest granulomatosis with polyangiitis (GPA). Over 90% of patients with GPA are antineutrophil cytoplasmic antibody positive (cANCA), with proteinase 3 (PR3) being the most common antigen targeted.

Question 40

B. (Hepatorenal syndrome) Abdominal bloating and fever for 12 hours, on the background of liver cirrhosis and a neutrophil count >250 cells/μL in the ascitic fluid with the rapid increase of the serum creatinine to more than the upper limit of normal after an acute event suggests type 1 hepatorenal syndrome. While peritonitis or sepsis remain important differentials in patients with liver cirrhosis and ascites, the rapid deterioration in renal function observed in this case is more consistent with hepatorenal syndrome, as sepsis and peritonitis would have a more gradual onset of renal failure.

Question 41

D. (X-linked dominant) Haematuria for a week, on the background of similar shorter episodes and wearing hearing aids since birth combined with a soft and non-tender abdomen and bilateral sensorineural hearing loss on examination and elevated serum urea and creatinine suggests Alport syndrome. Alport syndrome is an X-linked dominant condition, characterised by sensorineural deafness and often requiring renal transplantation as 50% develop end-stage renal failure.

Neurology 20

EXPLANATIONS

Question 1

E. (Tension headache) A dull, stress-related headache described as a tight band around the head combined with an unremarkable examination suggests a tension headache. Migraines are classically unilateral and described as a throbbing pain rather than a tight-band.

Question 2

E. (Tonic-clonic seizure) Syncope for 2 minutes before regaining consciousness suggests a generalised seizure over a focal one. The stiffening (tonic phase) followed by the jerking movements of her limbs (clonic phase), suggests a tonic-clonic seizure.

Question 3

C. (Partial anterior circulation infarct) Confusion, Wernicke aphasia (fluent but impaired comprehension) and right-sided hemiparesis, on the background of hypertension, suggests a partial anterior circulation infarct (2/3 of the Bamford Stroke Classification for anterior circulation infarcts). The Bamford stroke classification is as follows: unilateral weakness (and/or sensory deficit) of the face, arm and leg, homonymous hemianopia and higher cerebral dysfunction (dysphasia, visuospatial disorder).

Question 4

A. (Cluster headache) A severe left-sided headache, associated with stabbing pain, on the background of similar episodes for 2 months combined with a 15-pack-year smoking history, suggests a cluster headache.

Question 5

E. (Sumatriptan and paracetamol) Recurrent throbbing right-sided headache, preceded by jagged crescents in the vision (visual aura); improved in a dark, quiet room and worsened by stress, suggesting a migraine. The first-line management for migraine is an oral triptan, i.e., sumatriptan with paracetamol/NSAID.

Question 6

B. (Chronic subdural haematoma) Progressively worsening intermittent headaches, confusion and difficulty walking on the background of a minor fall on the background of hypertension and mild cognitive impairment combined with a hypodense crescentic collection suggest a chronic subdural haematoma. An acute subdural would present with an hyperdense crescentic collection.

Question 7

D. (IV thrombolysis and thrombectomy) Broca aphasia (non-fluent speech but intact comprehension) for 3 hours combined with left-sided hemiplegia and homonymous hemianopia suggests a proximal anterior circulation. As the man presented within 4.5 hours of symptoms, IV thrombolysis with alteplase within 4.5 hours of symptom onset and thrombectomy within 6 hours of symptom onset is the appropriate management.

Question 8

A. (Aspirin) Left-sided hemiparesis and speech impairment that lasted 30 minutes on a background of hypercholesterolaemia and hypertension suggest a transient ischaemic attack. Aspirin is the management of choice for a TIA unless there are contraindications, such as a history of a bleeding disorder or anticoagulant therapy.

Question 9

C. (CT head) Right-sided resolved hemiplegia for 30 minutes, on the background of pulmonary embolism suggests a transient ischaemic attack. Urgent CT head needs to be performed to exclude the possibility of a haemorrhage in people on anticoagulants (such as apixaban).

Question 10

D. (Posterior circulation infarct) Sudden loss of consciousness for 5 minutes and postrecovery cerebellar signs (slurred staccato-like speech, dysmetria, nystagmus and ataxia) suggests a posterior circulation infarct, which affects the vertebrobasilar arteries and can be characterized by cerebellar pathological signs.

Question 11

C. (Lewy body dementia) The triad of visual hallucinations, Parkinsonian features (shuffling gait and bilateral resting tremors, improved by voluntary movements) and mild cognitive impairment (MMSE between 21 and 26) suggests Lewy body dementia.

Question 12

B. (Cushing's triad) Nausea and headache after a car accident, on the background of meningioma combined with a widened pulse pressure, bradycardia and irregular breathing on observations and a reduced GCS, with dilated pupils that are nonreactive to light on examination suggests a raised intracranial pressure. The triad of widened pulse pressure, bradycardia and irregular breathing is called Cushing's triad. Gradenigo's triad is characterised by sixth nerve palsy, persistent ear discharge and deep-seated retroorbital pain and Trotter's triad is a complex constellation of symptoms associated with nasopharyngeal carcinoma.

Question 13

D. (Loss of neurons in the basal nucleus of Meynert) Amnesia and agnosia, combined with his moderative cognitive impairment on MMSE, suggest Alzheimer disease (AD). AD is associated with cerebrocortical atrophy with a particular loss of neurons in the basal nucleus of Meynert.

Question 14

A. (IV lorazepam) An episode of loss of consciousness, tongue biting, and body stiffness suggests a seizure. IV lorazepam was given per status epilepticus guidelines; however, this did not terminate the seizure. Although one dose of IV lorazepam has been given, another dose can be given 10–20 minutes after the first dose. If two doses of benzodiazepines have failed, then alternatives such as phenytoin or levetiracetam should be trialled.

Question 15

E. (Xanthochromia) Severe occipital pain 3 hours ago, on the background of adult polycystic kidney disease combined with photophobia and neck stiffness on examination, suggests a subarachnoid haemorrhage but her CT head is normal. The breakdown of red blood cells causes xanthochromia, which is representative of a subarachnoid haemorrhage on lumbar puncture.

Question 16

D. (Global aphasia) Sudden right-sided hemiplegia, only being able to communicate through gestures and laboured speech with impaired comprehension and repetition, suggests global aphasia (all aspects of speech affected).

Question 17

C. (Circle of Willis) Sudden, occipital thunderclap headache on the background of Ehlers-Danlos syndrome, combined with signs of meningism (neck stiffness and photophobia) and basal cistern hyperdensities on CT head, suggests subarachnoid haemorrhage. The circle of Willis would be affected in a subarachnoid haemorrhage, as it is the most common location for a berry aneurysm (the most common cause of SAH) to burst.

Question 18

D. (Duplex US) Left arm weakness on the background of hypercholesterolaemia combined with a carotid bruit and Broca's aphasia (non-fluent speech, with intact comprehension) and a well-defined area of low density in the right frontoparietal area on CT head, suggests a right middle cerebral artery infarct. The most appropriate investigation is duplex US to investigate the carotid bruit and ascertain whether the woman has carotid artery stenosis.

Question 19

A. (High-flow oxygen) Severe right-sided headache lasting for an hour, on the background of multiple episodes of similar severe pain for a month, combined with restlessness and right eyelid swelling and redness on examination, which suggests an acute cluster headache. High-flow oxygen is the management for an acute cluster headache, as it is thought that oxygen contracts cerebral vessels which alleviates the cerebral vessel dilation that a cluster headache causes.

Question 20

D. (Middle meningeal artery) Loss of consciousness after head trauma before a lucid interval and then deteriorating to a GCS of 11/15 with a hyperdense biconvex collection on CT head suggests an extradural haemorrhage. The middle meningeal artery is often affected as the pterion, commonly affected by low-impact trauma in an extradural haemorrhage, overlies the middle meningeal artery.

Question 21

A. (Aneurysm coiling) Severe, occipital headache that came on 2 hours ago with signs of meningism (photophobia and neck stiffness) on examination, and xanthochromia on LP suggests a subarachnoid haemorrhage (SAH). Guidelines indicate that once a spontaneous SAH is detected, a CT intracranial angiogram should be used to detect an intracranial aneurysm. The management for an intracranial aneurysm is an aneurysm coiling by an interventional neuroradiologist.

Question 22

E. (Perisylvian volume loss) Behaviour and personality change (more impulsive and less empathetic behaviour and being socially inappropriate) over a year combined with a normal MMSE suggests frontotemporal dementia (FTD). FTD has perisylvian (area in the lateral fissure associated with language) volume loss on MRI.

Question 23

E. (Temporal lobe) Zoning out of conversations and lip-smacking for a minute, combined with confusion and postictal dysphasia, suggests the temporal lobe is being affected. Temporal lobe seizures are associated with HELP (Hallucinations, Emotional, Lip-smacking, Postictal dysphasia) symptoms.

Question 24

B. (Propranolol) Severe, throbbing, unilateral headaches lasting between 6 and 8 hours at least twice a week, preceded by a visual aura and worsened by alcohol and the oral contraceptive pill, suggesting a migraine. Prophylaxis for migraine should be given if they occur more than once a week, and as she is of child-bearing age, propranolol is the correct prophylaxis, preferred over topiramate which is teratogenic and also shown to reduce the effectiveness of contraceptives.

Question 25

C. (Memantine) Progressively declining memory, aphasia and getting lost in familiar places combined with moderate cognitive impairment (10–18) on MMSE suggest Alzheimer disease. Although acetylcholinesterase inhibitors like donepezil are the first-line, they are contraindicated in patients with known bradycardia; hence, memantine is the management of choice.

Question 26

C. (Lamotrigine) Painful skin, mucosal rash, and fever for 6 days, on the background of generalized tonic-clonic seizures combined with being Nikolsky sign positive (when rash is rubbed, blisters appear on the skin), suggests Stevens-Johnson syndrome. Lamotrigine is the second-line treatment for generalized tonic-clonic seizures. Stevens-Johnsons syndrome is a type IV hypersensitivity reaction often to a drug, and is a less severe disease than toxic epidermal necrolysis (which presents similarly). However, in women of childbearing age, it is the first line and is one of the primary causes of Stevens-Johnson syndrome.

Question 27

A. (Bell's palsy) Left-sided facial discomfort, postauricular pain and noise irritability combined with resting facial symmetry, an inability to raise his left eyebrow, and an inability to smile or pucker his lips on examination suggest a lower motor neuron facial palsy (upper motor neuron would have forehead sparing) and as there is no apparent cause, suggests Bell palsy.

Question 28

B. (Long thoracic nerve) Generalized neck and scapula pain after a total right-sided mastectomy 3 weeks ago combined with right-sided scapula winging on examination, suggests a serratus anterior lesion, which is innervated by the long thoracic nerve, hence this is the nerve affected.

Question 29

B. (Levodopa) A progressively worsening tremor in the right hand, affecting her daily activities, on the background of recently diagnosed Parkinson's disease. Levodopa is the first-line treatment for Parkinson's disease, in which motor symptoms affect the quality of life.

Question 30

E. (Spasticity) Primary lateral sclerosis only affects upper motor neurons (UMN). Spasticity is also known as hypertonia, which refers to increased muscular tone, and out of the options given, is the only UMN symptom.

Question 31

B. (Guillain-Barré syndrome) Ascending lower limb weakness with bilateral diplopia and absent reflexes on examination suggests demyelination of the peripheral nervous system. This combined with a decreased motor nerve conduction velocity on nerve conduction studies suggests Guillain-Barré syndrome.

Question 32

A. (Accessory) Right shoulder pain radiating to the arm after a recent lymph node biopsy combined with right shoulder drooping, decreased power of the shoulder, and an inability to turn the head to the left-hand side on examination suggest problems with the trapezius and sternocleidomastoid muscles, which are innervated by the accessory nerve.

Question 33

B. (Idiopathic intracranial hypertension) Blurred vision and morning headaches on the background of doxycycline use (big risk factor) combined with obesity and raised ICP signs (papilloedema) on fundoscopy suggest idiopathic intracranial hypertension.

Question 34

C. (Striatum) Increased irritability and neglecting physical appearance associated with impaired speech and involuntary jerky movements combined with saccadic eye movements, an unsteady gait on examination, and his young age (38) suggest Huntington disease. Huntington disease is characterized by a degeneration of GABAergic neurons in the striatum, caudate and putamen.

Question 35

A. (*Campylobacter jejuni*) Bilateral, ascending leg weakness and pain after an episode of diarrhoea combined with absent reflexes and decreased power in the lower limbs, with downgoing plantars suggests Guillain-Barré syndrome. *Campylobacter jejuni* is the most common causative organism of Guillain-Barré syndrome.

Question 36

D. (Pyridostigmine) Muscle fatiguability, worsening vision and dysphagia on the background of pernicious anaemia combined with bilateral ptosis and diplopia on CN testing suggest myasthenia gravis. Long-term acetylcholinesterase inhibitors such as pyridostigmine are first line, thereby reducing acetylcholine breakdown in the neuromuscular junction.

Question 37

B. (Drug-induced parkinsonism) Sudden movement problems on the background of haloperidol usage combined with bradykinesia and bilateral tremors in the hands-on examination suggest parkinsonism. Drug-induced parkinsonism is more likely than idiopathic Parkinson disease due to bilateral parkinsonism features and a lack of rigidity.

Question 38

C. (Benzylpenicillin) A severe headache and fever, on the background of HIV combined with meningism (photophobia and neck stiffness) and a nonblanching rash on the left arm on examination, suggests meningococcal meningitis. The management of meningococcal meningitis is with benzylpenicillin or a third-generation cephalosporin such as ceftriaxone as soon as possible.

Question 39

D. (Radial) Problems with forearm extension and a right wrist drop after a motorcycle accident combined with a right humeral midshaft fracture on X-ray suggest radial nerve palsy. The radial nerve innervates the dorsal arm muscles (the triceps brachii and the anconeus) and the extrinsic extensors of the wrists and hands.

Question 40

D. (Oligoclonal bands) Blurred vision and extreme tiredness for a week combined with brisk lower leg reflexes on examination and high-density periventricular lesions on the MRI head suggest multiple sclerosis. Oligoclonal bands (specifically of IgG) are seen in 80% of patients with multiple sclerosis.

Question 41

A. (Common peroneal nerve) Foot drop after trauma to the lateral aspect of the left knee with sensation loss of the dorsum of the foot and lower lateral part of the leg on examination suggests a common peroneal nerve lesion. The common peroneal nerve is a branch of the sciatic nerve and it splits into the superficial and deep peroneal nerves; it is very commonly affected because it is unprotected as it traverses the lateral aspect of the head of the fibula.

Question 42

C. (High glucose, low protein, neutrophil predominance) A high-grade fever, severe headache and neck stiffness combined with tachycardia, nuchal rigidity and positive Kernig sign on examination and *Neisseria meningitides* on viral PCR suggest bacterial meningitis. Bacterial meningitis would have high protein, low glucose and neutrophil predominance in their CSF, whilst lymphocyte predominance would be expected with viral meningitis.

Question 43

E. (Trochlear) Poor vision causing falls while walking down the stairs combined with diplopia of the right eye when looking down and a deficit with the medial and downward movements of his right eye, suggests an issue with the superior oblique muscle, which is innervated by the trochlear nerve (CN IV).

Question 44

B. (Essential Tremor) A bilateral tremor exacerbated by outstretched arms for 4 years, finding it challenging to complete simple daily tasks on the background of a family history of a tremor suggests an essential tremor.

Essential tremor is an autosomal dominant condition, affecting the upper limbs predominantly.

Question 45

B. (IV acyclovir) A worsening fever and headache over 3 days with features of Broca aphasia (nonfluent speech but intact comprehension), and having an increased signal in the right mediotemporal lobe suggests encephalitis, which is caused by herpes simplex virus-1 primarily. IV acyclovir is the management of choice for all suspected cases of encephalitis initially, to reduce the risk of long-term sequelae.

Question 46

E. (Riluzole) A 3-month history of lower motor neuron signs (tongue fasciculations) and upper motor neuron signs (hypertonia, hyperreflexia) suggests motor neuron disease. Riluzole prevents the stimulation of glutamate receptors and is the first-line treatment for amyotrophic lateral sclerosis (ALS), the most common type of motor neuron disease. Riluzole has been shown to prolong life by 3 months.

Question 47

D. (Meniere's disease) Vertigo, hearing loss and tinnitus for an hour for 2 months combined with a positive Romberg's test and nystagmus on examination, with Rinne's test showing air conduction to be better than bone conduction in both ears, pointing to sensorineural hearing loss. The triad of vertigo, sensorineural hearing loss and tinnitus suggests Meniere disease.

Question 48

C. (Median) Wrist pain and swelling after falling on an outstretched right arm, with an inability to move the thumb away from the index finger (adductor pollicis brevis lesion) on examination combined with a distal radius fracture with dorsal displacement of fragments (Colles fracture), suggests the median nerve is affected.

Question 49

C. (L3–L4) Progressive lower limb weakness and dysphagia for 3 days, on the background of resolved gastroenteritis a week ago combined with diplopia and an absent knee reflex on examination, suggests Guillain-Barré syndrome. The knee reflex is associated with the L3 and L4 nerve roots.

Question 50

B. (Cerebellum) Ataxia and intention tremor, affecting the work combined with an abnormal heel-to-shin test and slurred staccato speech on examination suggest a cerebellar pathology (DANISH symptoms). DANISH symptoms: Dysdiachokinesia/Dysmetria, Ataxia, Nystagmus, Intention tremor, Slurred speech, Hypotonia.

Question 51

C. (Propranolol) Progressively worsening tremors in the upper limbs for 5 years, affecting daily living, with symptoms improving at rest combined with a bilateral tremor that worsens when outstretched on examination, suggesting an essential tremor. Propranolol is the management of choice for an essential tremor, reducing the tremor in 75% of patients.

Question 52

B. (Subacute combined degeneration of the spinal cord) Difficulty walking and leg numbness combined with impaired vibration and proprioception in the legs, Romberg's positive and wide-based, unsteady gait on examination suggests a spinal cord disorder. Megaloblastic anaemia after starting a vegetarian diet suggests Vitamin B12 deficiency, which combined with deficits with the dorsal columns, lateral corticospinal tracts and spinocerebellar tracts, suggests subacute combined degeneration of the spinal cord.

Question 53

E. (Temporal artery biopsy) A severe temporal headache, worse in the morning, associated diplopia and anterior ischaemic optic neuropathy (swollen pale disc caused by ischaemic of the optic nerve head) suggests temporal arteritis. Temporal artery biopsy is the diagnostic investigation for temporal arteritis, showing an inflammatory halo around the affected artery or a segmental stenosis.

Question 54

B. (Lambert-Eaton syndrome) Lower limb muscle weakness and problems walking, on the background of small-cell lung cancer combined with being Romberg's positive, suggests a neuromuscular junction disorder. Improved muscular strength after repeated muscle contractions, on the background of small-cell lung cancer suggests Lambert-Eaton syndrome (antibody directed against presynaptic voltage-gated calcium channel) over Myasthenia Gravis (antibodies to acetylcholine receptors).

Question 55

A. (Albuminocytologic dissociation) Rapidly progressing ascending lower extremity weakness with diplopia and absent deep tendon reflexes in the lower limb, suggests Guillain-Barré syndrome, a demyelinating disease in this case precipitated by the recent gastroenteritis. A lumbar puncture would show albuminocytologic dissociation (increased CSF protein with a normal white blood cell count). Lymphocytic pleocytosis would be associated with viral meningitis and Lyme disease whilst neutrophilic pleocytosis would be associated with bacterial meningitis.

Question 56

A. (Carbamazepine) Severe, unilateral electric shock pain multiple times a day, lasting for 30 seconds, precipitated by simple activities, suggests trigeminal neuralgia. The management for trigeminal neuralgia is carbamazepine unless there are red-flag features like early onset and optic neuritis, in which case prompt referral to neurology.

Question 57

D. (Relapsing-remitting disease) Right arm weakness and diplopia for 3 months, following similar episodes that self-resolved a year ago combined with hyperreflexia of the knees and ankles and Lhermitte's phenomenon on examination, suggests multiple sclerosis. Relapses of the MS symptoms with periods of remission in between these times of relapses suggest relapsing-remitting disease. Whilst cervical spondylosis can cause myelopathy, it is unlikely to have a relapsing pattern like in this scenario.

Question 58

E. (Wernicke's encephalopathy) Confusion on the background of binge drinking problems combined with bilateral horizontal nystagmus and ophthalmoplegia, inability to walk in a straight line, and confusion suggest Wernicke encephalopathy (Wernicke triad = confusion, ataxia, ophthalmoplegia/nystagmus). Wernicke's is caused by a thiamine deficiency causing atrophy of mammillary bodies. Korsakoff syndrome is the triad of Wernicke's with confusion and confabulation.

Question 59

B. (Bromocriptine) Impulse control and hallucinations since starting medication for Parkinson disease suggest that a dopamine receptor agonist, such as bromocriptine, was prescribed. Whilst levodopa is the first line for Parkinson's, the history of acute closed-angle glaucoma means that it is contraindicated, because it is known to increase intraocular pressure.

Question 60

A. (Baclofen) Leg stiffness and painful back spasms, which have not been improved by analgesia combined with a periventricular lesion on the MRI head, suggest MS associated with spasticity pointing to the appropriate management being baclofen or gabapentin. Baclofen is a $GABA_B$ receptor activation, blocking mono-and-polysynaptic reflexes by acting as an inhibitory ligand, inhibiting the release of excitatory neurotransmitters. If medications like baclofen are ineffective in stopping the spasticity, botulinum toxin (botox) injections can be indicated

Question 61

A. (*Borrelia burgdorferi*) Bilateral facial drooping on the background of a flu-like illness, associated with fever, myalgia and a bulls-eye rash growing in size combined with an inability to puff out cheeks or raise either eyebrow suggests a facial nerve palsy. A facial nerve palsy combined with the background of flu-like illness associated with a bulls-eye rash after hiking suggests Lyme disease. The causative organism for Lyme disease is *Borrelia burgdorferi*, with the vector of this being an Ixodes tick.

Question 62

E. (Uhthoff's phenomenon) Painful blurry vision that self-resolves before disappearing for months (relapsing-remitting pattern) combined with significantly reduced visual acuity in the left eye, and pain is exacerbated by warm temperatures. Uhthoff phenomenon describes the worsening of vision with increased body temperature and is seen in multiple sclerosis, which is the likely diagnosis given the relapsing-remitting pattern of optic neuritis. It is caused by heat may increase the time when voltage-gated sodium channels are inactivated, which delays further action potentials.

Question 63

E. (Klumpke's palsy) Clawing in his right hand and a hyperextended wrist after falling on an outstretched hand (FOOSH) combined with right upper eyelid ptosis and miosis (Horner syndrome) and weakness of finger flexion and extension on examination suggests brachial plexus injury. Klumpke palsy occurs due to damage to the lower part of the brachial plexus (C8, T1) which affects the intrinsic muscles of the hand and flexors of the wrist and fingers,

Question 64

D. (Multiple system atrophy) Multiple falls and erectile dysfunction for a month combined with postural hypotension, bradykinesia, cogwheel rigidity, and a unilateral resting tremor on examination suggests multiple system atrophy (Parkinson's + autonomic failure)

Question 65

A. (Brain abscess) The triad of fever, headache and focal neurological signs (right-sided ptosis) on examination and a ring-enhancing lesion on the left frontal lobe on CT head suggests a brain abscess. Whilst toxoplasmosis and tuberculoma can cause a ring-enhancing lesion, the lack of signs pointing to an alternative primary pathology (i.e. HIV for toxoplasmosis) and the onset of the patient's symptoms means we can exclude these.

Question 66

A. (Lacunar stroke) Complete loss of sensation in his upper and lower dermatomes of the left-sided limbs, with no signs of hemianopia, dysphasia or loss of right limb sensation combined with small vasculopathy in the basal ganglia on CT head suggests a lacunar stroke. Lacunar strokes present with isolated hemiparesis, hemisensory loss or hemiparesis with limb ataxia

Question 67

A. (Breast cancer) Progressive headaches and cognitive decline function, on the background of unintentional weight loss and multiple well-defined oedematous lesions on CT head, suggests a cerebral malignancy. Lung cancer is the most common cause of secondary brain tumours, in males whilst breast cancer is the most common in women.

Question 68

C. (Normal pressure hydrocephalus) Confusion and urinary incontinence combined with an abnormal gait on examination suggests normal pressure hydrocephalus (dementia, gait abnormality and urinary incontinence triad = Hakim triad)

Question 69

A. (Left posterior inferior cerebellar artery) The lateral medullary syndrome affects the posterior inferior cerebellar artery (PICA) and has ipsilateral facial numbness and contralateral loss of limb sensation, along with ipsilateral Horner syndrome (miosis and ptosis), hence the left PICA is the artery affected.

Question 70

A. (Acoustic neuroma) Progressively declining hearing for 3 years and vertigo, right-sided headaches and tinnitus combined with an absent corneal reflex (cranial nerve V palsy) and air conduction > bone conduction bilaterally (sensorineural hearing loss) on examination suggests an acoustic neuroma (vestibular schwannoma). Whilst this is a tumour of the vestibulocochlear nerve, if the tumour grows substantially it can cause impingement of the trigeminal nerve.

Question 71

C. (Epley manoeuvre) Sudden dizziness and vertigo on head movement upwards lasting only 15 seconds without tinnitus or hearing loss suggests benign paroxysmal positional vertigo (BPPV). The Epley manoeuvre is the first-line management option for BPPV and is 80% effective in removing canaliths from the semicircular canal. The Dix-Hallpike is diagnostic for BPPV (**Di**x = **Di**agnostic) and a positive test would show rotatory nystagmus.

Question 72

B. (IV ceftriaxone and metronidazole) The classic triad of fever, headache and focal neurological deficits (ptosis and mydriasis of the right eye) suggests a brain abscess. This is confirmed by papilloedema on fundoscopy and a ring-enhancing lesion in the right frontal lobe on the MRI head. Guidelines recommend an IV third-generation cephalosporin such as ceftriaxone and IV metronidazole as the first line for brain abscesses. Whilst toxoplasmosis is an important differential for a ring-enhancing lesion, we would expect a more subacute presentation and risk factors in the patients like HIV or immunocompromise.

Question 73

A. (Craniopharyngioma) Visual problems, fatigue, excessive urination and a small stature combined with bitemporal hemianopia, affecting mainly the lower quadrants on examination, and a suprasellar mass on CT head suggests a pituitary tumour. A craniopharyngioma is a solid tumour of the suprasellar region, which causes lower quadrant bitemporal hemianopia as the suprasellar tumour causes compression of the superior optic chiasm.

Question 74

D. (Medulloblastoma) A medulloblastoma is an aggressive paediatric tumour within the infratentorial compartment causing the raised ICP. Therefore it would present with headaches worse in the morning and vomiting combined with papilloedema on fundoscopy (raised intracranial pressure). The histology of rosette pattern of small, blue cells would be seen on the Haemotoxylin and Eosin (H+E) stain, which is further suggestive of medulloblastoma

Question 75

C. (Multiple sleep latency EEG) Daytime somnolence, cataplexy and severe daytime symptoms (ESS > 15), despite having a regular sleep schedule, suggest narcolepsy. Narcolepsy is caused by low levels of orexin, a hormone which regulates appetite and sleep patterns, with a multiple sleep latency EEG the investigation of choice for narcolepsy to establish a difference between physical tiredness and somnolence. Polysomnography is used for obstructive sleep apnoea and can be used for narcolepsy. It establishes apnoeic episodes in nighttime sleep rather than daytime, so would not be diagnostic for narcolepsy.

Question 76

E. (X-linked recessive) Duchenne muscular dystrophy is caused by a defect in the dystrophin gene, which is responsible for connecting the actin cytoskeleton of each muscle fibre to the underlying basal lamina, thereby causing Gower sign (difficulty getting up from the floor), frequent falls and calf muscle hypertrophy. Duchenne's is an X-linked recessive inherited disorder, hence making it more likely in boys.

Question 77

A. (Charcot-Marie-Tooth disease) Progressive lower leg weakness and wasting resulting in multiple ankle sprains with a lower extremity weakness, decreased vibration and proprioception and absent deep tendon reflexes on examination, suggests a hereditary motor and sensory neuropathy. The most common hereditary motor and sensory neuropathy is Charcot-Marie-Tooth disease, with presentation usually being in early adulthood.

Question 78

D. (Syringomyelia) The loss of temperature in the neck, shoulders and arms is described as a "cape-like" loss of sensation and patients commonly present after burning themselves without realising. This combined with upgoing plantars, spastic leg weakness and a history of Arnold-Chiari malformation is suggestive of syringomyelia. Syringomyelia is a CSF-filled cyst in the spinal cord, with the first symptom often being the "cape-like" loss of sensation because the crossing spinothalamic tracts in the anterior commissure of the spinal cord are first affected.

Question 79

E. (Neurogenic thoracic outlet syndrome) Left-sided neck pain and painless weakness in the left hand, noticeable after tennis training, on the background of a cervical rib combined with wasting and loss of sensation in the left hand on examination suggests neurogenic thoracic outlet syndrome, with the occupation precipitating his predisposition. Neurogenic thoracic outlet syndrome is the compression of the brachial plexus, subclavian artery or vein at the site of the thoracic outlet (ring formed by the top ribs) so the presence of a cervical rib makes this more likely.

Question 80

D. (Serum creatine kinase) Confusion and agitation after recently starting an atypical antipsychotic, with lead-pipe rigidity and a high-grade fever on examination, suggests neuroleptic malignant syndrome. Serum creatine kinase is raised in most cases of neuroleptic malignant syndrome, as antipsychotics can cause myonecrosis with more severe cases causing rhabdomyolysis.

Question 81

D. (Neurofibromatosis 2) Bilateral tinnitus, vertigo and sensorineural hearing loss with an absent corneal reflex bilaterally on examination suggest bilateral acoustic neuromas, which, combined with the family history (autosomal dominant) suggests neurofibromatosis 2. Neurofibromatosis 1 is caused by a gene mutation on chromosome 17 encoding neurofibromin and presents with café-au-lait spots, phaeochromocytomas and iris hamartomas, rather than bilateral vestibular schwannomas seen in neurofibromatosis 2, hence NF1 wouldn't present with hearing problems.

Question 82

D. (Repeated large-volume CSF taps) The triad of dementia, gait disturbances and urinary incontinence is suggestive of normal pressure hydrocephalus (Hakim's triad). Ventriculoperitoneal shunting is the first-line management for normal pressure hydrocephalus, however severe dementia contraindicates this as the amyloid-beta plaques cause poor shunt response. Therefore repeated large-volume CSF taps are preferred as they remove CSF flow obstruction at the aqueduct.

Question 83

C. (Sagittal sinus thrombosis) A sudden, severe headache, nausea and vomiting and left-sided hemiplegia suggest an intracranial pathology. The seizure two days ago and an empty delta sign on CT head, a triangular filling defect in the superior sagittal sinus, representing a thrombus, suggests sagittal sinus thrombosis. The condition is treated with anticoagulation to prevent further clot propagation and to facilitate recanalization of the occluded sinus.

Rheumatology 21

EXPLANATIONS

Question 1

B. (Osteoarthritis) Gradually worsening joint pain and stiffness in the hip, worsened by prolonged activity and weight-beating, on the background of hypercholesterolaemia, combined with a limited right hip ROM and crepitations heard on passive movement of the hip, suggests osteoarthritis. Osteoarthritis is caused by a loss of cartilage at synovial joints and is often accompanied by the degeneration of the underlying bone, with common risk factors including obesity and a previous history of trauma to the joint; on the other hand, osteoporosis has been shown to reduce the risk of osteoarthritis.

Question 2

D. (Rheumatoid arthritis) Intermittent pain and stiffness bilaterally of the hand joints, with the stiffness improving but the pain worsening during the day combined with swelling and tenderness of the PIPs and wrists bilaterally and a positive squeeze test on examination suggests rheumatoid arthritis. Rheumatoid arthritis can be diagnosed using the 2010 ACR/EULAR rheumatoid arthritis criteria, which include the following points: joint involvement (up to 5 points), positive RF and anti-CCP (up to 3 points), raised ESR/CRP (1 point) and symptoms longer than 6 weeks (1 point); a score of 6/10 suggesting definite RA.

Question 3

D. (X-ray of the hands) Increasing wrist pain for 5 months, improved by rest, on the background of hypertension, and Bouchard's nodes (bony enlargement of PIP joint) on examination suggest osteoarthritis. Although osteoarthritis is often a clinical diagnosis, an X-ray of the hands is indicated to visualize the LOSS symptoms of osteoarthritis (Loss of joint space, Osteophytes, Subchondral cysts, Subchondral sclerosis).

Question 4

C. (Female sex) Persistent back pain for a year with low-energy fractures, on the background of a family history of similar issues, premature menopause and alcohol excess combined with noticeable dorsal kyphosis suggest osteoporosis. The key risk factors for osteoporosis are female sex and advancing age.

Question 5

D. (Paracetamol) Gradually worsening joint pain and stiffness, with symptoms worsening with prolonged activity and weight-bearing, on the background of type 2 diabetes mellitus, combined with Heberden's nodes (bony enlargement of DIP joint) and a limited range of motion in his hip, suggests osteoarthritis. The first-line management of choice for osteoarthritis is paracetamol as analgesia.

Question 6

D. (Synovial fluid analysis) Acutely severe pain and swelling in the right big toe, causing difficulty walking combined with a low-grade fever with associated erythema and tenderness of his right first metatarsophalangeal joint on examination suggests acute gout (podagra). Synovial fluid analysis is the investigation of choice for gout, to look for negatively birefringent needle-shaped crystals.

Question 7

A. (Cholecalciferol) Bone pain and muscle weakness on the background of starting a vegan diet and a recent femoral neck fracture combined with rib tenderness and waddling gait suggest osteomalacia, which is vitamin D deficiency in adults. The management of choice for osteomalacia is cholecalciferol (vitamin D3) to correct the vitamin D deficiency.

Question 8

E. (<−2.5) Chronic bone pain affecting her ability to do her ADLs, on the background of recurrent falls and a smaller height than her most recently recorded on examination, suggests osteoporosis. The T score (a comparison of the patient's bone density with healthy, young adults) associated with osteoporosis on the DEXA scan is less than −2.5.

Question 9

C. (Methotrexate) Intermittent pain and morning stiffness bilaterally in the joints of the hands, on the background of Hashimoto thyroiditis combined with proximal interphalangeal joint (PIP) swelling and tenderness and a positive squeeze test on examination, suggests rheumatoid arthritis. The hand X-ray confirmed this by showing joint space narrowing and PIP osteopenia. The management of choice for rheumatoid arthritis is a disease-modifying antirheumatic drug (DMARD) like methotrexate with an adjuvant short-course of bridging prednislone on occasion.

Question 10

E. (Positively birefringent rhomboid-shaped crystals) Sudden pain and swelling in the left knee, on the background of haemochromatosis, combined with the knee being tender, erythematous and having a limited range of motion on examination with chondrocalcinosis (calcium crystals in the joint cartilage) on knee X-ray suggests pseudogout. Positively birefringent rhomboid-shaped crystals would be on synovial fluid analysis for pseudogout (**P**ositive = **P**seudogout)

Question 11

A. (N, N, N, N) A fall on the background of osteoporosis, with the hip being externally rotated and the right leg shortened on examination, suggests a neck of femur fracture. Osteoporosis is associated with a normal bone profile hence calcium, phosphate, ALP and PTH are all normal. On occasion, after a recent fracture ALP may be raised, with the other markers remaining normal, however this answer option is not provided.

Question 12

A. (Colchicine) Sudden severe pain and swelling in the left big toe, worsened after alcohol consumption combined with this toe being erythematous, warm to touch and extremely tender with synovial fluid analysis showing negatively birefringent needle-shaped urate crystals suggest gout. Colchicine or NSAIDs are the management of choice for acute gout; however, given the history of peptic ulcer disease, NSAIDs are contraindicated; hence, colchicine is preferred.

Question 13

C. (Still disease) Joint pain and swelling in multiple joints for 3 months, associated with morning stiffness that improves during the day combined with an axillary salmon-pink rash, temperature > 39°C for a week and splenomegaly, with negative antinuclear antibodies suggests Still disease (systemic juvenile idiopathic arthritis) as 5 of the Yamagushi criteria are met (with at least 2 major criteria – salmon-pink rash, fever and arthralgia for > 2 weeks).

Question 14

E. (HLA-DR4) Multiple joint pain and stiffness for a prolonged time, with symptoms worse in the morning and improved by activity combined with tenderness in the metacarpophalangeal joints and wrists bilaterally on examination and elevated anti-CCP antibodies suggest rheumatoid arthritis. HLA-DR4 is the HLA antigen associated with rheumatoid arthritis (4 DooRs in a rheum [room]).

Question 15

E. (Systemic lupus erythematosus) Arthralgia and fatigue on the background of Raynaud phenomenon combined with a malar rash, erythematous lesion on his limbs and joint tenderness on examination with positive antinuclear antibodies (ANA) suggest systemic lupus erythematosus. Systemic lupus erythematosus is an autoimmune condition, that is a type 3 hypersensitivity reaction causing immune complex formation in multiple organs such as the joints and kidneys.

Question 16

A. (Ankylosing spondylitis) Lower back pain and pleuritic chest pain, with these symptoms worse in the mornings combined with reduced lateral and forward flexion and sacroiliac joint tenderness on examination suggest ankylosing spondylitis. Syndesmophytes confirm this on an X-ray of the sacroiliac joints. Other X-ray changes that can be associated with ankylosing spondylitis is sacroiliitis, squaring of the lumbar vertebrae and a late sign can be a "bamboo spine."

Question 17

A. (Hydroxychloroquine) Bilateral arthralgia, joint swelling and a facial rash combined with joint tenderness and oral ulcers on examination suggest systemic lupus erythematosus (SLE). The DMARD hydroxychloroquine is the management of choice for SLE.

Question 18

C. (Polymyalgia rheumatica) Bilateral, dull shoulder and hip pain, worse in the morning and associated with stiffness with tenderness and limited range of motion of these joints on examination as well as raised inflammatory markers suggest polymyalgia rheumatica. Polymyalgia rheumatica is characterised by muscle stiffness and is commonly associated with temporal arteritis, hence it is proposed that IL-6, has a role in the pathophysiology of PMR.

Question 19

D. (Reactive arthritis) Unilateral joint pain and stiffness for a week after a resolved episode of diarrhoea a month ago associated with dysuria and bacterial conjunctivitis (purulent discharge) suggests reactive arthritis. Reactive arthritis is a HLA-B27 associated seronegative spondyloarthropathy, that classically presents with a triad of urethritis, conjunctivitis and arthritis.

Question 20

E. (Anti-Ro antibodies) Dry eyes and dry mouth in a middle-aged woman with a background of premature ovarian failure combined with sensory polyneuropathy and mild synovitis on examination suggests Sjögren syndrome. Anti-Ro antibodies are the primary antibody raised in Sjögren syndrome, raised in 70% of primary Sjögren syndrome cases, although anti-La antibodies can also be associated with Sjogren's.

Question 21

C. (Psoriatic arthritis) Joint pain and swelling of the fingers for 3 months, associated with developing plaque psoriasis on her knees and elbows combined with tenderness, swelling and erythema of her DIPs on examination suggests psoriatic arthritis. Psoriatic arthritis is also a seronegative (HLA-B27) spondyloarthropathy and often has characteristic nail changes: pitting and onycholysis.

Question 22

B. (Exercise and NSAIDs) Chronic lower back pain and stiffness, worse in the morning, on the background of anterior uveitis combined with reduced lumbar spine mobility and tenderness over the sacroiliac joints with an X-ray showing squaring of the lumbar vertebrae, suggest ankylosing spondylitis. Exercise and NSAIDs are the management of choice for ankylosing spondylitis to manage the pain.

Question 23

C. (Anti-dsDNA antibodies) Fatigue, pleuritic chest pain with a malar rash exacerbated by sunlight exposure, on the background of type 1 diabetes mellitus combined with mouth ulcers and joint pain on finger palpation and raised ESR and low complement levels on blood tests suggests systemic lupus erythematosus. Anti-dsDNA antibody is a highly specific antibody for SLE.

Question 24

B. (Schirmer test) Chronic dry mouth and dry eyes causing eye irritation, on the background of rheumatoid arthritis combined with generalized myalgia and arthralgia, suggest Sjögren syndrome. Schirmer test is the most appropriate investigation because it measures tear formation to prove the dryness of the eye, less than <10 mm of moisture is suggestive of Sjögren syndrome.

Question 25

E. (Prednisolone) Bilateral shoulder and hip pain and stiffness for 3 weeks, with the pain worse in the morning combined with shoulder and hip girdle tenderness on examination and raised inflammatory markers, suggesting polymyalgia rheumatica. Prednisolone is the management of choice for polymyalgia rheumatica, with a response to low-dose prednisolone seen in 24–72 hours (if this response is not seen consider potential other differentials).

Question 26

E. (Septic arthritis) An acutely swollen, painful left knee, on the background of being sexually active with multiple partners, combined with an erythematous, tender knee that has a limited range of motion on examination and an elevated ESR, suggests septic arthritis. Whilst reactive arthritis is an important differential to consider in a sexually active young person, it usually presents with a triad of urethritis, conjunctivitis and arthritis rather than just an acutely swollen joint.

Question 27

E. (X-ray of the sacroiliac joints) Chronic lower back pain and stiffness that is worse in the morning and improved by exercise in a young man combined with reduced lumbar spine mobility, sacroiliac joint tenderness and signs of anterior uveitis on examination suggest ankylosing spondylitis. An X-ray of the sacroiliac joints is the investigation of choice for ankylosing spondylitis, which can show the following: sacroiliitis, squaring of lumbar vertebrae, "bamboo spine" and syndesmophytes.

Question 28

E. (Pilocarpine) Persistently dry eyes and dry mouth with associated dysphagia and a reduced sense of taste and positive anti-Ro and anti-La antibodies, suggest Sjögren syndrome. Pilocarpine, a muscarinic receptor antagonist, is the management of choice for Sjögren syndrome to stimulate tear production.

Question 29

C. (Ibuprofen) Asymmetric arthritis and swelling in his knees and ankles after an episode of recent diarrhoea, combined with dysuria and bacterial conjunctivitis (purulent discharge) and keratoderma blenorrhagica on examination, suggest reactive arthritis. NSAIDs like ibuprofen are the management of choice for reactive arthritis. If the reactive arthritis is persistent, disease-modifying anti-rheumatic drugs (DMARDs) like methotrexate or sulphasalazine can be trialled.

Question 30

A. (Clindamycin) An acutely swollen, red and painful right knee, on the background of poorly controlled type 2 diabetes mellitus combined with a fever and limited range of motion in the knee and positive *Staphylococcus aureus* cultures, suggests septic arthritis. Flucloxacillin is the management of choice for septic arthritis, given the *Staphylococcus aureus* infection, however given the penicillin allergy, clindamycin should be preferred.

Question 31

D. (Methotrexate) Bilateral joint pain, swelling and stiffness of the DIPs associated with plaque psoriasis of the extensor and psoriatic nail changes (pitting and onycholysis) suggest psoriatic arthritis. Methotrexate is the management of choice for moderate/severe psoriatic arthritis (shown by x-ray changes). If methotrexate doesn't work then monoclonal antibodies such as ustekinimab and secukinimab can be trialled.

Question 32

B. (Isoniazid) Fatigue and pleuritic chest pain after being started on TB treatment combined with generalized arthralgia and a butterfly-shaped facial rash on examination and elevated antihistone antibodies suggest drug-induced lupus. Out of the management options for tuberculosis, isoniazid is known to cause drug-induced lupus due to the inhibitory reaction of isoniazid with complement component C4.

Question 33

C. (Kocher criteria) An acutely severely painful, swollen hip combined with a high-grade fever and with the hip having a limited range of motion and being unable to bear weight on examination suggests septic arthritis. Kocher's criteria assess the likelihood of septic arthritis in children by differentiating between septic arthritis and transient synovitis and consists of four criteria: fever > 38.5 degrees C, non-weight bearing, raised ESR and raised WCC.

Question 34

B. (Fibromyalgia) Chronic generalized muscular pain, fatigue and sleep disturbances, with the pain being a constant dull ache exacerbated by physical activity combined with no signs of joint swelling, but forgetfulness on examination with normal inflammatory markers suggests fibromyalgia.

Question 35

B. (N, N, Elevated, N) Chronic intermittent back pain, with hearing loss and head enlargement combined with lumbar spine tenderness and limited range of motion on examination suggests Paget disease of bone. Paget causes thickening of the calvarium and hence presents with bossing of the skull and the hearing loss is caused by cranial nerve entrapment. The bone profile of Paget would show an isolated rise in ALP. Heightened osteoblastic activity in Paget's disease leads to increased ALP production, contributing to elevated serum ALP levels.

Question 36

C. (Limited cutaneous systemic sclerosis) Finger swelling and dysphagia for 3 months, combined with Raynaud phenomenon, sclerodactyly and telangiectasia on examination, suggest CREST (Calcinosis, Raynaud phenomenon, Esophageal dysmotility, Sclerodactyly, Telangiectasia) syndrome, a limited cutaneous systemic sclerosis. Whilst the pathophysiology is not fully understood, it is thought to be due to a complex interplay of fibrosis, vascular dysfunction and immune system dysregulation.

Question 37

E. (Triamcinolone) Genital and oral ulcers on the background of multiple sexual partners combined with anterior uveitis and erythema nodosum on examination suggests Behçet disease (**Behçet triad**: oral ulcers, genital ulcers and anterior uveitis). Triamcinolone paste, a topical corticosteroid, is usually the first line management of Behçet mucocutaneous ulcers because it has shown greater efficacy than other corticosteroids in treating aphthous ulcers.

Question 38

B. (Dermatomyositis) Proximal muscle weakness and a facial rash, on the background of ovarian cancer with Gottron papules, suggest dermatomyositis. Dermatomyositis can be idiopathic but can be linked to malignancy (typically ovarian, breast and lung cancer).

Question 39

A. (Ewing sarcoma) A growing radial lump that is increasingly painful, especially worse at night in a young child, combined with systemic features of malignancy, i.e., unintentional weight loss and an onion-skin appearance of the radius, suggests Ewing's sarcoma. Ewing sarcoma is seen mainly in children and adolescents and mainly causes increasingly severe pain in the pelvis or long bones. Osteosarcoma is the other main paediatric tumour to exclude; however it would present with a sunburst pattern and is commonly associated with retinoblastoma (due to both being associated with a mutation in the Rb gene).

Question 40

D. (Anti-Jo-1 antibodies) Proximal muscle weakness in upper arms and a reddish-purple facial rash on the background of Ehlers-Danlos syndrome, combined with Gottron papules on examination and elevated creatine kinase and aldolase levels suggest dermatomyositis. Anti-Jo-1 antibodies are the primary antibody raised in dermatomyositis, with the main antigen Histidyl-tRNA synthetase.

Question 41

C. (Polymyositis) Proximal symmetrical muscle weakness (reduced power in the hip flexors and shoulder abductors) with systemic features and elevated lactate dehydrogenase and creatine kinase in a middle-aged woman suggests polymyositis. Polymyositis is caused by a T-cell-mediated cytotoxic process against muscle fibres causing symmetrical, proximal muscle weakness. Dermatomyositis would present similarly to polymyositis but would have dermatological manifestations such as a rash.

Question 42

B. (Amitriptyline) Widespread muscular pain that is a constant dull ache that worsens with physical activity and fatigue for 6 months combined with difficulty concentrating in a middle-aged woman and inflammatory markers that are not elevated suggest fibromyalgia. Tricyclic antidepressants, i.e., amitriptyline, are beneficial in fibromyalgia for neuropathic pain management, through the inhibition of serotonin and noradrenaline reuptake.

Question 43

A. (Chronic fatigue syndrome) Persistent fatigue, not improved by rest and generalized muscle pains, worsened by activity for 8 months combined with poor sleep and difficulty concentrating with normal LFTs and TFTs, and negative ANA suggests chronic fatigue syndrome (CFS), also known as myalgic encephalomyelitis. The main sign of CFS is post-exertional malaise/fatigue for >6 months.

Question 44

D. (Osteoma) Worsening headache feeling like pressure against the left eyeball, on the background of Gardner syndrome (a variant of familial adenomatous polyposis) combined with cortical irregularity in the left maxillary sinus suggests an osteoma of the skull, which is a benign overgrowth of bone. Ewing's sarcoma is a primarily paediatric tumour, that would present with an "onion skin" appearance on CT and a giant cell tumour would present with a "soap-bubble" appearance and occurs in the long bones.

Question 45

B. (Anticentromere antibodies) Raynaud phenomenon and dysphagia on the background of rheumatoid arthritis combined with sclerodactyly and telangiectasia on examination suggest limited systemic sclerosis, also known as CREST syndrome. Anticentromere antibodies are the primary antibody raised in CREST syndrome, are found in 60% of these patients and affect centromere and kinetochore function.

Endocrine and diabetes 22

EXPLANATIONS

Question 1

C. (Iatrogenic goitre) Smooth swelling in her neck, increasing in size, on the background of bipolar disorder, managed with lithium. Medications such as amiodarone and lithium can form goitre, as lithium can cause the inhibition of thyroid hormone uptake, inhibiting iodotyrosine coupling, altering thyroglobulin structure and thereby inhibiting thyroid hormone secretion. As no other history clues suggest an alternative diagnosis, this suggests iatrogenic goitre.

Question 2

C. (42–47 mmol/mol) A recent HbA1c test results in a diagnosis of prediabetes. The HbA1c limits for prediabetes mellitus are 42–47 mmol/mol, as 48 mmol/mol is the threshold for a diabetes mellitus diagnosis.

Question 3

E. (IV 0.9 NaCl) Abdominal pain and vomiting on the background of type 1 diabetes mellitus and hyperglycaemia and ketonaemia suggest DKA. DKA is caused by uncontrolled lipolysis causing an excess of free fatty acids that are ultimately converted to ketone bodies (causing ketonaemia). The first-line management for a patient with DKA is IV fluids, typically 0.9% NaCl, typically 1L over an hour because it reduces blood glucose and begins to correct the acidosis caused by the ketonaemia. After starting fluids, an IV insulin infusion of 0.1 units/kg/hour should be started.

Question 4

C. (Metformin) A diabetic review after being started on lifestyle interventions to manage his type 2 diabetes mellitus, shows his HbA1c reading in the clinic was 55 mmol/mol, which prompts pharmacological management. Metformin is the first-line management of type 2 diabetes mellitus when lifestyle modifications cannot keep the HbA1c under 48 mmol/mol. Metformin inhibits cyclic AMP production, blocking the action of glucagon, and thereby reducing fasting glucose levels.

Question 5

E. (Oral GlucoGel) The management of hypoglycaemia is dependent on three factors: the setting, the alertness and the ability to swallow the patient. In this scenario, the woman is alert, in a hospital setting and with no indication of difficulty swallowing, which suggests the need for a quick-acting carbohydrate orally such as an oral GlucoGel.

Question 6

E. (35–40 kg/m^2) A BMI >30 kg/m^2 suggests obesity, which can then further be classified into obesity stages 1, 2 and 3. Obesity stage 1 (30–35 kg/m^2), stage 2 (35–40 kg/m^2) and stage 3 (>40 kg/m^2).

Question 7

C. (Cushing syndrome) Despite a balanced diet and exercise for 6 months, weight gain associated with muscle weakness and easy bruising combined with purple striae and hypertension suggests Cushing syndrome. Cushing syndrome is often caused endogenously by a pituitary tumour secreting ACTH resulting in increased secretion of glucocorticoids, causing the symptoms in this scenario.

Question 8

B. (Cerebral oedema) Severe abdominal pain and vomiting for 10 hours, on the background of type I diabetes mellitus combined with Kussmaul respiration and ketones +++ on urine dipstick, suggests DKA. He is treated per the DKA guidelines but suffers a seizure. This is likely due to cerebral oedema, because, occasionally, rapid fluid resuscitation in DKA can result in cerebral oedema. It is thought that cerebral oedema occurs as extracellular osmolality decreases rapidly with treatment, water flows rapidly onto these cells causing the brain to swell.

Question 9

B. (Laparoscopic sleeve gastrectomy) Struggles with weight loss despite conservative measures (exercise/reducing calorie intake) and pharmacological measures (orlistat), indicates surgical options; with a BMI of 38 kg/m^2, the first-line surgical option is a laparoscopic sleeve gastrectomy. If the patient has stage 3 obesity (>40 kg/m^2), surgical options are indicated first-line instead of trialling conservative options.

Question 10

D. (Reduced, Reduced, Reduced) Severe abdominal pain for 6 hours, on the background of type 1 diabetes mellitus combined with an abnormal breathing pattern on examination with ketones +++ on urine dipstick and acidotic pH and elevated blood glucose suggests DKA. The abnormal breathing pattern associated with DKA is Kussmaul respiration, which describes a pattern of deep, laboured hyperventilation, that is a compensatory mechanism for the metabolic acidosis caused by DKA (deeper ventilation expels more CO_2), thereby there would be a decrease in pH, bicarbonate and pCO_2.

Question 11

D. (Hypokalaemic metabolic alkalosis) Muscle weakness and a dorso-cervical hump combined with reduced power in the upper arms and thighs, purple striae and hypertension on examination suggest Cushing syndrome. Cushing syndrome is associated with hypokalaemic metabolic alkalosis, thought to be due to increased ACTH levels resulting in elevated levels of cortisol and aldosterone.

Question 12

D. (Increases insulin sensitivity) Persistent diarrhoea for a month, on the background of type 2 diabetes mellitus that was previously managed conservatively, combined with mild tenderness over the abdomen and lactic acidosis. Metformin is a biguanide known to cause lactic acidosis (inhibition of gluconeogenesis by blocking pyruvate carboxylase causes lactate build-up) and cause gastrointestinal upset and is the first-line pharmacological management for type 2 diabetes, which functions by increasing insulin sensitivity.

Question 13

A. (J waves) Confusion with noticeable shivering and disorientation to time and placed mild hypothermia (28-32°C) and a reduced GCS suggest the ECG would show J waves (a deflection where the QRS complex joins the ST segment associated with hypothermia). Hypothermia causes exaggerated outward potassium currents leading to repolarisation abnormalities.

Question 14

C. (Prolonged QT interval) Weight gain and fatigue combined with purple striae, buffalo hump and a high BP on examination suggest Cushing syndrome, which is associated with hypokalaemic metabolic acidosis. A hypokalaemic metabolic acidosis is associated with a prolonged QT interval because hypokalaemia prolongs action potential duration by reducing outward current through both K^+ channels and Na^+-K^+ ATPase.

Question 15

B. (Graves disease) The triad of exophthalmos, pretibial myxoedema and thyroid acropachy (clubbing in both hands), known as Diamond triad is diagnostic of Graves disease despite all three only being present in 1% of patients. A diffuse, homogenous, increased uptake on scintigraphy due to substantially increased thyroid hormone synthesis throughout the thyroid gland. Toxic multinodular goitre would show patchy uptake on scintigraphy, with a toxic adenoma showing a singular "hot" nodule.

Question 16

C. (Low-dose dexamethasone suppression test) Unintentional weight gain and muscle weakness combined with thin, fragile skin with multiple bruises, purple skin and a swollen face with a high BP suggest Cushing syndrome. The most appropriate subsequent investigation is the low-dose (overnight) dexamethasone suppression test to see if their morning cortisol spike is suppressed.

Question 17

A. (Addison disease) Addison disease is characterised by increasing fatigue and unintentional weight loss combined with hyponatraemia and hyperkalaemia. The electrolyte abnormalities are caused by hypoaldosteronism, with patients often having hyperpigmentation of palmar creases caused by increased ACTH causing increased melanocyte-stimulating hormone (MSH).

Question 18

E. (Inhibits reabsorption of glucose in the kidney) Fever and urinary frequency for 2 days on the background of type 2 diabetes mellitus combined with hypogastric abdominal pain and nitrites and leucocytes on urine dipstick suggest a urinary tract infection. SGLT-2 inhibitors such as empagliflozin are known to cause urinary tract infections (due to glycosuria) and work by inhibiting glucose reabsorption in the kidney.

Question 19

A. (Fludrocortisone and hydrocortisone) Unintentional weight loss and weakness for 5 months with hyperpigmentation of the palmar creases and weakness, specifically of the proximal muscles of the limbs with hyponatraemia and hyperkalaemia suggest Addison disease. Patients with Addison disease need both glucocorticoid and mineralocorticoid replacement; hence, the management of choice is fludrocortisone and hydrocortisone.

Question 20

C. (Bendroflumethiazide) Dry mouth and polyuria, with an elevated fasting plasma glucose and 2-hour plasma glucose from her oral glucose tolerance test, suggest impaired glucose tolerance. Bendroflumethiazide is known to cause impaired glucose tolerance due to reduced glucose-stimulated insulin release.

Question 21

A. (High cortisol and high ACTH) Unintentional weight loss and a haemoptysis episode a week ago, on the background of a 30-pack year smoking history (lung cancer signs) combined with purple abdominal striae and clubbing on examination and hypokalaemia and hyponatraemia suggest small cell lung cancer causing Cushing syndrome as a paraneoplastic feature. This would cause high cortisol and high ACTH on high-dose dexamethasone suppression test.

Question 22

E. (Waterhouse-Friderichsen syndrome) Severe headaches, neck stiffness and purpuric rash combined with a fever, hypotension, tachycardia and tachypnoea suggest meningococcal meningitis. The combination of meningococcal meningitis, hyponatremia, hyperkalaemia and bilateral adrenal enlargement on the CT abdomen suggests Waterhouse-Friderichsen syndrome. This is caused by Neisseria meningitides causing haemorrhage into the adrenal cortex.

Question 23

A. (Acromegaly) Shoes no longer fitting and joint pain in the wrists and knees for a year; on the background of hypertension combined with macroglossia and bilateral hemianopia on visual field examination suggests acromegaly. Acromegaly is caused by a pituitary adenoma secreting excessive growth hormone, with the pituitary adenoma compressing the optic chiasm and causing bitemporal hemianopia. Gigantism refers to excessive growth hormone production before the closure of the epiphyseal growth plates.

Question 24

C. (Primary hyperparathyroidism) The mnemonic "stones, bones, abdominal groans and psychic moans" describes the symptoms that would be seen in primary hyperparathyroidism, which is caused by increased calcium and PTH. Multiple endocrine neoplasia type 1 would present with pituitary tumour, pancreatic tumours like an insulinoma and parathyroid hyperplasia.

Question 25

C. (Plasma aldosterone: renin ratio) Fatigue with muscular weakness and hypertension, combined with hypokalaemia, suggests primary hyperaldosteronism. The first-line investigation for primary hyperaldosteronism is the plasma aldosterone: renin ratio, with the high aldosterone causing sodium retention hence causing a low renin through negative feedback.

Question 26

B. (Nephrogenic diabetes insipidus) Excessive thirst and poor sleep as a result of nocturia, on the background of bipolar disorder combined with low urine osmolality initially and after the administration of desmopressin suggests nephrogenic diabetes insipidus. Nephrogenic diabetes insipidus is caused by the kidney's insensitivity to antidiuretic hormone (ADH), unlike cranial diabetes insipidus caused by insufficient production of ADH, which is why urine osmolality did not increase after desmopressin (synthetic ADH) administration.

Question 27

E. (IV Fluids) Fatigue and constipation for 2 weeks, on the background of breast cancer for which she recently finished chemotherapy combined with pallor and hypercalcaemia, suggest hypercalcemia of malignancy. The immediate management of hypercalcaemia of malignancy is IV fluids because they provide oral hydration, promotes calcineuresis and reverse dehydration, which be caused by hypercalcaemia-induced nephrogenic diabetes insipidus. Following fluid therapy, bisphosphonates are indicated to inhibit bone resorption.

Question 28

A. (Levothyroxine) Hyperthyroidism (dysphagia and unintentional weight loss) 2 months ago on the background of flu-like symptoms for the week prior combined with hypothyroid investigation results (high TSH and low T4 and reduced uptake globally on thyroid scintigraphy) suggests de Quervain thyroiditis. De Quervain is characterised by a thyrotoxic phase (thyroid follicular damage and release of thyroid hormone and then period of hypothyroidism. The management for de Quervain thyroiditis in the hypothyroid phase is levothyroxine, however, in cases of severe thyrotoxicosis the management is potassium iodide with prednisolone to reduce the conversion of T4 to T3.

Question 29

C. (Klinefelter syndrome) Abnormally large stature and bilateral gynaecomastia combined with small and firm testes and a lack of pubic hair on examination with an elevated LH and FSH and decreased testosterone suggest gonadal dysgenesis. Klinefelter syndrome (47, XXY) is caused by a nondisjunction event during paternal meiosis I and presents in genetic males with features of small testicles and a lack of secondary sexual characteristics. Kallmann syndrome would cause low LH and FSH (hypogonadotropic hypogonadism) with problems with their smell (anosmia).

Question 30

A. (Increased, Increased, Increased) Signs of hypercalcaemia (bone pain and low mood), on the background of chronic kidney disease suggest tertiary hyperparathyroidism. It occurs as a result of ongoing hyperplasia of the parathyroid glands after correction of underlying chronic kidney disease, which is why there is an elevated PTH and calcium. Due to prolonged hyperparathyroidism, PTH increases renal tubular reabsorption of phosphate, leading to decreased phosphate excretion in the urine, and thereby increased serum phosphate.

Question 31

B. (Phenoxybenzamine) Episodic headaches and palpitations combined with a very high BP and increased levels of 24-hour urinary collection of metanephrines with right adrenal medulla mass on CT abdomen suggest a phaeochromocytoma, an adrenal medulla tumour. Management of a phaeochromocytoma requires alpha-blockade first-line prior to surgery; hence, phenoxybenzamine is the management of choice. Administering alpha-blockers before beta-blockers allows for the blockade of alpha-adrenergic receptors first, which prevents unopposed alpha-adrenergic vasoconstriction. Once alpha-blockade has been established, beta-blockers can be safely introduced to further control tachycardia and other symptoms of catecholamine excess without the risk of exacerbating hypertension.

Question 32

C. (Low urine osmolality after water deprivation but high urine osmolality after desmopressin) Nocturia and polydipsia, on the background of a concussion during a rugby match 3 weeks combined with normal blood glucose, suggest cranial diabetes insipidus. Cranial diabetes insipidus is caused by decreased ADH secretion from the pituitary gland. A water deprivation test would show low urine osmolality after water deprivation but high after desmopressin is administered because it is not a sensitivity issue.

Question 33

E. (Urinary metanephrines) Worsening headache associated with anxiety and palpitations combined with a bilateral fine tremor and high BP on examination with normokalaemia and normonatraemia suggests phaeochromocytoma. A 24-hour urinary metanephrines (breakdown product of catecholamines) collection is preferred over the former first-line urinary catecholamines because it has a higher sensitivity for phaeochromocytomas.

Question 34

D. (Prolactinoma) A car accident after suffering intermittent headaches and amenorrhoea for 4 months combined with bilateral hemianopia on visual field examination suggests prolactinoma. Craniopharyngioma would most likely present in children, acromegaly would have signs of growth hormone excess such as a coarse facial appearance and a pituitary apoplexy would present with sudden onset headache similar to a subarachnoid haemorrhage, rather than a history of intermittment headaches. The excess prolactin causes amenorrhoea by inhibiting gonadotropins, along with causing galactorrhoea and osteoporosis in women.

Question 35

C. (Mumps) Gynaecomastia and signs of orchitis (severe testicular pain with a swollen, tender testicle that is Prehn's sign positive), on the background of parotitis and myalgia three months prior, suggests mumps. Orchitis is a common complication of mumps, a few weeks after the peak of parotitis and mumps has been shown to decrease the production of testosterone, which causes an imbalance in oestrogen:testosterone levels in the body and causes gynaecomastia.

Question 36

E. (Proliferative retinopathy) Blurred vision and floaters in the right eye, on the background of poorly controlled type 2 diabetes mellitus combined with neovascularization, intraretinal haemorrhages and cotton-wool spots in the right eye on fundoscopy suggest proliferative retinopathy. Proliferative retinopathy is a more severe form of diabetic retinopathy requiring either neovascularization or vitreous/preretinal haemorrhage to be diagnosed.

Question 37

E. (TSH receptor-stimulating antibodies) Signs of hyperthyroidism (unintentional weight loss, palpitations and heat intolerance) for 3 months combined with diffusely enlarged thyroid gland with a low TSH and a high serum T4 suggest Graves disease. The antibodies most commonly associated with Graves are TSH receptor-stimulating antibodies.

Question 38

E. (Trans-sphenoidal surgery) Progressively enlarging hands and feet and joint pain in the wrists and knees for 2 years associated with coarsening facial features combined with macroglossia suggests acromegaly. The first-line management for acromegaly is trans-sphenoidal surgery to remove the pituitary adenoma releasing excess GH causing the acromegaly. If surgery is not possible, a somatostatin analogue like octreotide is indicated.

Question 39

D. (Hypoparathyroidism) Muscular cramps and facial twitching on the background of thyroidectomy combined with positive Chvostek sign, hypocalcaemia, high phosphate and decreased PTH, suggest hypoparathyroidism. The symptoms of hypoparathyroidism are secondary to hypocalcaemia and are caused often by thyroid surgery due to reduced functional total parathyroid parenchyma volume causing reduced PTH.

Question 40

D. (Gastroparesis) Abdominal pain, bloating and vomiting after eating, on the background of poorly controlled type 2 diabetes mellitus with erratic blood glucose measures combined with abdominal distension and generalized abdominal pain and glycosuria suggests a gastrointestinal autonomic neuropathy secondary to poorly controlled diabetes. Gastroparesis is delayed emptying of solids by the stomach in the absence of any mechanical obstruction, with diabetes, affecting the vagal nerve, resulting in reduced frequency of antral contractions and decreased gastric tone.

Question 41

D. (Spironolactone) Fatigue and muscle weakness for 3 months combined with hypertension on examination, hypokalaemia, and bilateral adrenocortical hyperplasia (adrenal gland limb >10mm thick) on CT abdomen suggest primary hyperaldosteronism. As bilateral adrenocortical hyperplasia is the cause of his primary hyperaldosteronism, aldosterone antagonists such as spironolactone are needed to treat the hyperkalaemia.

Question 42

E. (Toxic multinodular goitre) Oligomenorrhea for 6 months on the background of iodine deficiency combined with an irregular goitre, bilateral lid lag and tachycardia on examination and patchy uptake on thyroid scintigraphy suggests toxic multinodular goitre. The symptoms of toxic multinodular goitre are more insidious and symptoms less dramatic than for Graves disease.

Question 43

D. (Insulin) Gestational diabetes is diagnosed after a fasting glucose > 5.6 mmol/mol or an OGTT 2-hour plasma glucose > 7.8 mmol/l (5678 rule). A fasting plasma glucose >7.0 mmol/mol indicates insulin for gestational diabetes. Otherwise, dietary interventions should be trialled for two weeks. Glibencamide is indicated if metformin is contraindicated or if insulin is refused and metformin fails to control glucose levels.

Question 44

D. (Regular observation) Microaneurysms, blot haemorrhages and hard exudates on the background of poorly controlled type 2 diabetes mellitus suggest background retinopathy, which is an early, less serious form of nonproliferative diabetic retinopathy. The management for background retinopathy is regular observation until neovascularization is present, when panretinal laser photocoagulation would be indicated.

Question 45

B. (Hyperosmolar hyperglycaemic state) Confusion and polydipsia on the background of type 2 diabetes mellitus combined with significantly elevated blood glucose (37.5 mmol/L) and serum osmolality (341 mOsmol/kg) but no significant ketonaemia (pH = 7.32) suggest hyperosmolar hyperglycaemic state. The criteria for HHS are profound hyperglycaemia (glucose ≥30 mmol/L), hyperosmolality (effective serum osmolality usually ≥320 mOsm/kg), and volume depletion in the absence of significant ketoacidosis (pH ≥7.3 and bicarbonate ≥15 mmol/L [≥15 mEq/L]).

Question 46

A. (Cardiomyopathy) Increased sweating and joint pain for a year combined with facial features with frontal bossing, enlargement of the hands and feet, hypertension on examination and an elevated serum IGF-1 suggest acromegaly. The main complications asociated with acromegaly are type 2 diabetes mellitus, hypertension and cardiomyopathy.

Question 47

D. (Oral glucose tolerance test) Weight gain during pregnancy that is more compared to a previous one 2 years ago on the background of both first-degree relatives having type 2 diabetes mellitus with a normal BP and no signs of proteinuria or haematuria necessitates an oral glucose tolerance test at 24-28 weeks (due to the risk factor of first-degree relative with diabetes).

Question 48

A. (Cabergoline) Loss of libido and occasional headaches combined with galactorrhoea on examination and significantly elevated prolactin suggest prolactinoma. The management of choice for a prolactinoma is a dopamine agonist like cabergoline, which inhibits prolactin secretion and shrinks the tumour size.

Question 49

C. (Congenital adrenal hyperplasia) Vomiting and poor feeding in a baby girl, combined with an enlarged labia and a mild salt-wasting crisis (hypotension and hyponatraemia), suggest congenital adrenal hyperplasia. The majority of the cases of congenital adrenal hyperplasia are caused by 21-hydroxylase deficiency and often present with virilisation of female genitalia and a salt-wasting crisis within the first three weeks of life.

Question 50

B. (Fluid restriction) Generalized weakness and nausea and vomiting for a week, on the background of small-cell lung cancer, combined with orthostatic hypotension, signs of dehydration (dry mucous membranes and decreased skin turgor) and a low serum sodium and serum osmolality, suggest SIADH. The management of choice for SIADH is a fluid restriction if the symptoms are mild or moderate (lack of neurological signs), with IV hypertonic saline indicated for severe SIADH and tolvaptan indicated for chronic SIADH if fluid restriction does not work.

Question 51

E. (Thyroid lymphoma) Rapidly growing mass in her neck region with a large, tender mass in the neck and dysphagia on examination on the background of the hypothyroid phase of Hashimoto's thyroiditis (positive anti-TPO and amenorrhoea), suggests thyroid cancer. Guidelines suggest suspecting thyroid cancer if there is a sudden onset of a rapidly expanding painless thyroid mass, significantly increasing in size over days and weeks. Thyroid lymphoma is a rare thyroid cancer associated with Hashimoto's thyroiditis, as the B cells that form the anti-TPO antibodies undergo clonal expansion and can accumulate genetic mutations that predispose them to malignant transformation into lymphoma cells.

Question 52

D. (Squamous cell carcinoma) Systemic signs of lung cancer (chronic cough with haemoptypsis, unintentional weight loss), and hypercalcaemia, suggest squamous cell carcinoma. Squamous cell carcinoma causes hypercalcaemia through the production of PTH-rp protein, which has the same N-terminal end as PTH and therefore it can bind to the same receptor, the Type I PTH receptor and exhibit the same effects.

Question 53

C. (Medullary thyroid cancer) Diarrhoea, fine tremors, palpitations and hypertension (phaeochromocytoma) with a rapidly, growing neck lump, hypercalcaemia, low phosphate and high PTH (parathyroid hyperplasia), suggest multiple endocrine neoplasia type 2a (phaeochromocytoma and parathyroid hyperplasia). Medullary thyroid cancer is the type of cancer associated with multiple endocrine neoplasia type 2a.

Question 54

E. (Tamoxifen) Left breast enlargement, without discharge and reduced testicle volume, on the background of being a young gym user suggests gynaecomastia secondary to anabolic steroid use, should be managed with selective oestrogen receptor modulators such as tamoxifen. Reassurance would be inappropriate given his embarrassment to exercise. More often than not, gynaecomastia secondary to anabolic steroid usage requires surgical intervention, but medical management should be trialled first.

Question 55

E. (Serum thyroglobulin) Papillary thyroid cancer has the best prognosis out of all the thyroid cancers, with thyroglobulin being used postthyroidectomy to monitor the completeness of removal of the thyroid cells. Persistently elevated or rising levels of thyroglobulin after thyroidectomy suggest the presence of residual thyroid tissue or recurrence of cancer. Serum calcitonin can be used to measure recurrence of medullary thyroid cancer because it is a cancer of the parafollicular cells, also known as C cells.

Question 56

E. (Smoking) Eye discomfort and protrusion on the background of poorly controlled Graves disease combined with bilateral eyelid retraction and proptosis, with normal visual acuity, suggests thyroid eye disease. The strongest risk factor for thyroid eye disease that is modifiable is smoking.

Question 57

D. (Urinary 5-HIAA) Diarrhoea, abdominal pain and facial flushing for 3 months combined with a pulmonary stenosis murmur and hypotension on examination suggest carcinoid syndrome. The investigation of choice for carcinoid syndrome is urinary 5-HIAA, which is the main metabolite of serotonin, with the pathway going from serotonin to 5-hydroxyindole-3-acetaldehyde by monoamine oxidase, which then is oxidized into 5-HIAA.

Question 58

D. (Surgical resection) Racing heartbeat and headaches combined with sweating profusely and elevated blood pressure on examination with an elevated 24-hour urinary collection of metanephrines and a left adrenal mass on the CT abdomen suggest phaeochromocytoma. The definitive management for phaeochromocytoma is surgical resection of the adrenal mass unless the patient is at high surgical risk due to causes such as heart failure, in which medical management with anti-hypertensives is indicated.

Question 59

B. (Pepperpot skull) Generalized weakness and bilateral loin to groin pain for a year combined with hypercalcaemia, low phosphate and high PTH suggest primary hyperparathyroidism. Out of the potential options, pepperpot skull is associated with primary hyperparathyroidism. Pepperpot skull refers to multiple well-defined lucencies in the calvaria (uppermost part of the skull) caused by resorption of trabecular bone causing spotty deossification.

Question 60

D. (Diabetic ulcer) Lesion on left foot after stepping on a glass a month ago associated with pain and erythema, on the background of type 2 diabetes mellitus and pain and erythema combined with a deep, necrotic ulcer on the plantar surface of the left foot suggests a diabetic ulcer. Diabetic ulcers most often occur on the feet and lower extremities due to reduced sensation, impaired blood flow, and increased susceptibility to trauma in these areas.

Question 61

B. (Bartter syndrome) Bartter syndrome is caused by defective chloride absorption at the Na^+ K^+ $2Cl^-$ cotransporter (NKCC2) in the ascending loop of Henle, thereby causing hypokalemia features (muscle weakness) along with failure to thrive. What differentiates Bartter syndrome from other causes of hypokalaemia like as primary hyperaldosteronism is the presence of normotension, whilst the other listed options would present with hypertension.

Question 62

C. (Octreotide) Diarrhoea and flushing occurring more frequently combined with flushed skin, a wheeze on examination, and a raised level of 5-HIAA suggests carcinoid syndrome. The management for carcinoid syndrome are somatostatin analogues such as octreotide. Octreotide works by binding to somatostatin receptors on the surface of carcinoid tumour cells, thereby it suppresses the release of serotonin and other vasoactive substances from the tumour cells providing symptomatic relief for patients.

Question 63

D. (Surgical excision) Recurrent neck lump after an upper respiratory infection, combined with a midline mass found over the anterior neck around 2 cm below the hyoid bone that is painless and mobile on swallowing suggests a thyroglossal cyst. A thyroglossal cyst is the most common cause of a midline neck mass and occurs due to the presence of an embryological remnant, the thyroglossal tract. The thyroglossal tract arises from the foramen caecum at the junction of the anterior two-thirds and posterior one-third of the tongue. Inflammation of the tract remnant occurs commonly after infection such as an upper respiratory tract infection. The definitive management is the surgical excision of the cyst, often using the Sistrunk procedure.

Question 64

A. (Autosomal dominant) Hypertension and palpitations (phaeochromocytoma) with bilateral loin to groin pain, hypercalcaemia, low phosphate and high PTH (parathyroid hyperplasia) and a small, well-defined lesion in the head of the pancreas (pancreatic tumour) suggests multiple endocrine neoplasia type I (3 Ps: Parathyroid hyperplasia, phaeochromocytoma and pancreatic tumours). The mode of inheritance for multiple endocrine neoplasia type I is autosomal dominant.

Question 65

D. (Iron-deficiency anaemia) HbA1c can be inaccurate, higher than expected because of an increased red blood cell lifespan. Out of the potential options, iron-deficiency anaemia is the only one that increases the red blood cell lifespan. In iron deficiency, red cell production decreases consequently an increased average age of circulating red cells ultimately leads to elevated HbA1c levels. Furthermore, reduced iron stores have a link with increased glycation of haemoglobin, leading to false-high values of HbA1c in nondiabetic individuals.

Question 66

E. (Topical lubricants) Eye redness and insecurities over eye protrusion, on the background of poorly controlled Graves disease combined with bilateral eyelid retraction and conjunctival injection, suggest thyroid eye disease. The most appropriate management for thyroid eye disease is topical lubricants.

Question 67

B. (Failure of gonadotrophin-releasing hormone-secreting neurons to migrate to the hypothalamus) Poor physical development and anosmia combined with abnormal descent of the testes, a reduced LH and FSH, and a reduced testosterone suggests Kallmann syndrome. Kallmann syndrome is caused by the failure of the gonadotrophin-releasing hormone (GnRH)-secreting neurons to migrate to the hypothalamus, with the anosmia caused by the failure of migration of olfactory nerve cells.

Question 68

D. (RET) Headaches and palpitations on the background of a family history of medullary thyroid cancer combined with hypertension and elevated serum calcitonin levels, and multiple thyroid nodules on thyroid US suggest multiple endocrine neoplasia type IIb (medullary thyroid cancer and phaeochromocytoma). The oncogene associated with multiple endocrine neoplasia type IIb is the RET oncogene, with mutations leading to constitutive activation of the RET signalling pathway, resulting in uncontrolled cell proliferation and tumour formation in the thyroid gland.

Question 69

C. (Gliclazide) This patient has Maturity Onset Diabetes of the Young (MODY) due to the young age of onset (<25), family history of diabetes (in two consecutive generations), normal BMI, absence of typical type 2 diabetes symptoms, normal C-peptide level (indicating preserved beta-cell function unlike in type 1 diabetes), and known HNF1A gene mutation.
HNF1A gene mutation patients are particularly sensitive to sulfonylureas (gliclazide), which can effectively control their blood glucose levels at lower doses compared to those used in type 2 diabetes. Metformin, a common first-line treatment for type 2 diabetes would not be appropriate for MODY patients. GCK mutation patients can be managed conservatively. INS mutation patients can be managed by insulin.

Haematology 23

EXPLANATIONS

Question 1

C. (Hodgkin lymphoma) A painless, rubbery, nontender lymph node in the right neck and pruritus for 2 months, on the background of HIV combined with axillary lymphadenopathy on examination, normocytic anaemia and Reed-Sternberg cells on lymph node biopsy suggest Hodgkin lymphoma. Hodgkin lymphoma is defined by the presence of Reed-Sternberg cells on lymph node biopsy, which none of the non-Hodgkin's lymphomas would present with. Hodgkin lymphoma would also present with a raised LDH and eosinophilia (due to the production of IL-5).

Question 2

A. (Acute lymphoblastic leukaemia) Bone pain and fatigue in a child combined with multiple petechiae and ecchymoses on the skin and lymphadenopathy and hepatosplenomegaly on examination, neutropenia and thrombocytopenia suggest acute lymphoblastic leukaemia. Acute lymphoblastic leukaemia (ALL) is the most common malignancy affecting children and occurs when lymphoid progenitor cells become altered causing uncontrolled proliferation and infiltrates various body organs, causing signs of bone marrow failure such as anaemia.

Question 3

E. (Intrinsic factor antibodies) Dyspnoea and fatigue for a year, on the background of type 1 diabetes mellitus, combined with macroglossia and impaired vibration in the leg on examination combined with macrocytic anaemia suggest pernicious anaemia (the most common cause of vitamin B12 deficiency), given the autoimmune history. Intrinsic factor antibodies are associated with pernicious anaemia.

Question 4

A. (Acute myeloid leukaemia) Fatigue, unintentional weight loss and dyspnoea for 2 months combined with petechiae and hepatosplenomegaly on examination, anaemia and neutropenia on blood and pleomorphic myeloblasts on blood film suggest acute myeloid leukaemia. Acute myeloid leukaemia is associated with bone marrow failure such as pallor (anaemia), bleeding (thrombocytopenia), splenomegaly and neutropenia, as well as pleomorphic myeloblasts which are not seen in the other leukaemias.

Question 5

E. (X-linked recessive) An 8-year-old-girl has prolonged bleeding after tooth extraction. She has multiple minor bruises on her arms and legs but no joint pain, suggesting haemophilia, which is an X-linked recessive condition. An X-linked condition it is more likely to present in males as only one defective copy is needed, however can present in females with an affected father and a carrier/affected female.

Question 6

B. (Chronic myeloid leukaemia) Fatigue, night sweats and weakness for 5 months combined with pallor, splenomegaly and petechiae on examination, anaemia and thrombocytosis and cytogenetic analysis show the presence of the Philadelphia chromosome (t(9;22)) suggest chronic myeloid leukaemia.

Question 7

D. (Hydroxyurea) Severe joint pain and dyspnoea for 2 hours, on the background of similar back pain combined with splenomegaly and scleral icterus, anaemia with increased reticulocytes and sickle-shaped red blood cells suggest a vaso-occlusive crisis. Hydroxyurea is the management of choice for sickle cell anaemia to prevent painful episodes, which works by increasing the levels of HbF in the blood, thereby preventing painful episodes. For an acute crisis, management involves analgesia, antibiotics if signs o infection and a blood transfusion if there are neurological complications.

Question 8

A. (Activated partial thromboplastin time) A fall during football, injuring the right knee, causing the knee to swell up significantly and be associated with prolonged severe bleeding combined with a large right knee effusion and a limited ROM due to pain, suggests haemophilia. Activated partial thromboplastin time is the investigation of choice for haemophilia as it is increased in isolation, unlike other clotting tests for haemophilia.

Question 9

D. (Haemoglobin electrophoresis) Recurrent joint and bone pain associated with fatigue and dyspnoea combined with pallor, scleral icterus and multiple joint tenderness on examination, and a high reticulocyte count and anaemia on blood suggest sickle cell anaemia. Haemoglobin electrophoresis is the investigation of choice for sickle cell anaemia, to look for HbSS (homozygous) or sickle cell trait (HbAS).

Question 10

C. (Factor VIII concentrate) Left elbow swelling suggests haemarthrosis, prolonged bleeding, and a raised aPTT is indicative of haemophilia. Haemophilia A is caused by a deficiency of Factor VIII is more prevalent, so administering Factor VIII concentrate is the appropriate treatment choice.

Question 11

D. (Imatinib) Fatigue and weakness with systemic signs of malignancy for 6 months combined with pallor, splenomegaly and petechiae on examination, anaemia and thrombocytosis and blast cells on blood film suggest chronic myeloid leukaemia. Imatinib is the first-line management for chronic myeloid leukaemia, which works by binding to BCR-ABL kinase domain thereby inducing leukaemic cells apoptosis.

Question 12

B. (Burkitt lymphoma) Fatigue and night sweats for 3 months, on the background of SLE combined with hepatosplenomegaly and lymphadenopathy on examination, normocytic anaemia on blood and a starry sky appearance (lymphocyte sheets interspersed with macrophages) on lymph node biopsy suggest Burkitt's lymphoma, a type of Non-Hodgkin lymphoma.

Question 13

A. (ABVD regimen) Painless, rubbery, nontender lymph node in the neck that's painful on alcohol consumption with associated night sweats and unintentional weight loss combined with multiple lymph nodes in the axilla and groin on examination, normocytic anaemia and eosinophilia in the bloods and Reed-Sternberg cells on lymph node biopsy suggest Hodgkin's lymphoma. ABVD regimen (doxorubicin, bleomycin, vinblastine and dacarbazine) is the standard chemotherapy regimen for Hodgkin's lymphoma.

Question 14

D. (Richter transformation) Acute onset night sweats and unintentional weight loss, on the background of chronic lymphocytic leukaemia combined with lymphadenopathy and abdominal pain on examination and large atypical lymphoid cells on lymph node biopsy, suggest the CLL has transformed to non-Hodgkin's lymphoma, known as the Richter transformation.

Question 15

A. (Howell-Jolly bodies) A routine blood test for coeliac disease shows anaemia; hyposplenism is a well-known complication of coeliac disease; hence, the most likely thing to be seen would be Howell-Jolly bodies. Howell-Jolly bodies are basophilic nuclear remnants in circulating erythrocytes, which are meant to be expelled as part of bone marrow maturation, however, a damaged spleen would mean that these cells aren't filtered out.

Question 16

B. (Direct pressure and nose pinching) Recurrent spontaneous epistaxis for a week with no precipitating factors combined with active bleeding from the nasal septum suggests direct pressure and nose pinching are the most appropriate management. This is the management outlined by the guidelines in active epistaxis with no signs of major haemorrhage, with a vasoconstrictor being considered if nose pinching does not stop the bleeding.

Question 17

B. (Beta-thalassaemia) Failure to thrive with pallor, fatigue and hepatosplenomegaly, combined with microcytic hypochromic anaemia on blood film and raised HbA2 and HbF on haemoglobin electrophoresis, suggests beta-thalassaemia.

Question 18

B. (Factor V Leiden) Factor V Leiden mutation is the most common inherited risk factor for venous thromboembolism (VTE), including deep vein thrombosis (DVT) and pulmonary embolism (PE). It results from a single-point mutation in the factor V gene, leading to resistance to inactivation by activated protein C and predisposing individuals to excessive blood clotting. Patients with factor V Leiden mutation have an increased risk of developing DVT, particularly in the absence of other known risk factors.

Question 19

A. (Anaemia of chronic disease) Anaemia of chronic disease is a common cause of anaemia in patients with chronic inflammatory conditions, such as rheumatoid arthritis, and is characterized by impaired iron utilization despite adequate iron stores. Inflammation-induced cytokines, such as interleukin-6 (IL-6), suppress erythropoiesis and impair iron metabolism, hence causing high ferritin and low TIBC.

Question 20

B. (Lifelong blood transfusion) A young girl in the first year of her life with failure to thrive, pallor, jaundice and hepatosplenomegaly combined with an elevated HbF and HbA2 suggests beta-thalassaemia. The management of choice for beta-thalassaemia is lifelong blood transfusions.

Question 21

A. (Aplastic anaemia) Recurrent epistaxis and menorrhagia, with multiple petechiae and ecchymoses over the limbs on examination combined with pancytopenia and a hypocellular marrow on bone marrow biopsy, suggest aplastic anaemia. To diagnose aplastic anaemia at least two of the following peripheral cytopenias must be present: haemoglobin <100 g/L, platelets $<50 \times 10^9$/L, absolute neutrophil count $<1.5 \times 10^9$/L.

Question 22

E. (Splenectomy) Pallor and jaundice, on the background of acute cholecystitis associated with black pigmented gallstones combined with splenomegaly and scleral icterus on examination and severe anaemia, reduced reticulocyte count and increased MCHC, suggest hereditary spherocytosis. Splenectomy is the definitive management for hereditary spherocytosis.

Question 23

E. (Prednisolone) Easy bruising, epistaxis and bleeding gums combined with multiple petechiae and ecchymoses on the legs on examination and isolated thrombocytopenia suggest immune thrombocytopenia. Prednisolone is the first-line management for immune thrombocytopenia with symptoms of bleeding such as oral mucosal bleeding because corticosteroids prevent immune-mediated destruction of platelets.

Question 24

E. (Multiple myeloma) Bone pain worse in the spine and ribs, on the background of a family history of malignancy combined with mild pallor and generalized bruising on examination, anaemia and hypercalcaemia and Rouleaux formation on blood film suggest multiple myeloma. Multiple myeloma is associated with CRABBI (calcium, renal, anaemia, bleeding, bones, infection) symptoms.

Question 25

B. (Aspirin and venesection) Fatigue, worsening headache and pruritus after hot showers for 5 months combined with hypertension, splenomegaly and excoriations all over the body on examination and polycythaemia and thrombocytosis suggests polycythaemia vera. Aspirin and venesection is the management of choice for polycythaemia vera to reduce the risk of thrombotic events, in patients with a platelet count $<1500 \times 10^9$/L and those that are low-risk (aged <60 years with no history of thrombosis)

Question 26

A. (Haemolytic uraemic syndrome) Bloody diarrhoea combined with renal failure (elevated urea and creatinine), thrombocytopenia and schistocytes on blood film suggest haemolytic uraemic syndrome. It is caused by E. coli 0157:H7 forming a Shiga toxin which damages renal glomerular endothelial cells, causing cell damage and detachment, exposing the basement membrane with resultant microvascular thrombosis.

Question 27

E. (Von Willebrand Factor [vWF] assay) Severe menorrhagia on the background of similar episodes in the past, on the background of both her mother and maternal aunt having menorrhagia combined with normal platelet counts and prothrombin time, suggests Von Willebrand disease. Von Willebrand Factor (vWF) assay is the investigation of choice for Von Willebrand disease.

Question 28

C. (*Escherichia coli* 0157:H7) The triad of bloody diarrhoea after food poisoning associated with renal failure and thrombocytopenia suggests haemolytic uraemic syndrome (HUS). *Escherichia coli* 0157:H7 is indicated in 90% of cases of HUS.

Question 29

C. (Desmopressin) Prolonged bleeding after surgery on the background of his mother having menorrhagia combined with a normal prothrombin time and platelet count but decreased von Willebrand factor suggests von Willebrand disease. Desmopressin is the management of choice for von Willebrand disease to raise levels of vWF.

Question 30

A. (Fresh frozen plasma) Dysuria and confusion after recent surgery combined with hypotension, tachycardia and evidence of bleeding (petechial bruising and from cannula) on examination along with a low platelet count and prolonged PT and aPTT suggest disseminated intravascular coagulation (DIC). The management of choice for DIC is fresh frozen plasma to replace the lost clotting factors. Surgery can predispose individuals to DIC through multiple mechanisms involving tissue injury, activation of the clotting cascade, inflammatory response, and blood transfusion reactions.

Question 31

A. (Allopurinol) Fatigue, generalized weakness and oliguria after recent chemotherapy combined with confusion and lethargy on examination, with hyperkalaemia, hypocalcaemia, hyperuricaemia and raised creatinine suggest tumour lysis syndrome. Allopurinol can be given prophylactically for tumour lysis syndrome to reduce uric acid production, as it is a xanthine oxidase inhibitor which blocks the purine to urate conversion pathway.

Question 32

D. (JAK2) A worsening headache and pruritus episodes after a hot bath, on the background of a pulmonary embolism, combined with hypertension, splenomegaly and excoriation on the arms and torso on examination with polycythaemia and thrombocytosis, suggest polycythaemia vera, which is associated with the Janus Kinase 2 (JAK2) mutation in 95% of cases. JAK2 is implicated in the signalling by temperatures in the type II cytokine receptor family.

Question 33

C. (Bortezomib + stem cell transplant) Polyuria and back pain on the background of recurrent infections combined with bone tenderness and pallor on examination, hypercalcaemia, and renal failure suggest multiple myeloma. Multiple myeloma is associated with CRABBI (calcium, renal, anaemia, bleeding, bones, infection) symptoms, and the definitive management of choice is an induction therapy such as Bortezomib before stem cell transplant.

Question 34

B. (Neutropenic sepsis) Chills, high-grade fever and generalized weakness, on the background of recent chemotherapy combined with tachycardia and mild pallor on examination, suggest neutropenic sepsis. For neutropenic sepsis to be diagnosed two of the following criteria need to be met: neutrophil count of $<0.5 \times 10^9$/l and either a fever of >38.0°C or other signs and symptoms consistent with clinically significant sepsis.

Question 35

E. (Stop blood transfusion) Dyspnoea and orthopnoea after a blood transfusion combined with hypertension, tachycardia, bibasal crepitations and raised JVP on examination suggest transfusion-associated circulatory overload (TACO). TACO refers to features of heart failure precipitated by an excessive rate of transfusion and management should be to initially stop the blood transfusion.

Question 36

B. (Bone marrow biopsy) Fatigue and unintentional weight loss for 6 months, associated with appetite loss and night sweats, on the background of polycythaemia vera combined with splenomegaly and multiple bruises and tear-drop poikilocytes on a blood smear, suggest myelofibrosis. Bone marrow biopsy is the investigation of choice for myelofibrosis and should be a dry tap.

Question 37

E. (Transfusion-related acute lung injury) Dyspnoea and fever whilst receiving a blood transfusion combined with tachycardia, hypotension and bilateral crepitations on examination and bilateral pulmonary infiltrates suggest transfusion-related acute lung injury (TRALI). TRALI is defined as non-cardiogenic pulmonary oedema secondary to host neutrophil activation in donor blood causing increased vascular permeability. The hypotension is caused by the increased vascular permeability, causing rapid and large increases in blood flow to peripheral tissue leading to a decrease in the volume of circulating blood and subsequent hypotension.

Question 38

A. (Blood transfusion and folic acid) Sudden haematuria with scleral icterus and splenomegaly on examination and Heinz bodies on peripheral blood smear suggests glucose-6-phosphate dehydrogenase (G6PD) deficiency. This is due to primaquine causing premature splenic sequestration of intact erythrocytes.

Question 39

E. (Waldenstrom macroglobulinaemia) Systemic signs of malignancy, on the background of upper respiratory tract infection, combined with hepatosplenomegaly and lymphadenopathy with lymphoplasmacytic lymphoma cells on bone marrow biopsy suggest Waldenstrom macroglobulinaemia. Waldesntrom macroglobulinaemia is a lymphoplasmacytoid malignancy caused by monoclonal IgM paraprotein secretion.

Question 40

D. (Piperacillin-tazobactam) Signs of sepsis on the background of recent chemotherapy for breast cancer with neutropenia suggest neutropenic sepsis. For neutropenic sepsis to be diagnosed two of the following criteria need to be met: neutrophil count of $<0.5 \times 10^9$/l and either a fever of >38.0°C or other signs and symptoms consistent with clinically significant sepsis. Piperacillin with tazobactam (Tazocin) is the immediate management for neutropenic sepsis due to its broad-spectrum nature.

Question 41

A. (ADAMTS13) Recurrent abdominal pain and fever in a woman, on the background of SLE, combined with multiple petechiae and ecchymoses on examination with haemolytic anaemia and thrombocytopenia suggest thrombotic thrombocytopenic purpura (TTP). ADAMTS13 is the enzyme deficiency associated with TTP, causing large sticky multimers of von Willebrand's factor, thereby causing the thrombotic effects of TTP.

Question 42

C. (Glucose-6-phosphate dehydrogenase [G6PD] deficiency enzyme assay) An episode of haematuria and generalized weakness with scleral icterus and splenomegaly and peripheral blood smear showing Heinz bodies (small round inclusions within the RBC), suggest glucose-6-phosphate dehydrogenase (G6PD) deficiency. A G6PD deficiency enzyme assay is the investigation of choice for G6PD deficiency.

Question 43

D. (Myelodysplasia) Fatigue bleeding gums and easy bruising combined with multiple petechiae and ecchymoses on her arms and torso, with pancytopenia and 5q deletion, suggest myelodysplasia. Myelodysplasia is a clonal haematopoietic neoplasm characterised by cytopenias with cytogenetic abnormalities like 5q deletion, which is a loss of the q arm of human chromosome 5 in bone marrow myelocyte cells.

Question 44

E. (*Staphylococcus epidermidis*) Staphylococcus epidermidis, a commensal skin flora is the most likely cause of the high-grade fever and generalized weakness in this neutropenic patient with acute lymphoblastic leukaemia who has recently undergone induction chemotherapy. It is a common cause of catheter-related bloodstream infections, which are prevalent in patients with indwelling medical devices (used in chemotherapy).

Question 45

D. (Nonmyeloablative stem cell transplant) Myelofibrosis is a rare blood cancer characterized by bone marrow fibrosis, leading to disrupted blood cell production, anaemia, and splenomegaly. It may develop on its own (primary) or from other myeloproliferative diseases. Common mutations include JAK2, CALR, and MPL. Diagnosis involves clinical evaluation, blood tests, bone marrow biopsy, and genetic testing. The management of myelofibrosis depends on the patient's risk (using the Dynamic International Prognostic Scoring System (DIPSS)) and age. The DIPSS score comprises five scoring points: >65 years old, WCC: >25 × 109 cells/dl, haemoglobin: <100 g/L, peripheral blasts ≥1% and constitutional symptoms. Nonmyeloablative stem cell transplant is the management of choice for myelofibrosis in patients over 50 with a DIPSS score > 1, with no contraindications to stem cell transplant.

Section 4
SURGERY ANSWERS

Trauma and surgical emergencies 24

Question 1

D. (Needle decompression in the 2nd intercostal space) Tension pneumothorax presents with respiratory distress, reduced breath sounds, hyperresonance to percussion and tracheal deviation away from the affected side. Emergency management with needle decompression is appropriate in haemodynamic instability. Following this, definitive chest drain placement can occur. Finger thoracostomy is used in peri-arrest situations.

Question 2

D. (Subdural haematoma) Headache, confusion and gait ataxia following a fall are classical features of subdural haematoma, common in elderly patients, those with hypertension, and alcoholics with recurrent falls. Intracerebral haemorrhage only occurs in severe uncontrolled hypertension. Wernicke encephalopathy presents with gradual onset of confusion, gait ataxia and ophthalmoplegia in those with a history of alcohol excess.

Question 3

C. (Haematoma evacuation) Craniotomy and haematoma evacuation is the most appropriate management of an extradural haematoma, which can occur following acute head injury and rupture of the middle meningeal artery over the temporal lobe. Initial loss of consciousness followed by a lucid interval before progressive GCS deterioration is the typical presentation. Burr hole surgery can be used as a temporary emergency measure in patients with GCS <8. Mannitol and Tranexamic acid can be considered as adjunctive measures.

Question 4

C. (Lumbar puncture) A young woman with a sudden, severe headache is the classical presentation of a subarachnoid haemorrhage. If CT is nondiagnostic, a lumbar puncture after 12 hours should be performed, to detect xanthochromia of the CSF, indicating bilirubin from breakdown of red blood cells. Meningeal symptoms are common, from blood irritating the meninges.

Question 5

C. (CT scan of head) Following significant polytrauma, extensive imaging is required. A CT head is the most important immediate investigation to obtain, as there is evidence of potential traumatic brain injury with occipital laceration, loss of consciousness and respiratory depression, which must be urgently identified and treated to avoid long-term neurological impairment.

Question 6

B. (Fasciotomy) Compartment syndrome can occur following limb trauma and bleeding into the fixed limb compartment spaces, increasing intracompartmental pressure and leading to tissue ischaemia. It presents with pain out of proportion to clinical signs and leg swelling, paralysis and neurovascular impairment. Urgent fasciotomy is required to reduce intracompartmental pressures and tissue necrosis.

Question 7

E. (Transfusion-related circulatory overload) Acute transfusion reactions may develop as a result of ABO incompatibility, allergy to blood products, systemic inflammatory responses or volume overload. Transfusion-associated circulatory overload presents following rapid transfusion of large volumes of blood, with symptoms of acute heart failure.

Question 8

B. (Flail chest) Flail chest occurs when three or more adjacent ribs are fractured in multiple places, typically following blunt chest wall trauma. Respiratory distress, palpable crepitus and paradoxical chest wall movement during respiration are typical features.

Question 9

D. (Splenectomy) There is evidence of splenic rupture, with a LUQ laceration, diffuse abdominal pain, guarding and dullness to percussion on the left-hand side. Definitive management of splenic rupture with haemodynamic instability is with urgent splenectomy. Arterial embolization can be considered in low-grade injuries with haemodynamic stability.

Question 10

C. (Intraosseous access in the proximal tibia) Intraosseous access is used following multiple failed attempts at peripheral IV access. In severe haemodynamic instability there is a risk of cardiac arrest without urgent fluid resuscitation; hence IO access is appropriate.

Question 11

C. (Large volume fluid resuscitation) Following crush injuries, rhabdomyolysis of muscle tissue can occur, with release of creatine phosphokinase and myoglobin leading to acute tubular necrosis, myoglobinuria and AKI. Hypovolaemic shock can occur if muscle breakdown is significant; hence large-volume fluid resuscitation is the mainstay of treatment.

Question 12

E. (Point-of-care FAST scan) Intra-abdominal bleeding presents with abdominal bruising, pain and peritoneal signs (guarding, reduced bowel sounds). Haemodynamic instability indicates major bleeding. The diagnosis can be urgently confirmed with bedside ultrasonography, with a Focused Assessment with Sonography for Trauma (FAST) scan.

Question 13

B. (Debridement and skin graft) Third-degree full-thickness burn present with painless, nonblanching skin and white waxy discoloration of the burnt area. Management involves debridement of necrotic tissue and reconstruction, typically skin grafting. Topical moisturizers, antiseptic ointments and silver dressings are used for first or second-degree injuries.

Question 14

C. (Disseminated intravascular coagulation) DIC can occur following significant blood loss and presents with uncontrolled bleeding and coagulopathy, classically with elevated APTT, PT and fibrinogen. Overactivation of the clotting cascade leads to clotting factor consumption and massive haemorrhage. Management involves transfusions of blood products and treatment of the underlying cause.

Question 15

A. (Chest drain insertion) Haemothorax can develop following penetrating chest wall injuries and presents with chest pain, dyspnoea, reduced breath sounds and dullness to percussion, with a total white out and meniscus level on CXR. Management involves chest drain placement. Thoracotomy is indicated if the chest drain output is significant or if multiple blood transfusions are required.

Question 16

B. (Hemisection of the spinal cord) Hemisection of the cord can occur following a penetrating injury, presenting with ipsilateral paralysis and proprioceptive loss below the lesion, with contralateral loss of pain and temperature sensation, due to lesion of the spinothalamic tract with decussates in the spinal cord. Loss of sphincter control can also occur.

Question 17

A. (Analgesia) Flail chest presents with chest wall tenderness, respiratory distress, palpable crepitus and paradoxical movement of the chest wall during respiration. Flail chest occurs when three or more adjacent ribs are fractured in multiple places. Typically surgery is not required unless there is significant chest wall deformity or rib nonunion. Patients can be managed with strong NSAIDs and opiate analgesia.

Question 18

E. (Spondylodesis) Spinal fractures present with focal spinal tenderness following a fall. The presence of lower limb neurological symptoms indicates an unstable fracture, which should be managed with spondylodesis, involving vertebral body fusion via internal fixation.

Question 19

C. (Postburn hypermetabolism) Following a severe burn injury, postburn hypermetabolism can occur. Initially a hypermetabolic phase occurs, with decreased cardiac output and metabolic rate. Subsequently a hypermetabolic, catabolic state occurs, presenting with hyperdynamic circulation, weight loss, hyperthermia and multiorgan dysfunction. Management involves nutritional support, anabolic steroids and effective management of the burn areas with excision and grafting.

Question 20

A. (Diaphragmatic rupture) Diaphragmatic rupture can occur following penetrating trauma and presents with audible bowel sounds in the chest. The CXR demonstrates herniation of bowel loops into the chest and mediastinal shift.

Perioperative care 25

Question 1

B. (Codeine) Paracetamol is the first step on the WHO analgesic ladder. NSAIDs are appropriate adjunctive measures at each step - however, this patient has contraindication to NSAID use (peptic ulcer disease), hence stepping up to weak opioids such as codeine is appropriate. Co-codamol contains paracetamol, so it must be used in place of, not alongside, paracetamol.

Question 2

B. (CPR) Patients are at increased risk of myocardial infarction in the perioperative period due to increased myocardial oxygen demand and ischaemia. The initial management of acute myocardial infarction may include aspirin, GTN spray, morphine and clopidogrel – however, unresponsiveness and unrecordable BP and oxygen saturations suggests acute cardiac arrest, meaning CPR should be initiated immediately as per ALS.

Question 3

E. (Treatment dose low-molecular-weight heparin) DVTs present with leg pain, swelling and erythema, with risk factors including malignancy, pelvic surgery and immobility. Management is with anticoagulation. Apixaban is first line in patients without renal impairment. Given CKD 3 and hypertension, treatment-dose low-molecular-weight heparin (LMWH) is preferred in this case.

Question 4

E. (NG tube and IV fluids) Postoperative ileus present with nausea and vomiting, abdominal pain and distension, obstipation and absent bowel sounds. Management involves NG tube insertion with free drainage, IV fluids, bowel rest and nutritional support.

Question 5

A. (Fixed rate insulin infusion) Diabetic ketoacidosis which can occur during a preoperative fasting without appropriate management of blood glucose. Management is with fluid resuscitation and fixed-rate insulin infusion.

Question 6

C. (IM adrenaline 1:1000) Warning signs of anaphylaxis include acute development of an itchy urticaria rash minutes after anaesthetic administration. NMDA antagonists such as suxamethonium are a common cause. IM adrenaline 1:1000 should be immediately given.

Question 7

C. (Surgical site infection) Five days post-operatively, the most common cause of fever is surgical site infection. She has worsening pain in her hip, suggesting local wound infection, and no other localizing symptoms.

Question 8

E. (Septic shock) Pyrexia, tachycardia and hypotension, with elevated white cells and CRP, suggest septic shock. Tachypnoea is one of the earliest signs of sepsis.

Question 9

C. (Capillary blood glucose) Insulin-controlled diabetes increases the risk of perioperative hypoglycaemia. Drowsiness, confusion, tachycardia and tachypnoea are typical features. Management in drowsy patients is with IV dextrose or glucogel.

Question 10

A. (Acute tubular necrosis) An AKI is diagnosed when creatinine rises above 1.5 × the baseline level. All answers are important causes of AKI. In this case, the medication history includes ramipril and aspirin, which can cause acute tubular necrosis and AKI if not held in the perioperative period. Contrast nephropathy is rare.

Question 11

B. (Atelectasis) Postoperatively, pain and immobility can cause patients to inadequately ventilate their lungs, causing alveolar collapse and atelectasis. Decreased breath sounds, cough, lower-grade fever and new oxygen requirement are typical features. Good pain relief and early mobilization are the most effective management.

Question 12

D. (CT of abdomen) Peritonitis presents with pyrexia, shock and abdominal guarding and rebound tenderness. An anastomotic leak is the likely cause. CT abdomen will demonstrate abnormal peritoneal fluid collection.

Peritoneal fluid analysis can help distinguish SBP and secondary peritonitis, but there is no indication this patient had preexisting ascites risking development of SBP.

Question 13

B. (Echocardiogram) Aortic stenosis presents with palpitations and an ejection systolic murmur in the aortic area. This should be confirmed on echocardiogram prior to surgery so an appropriate anaesthetic plan can be made, given increased perioperative cardiac risk.

Question 14

B. (CT scan of pulmonary arteries) PEs present with dyspnoea, tachycardia, haemoptysis and chest pain. Orthopaedic surgery is a significant risk factor for VTE. Her Wells score is 7, indicating PE is likely. A CTPA will confirm the diagnosis.

Question 15

E. (Naloxone) Opiate overdoses present with reduced GCS, respiratory depression, with pinpoint pupils. Stridor can occur due to airway collapse. Naloxone should be administered to rapidly reverse the opiates, and his analgesia regimen reviewed to prevent further episodes.

Question 16

B. (Aspiration pneumonia) Pneumonia presents with cough, dyspnoea, pyrexia, tachypnoea and hypoxia. The chest X-ray demonstrates the NG tube has been placed in the lungs, resulting in aspiration of feed and development of infection. The NG tube should be removed and antibiotics prescribed.

Question 17

D. (Paracetamol) Febrile nonhaemolytic transfusion reactions present with fever during transfusion administration. There is no evidence of acute haemolysis requiring adrenaline or pulmonary complications requiring diuresis. The transfusion should be stopped, antipyretics given, and the transfusion restarted at a slower rate if he remains stable.

Question 18

D. (Refeeding syndrome) Refeeding syndrome results from rapid reintroduction of nutrition in chronic, severe malnourishment. Symptoms include tachycardia, oedema and tremor. The electrolyte derangement (low potassium, phosphate and magnesium) is diagnostic. There is a risk of seizures, arrhythmias and acute renal failure with urgent electrolyte replacement.

Question 19

A. (Accept her decision and cancel the surgery) The patient has demonstrated the ability to understand, retain, weigh up and communicate her decision not to have surgery, indicating she has capacity to refuse. Detention under the Mental Health Act is not an automatic indication that she lacks capacity.

Question 20

B. (Coagulation screen) DIC presents with bleeding from multiple sites, confusion and hypotension, which can occur perioperatively due to significant clotting factor consumption. Coagulation screen will demonstrate anaemia, thrombocytopenia and elevated APTT and PT. Management involves transfusion of blood products.

Gastrointestinal surgery 26

Question 1

E. (Peptic ulcer disease) Gastric ulcers present with epigastric pain worse after eating and weight loss (due to food avoidance). Anxiety and alcohol use are risk factors, as well as NSAID use and smoking. Management is with H. pylori testing and treatment if present, and acid-reducing therapies.

Question 2

A. (Bleeding oesophageal varices) Haematemesis and evidence of chronic liver disease, with jaundice, pruritus, abdominal distention and caput medusa, suggest portosystemic anastomoses, which can include oesophageal varices. Oesophageal varices are at high risk of bleeding. Management is with endoscopic haemostasis, antibiotics and terlipressin, which reduces portal pressures.

Question 3

D. (Diverticular disease) Diverticular disease presents with constipation and left lower quadrant tenderness. Chronic constipation and smoking are risk factors. Colonoscopy demonstrates the classic outpouchings of colonic mucosa. Management is with lifestyle modifications to reduce constipation and smoking cessation.

Question 4

D. (Intravenous fluids) Severe epigastric pain radiating to the black, vomiting and fever are features of pancreatitis. Gallstones are the likely underlying aetiology, given preceding symptoms of biliary colic. Intravenous fluids are the mainstay of treatment unless there is evidence of associated superinfection. Antiemetics and analgesia are important adjunctive measures. Antibiotics are not recommended.

Question 5

C. (Omeprazole) GORD presents with burning chest pain, nausea and swallowing discomfort. Management involves either trial of PPI or H. pylori testing and treatment. You should not treat empirically for H. pylori without a confirmed positive result, hence omeprazole is the correct answer

Question 6

B. (Emergency appendectomy) Migratory abdominal pain, nausea and vomiting and low-grade fever are classic features of appendicitis. RLQ pain on palpation of the LLQ is Rovsing sign, highly suggestive of appendicitis. Management is with emergency appendectomy. Preoperative antibiotic therapy is indicated in most cases, with coverage for gram-negative and anaerobic organisms, but appendectomy is definitive.

Question 7

E. (Urea breath test) PUD presents with epigastric pain, nausea and indigestion. Pain worse at night and relieved by eating suggests a duodenal ulcer. Initial investigation is with urea breath test or stool testing to diagnose H. pylori infection, which if found, can be eradicated. Endoscopy is reserved for those with red flags for malignancy (appetite and weight loss, anaemia, recent onset of symptoms or with rapid progression, or melaena) or complications including bleeding or perforation.

Question 8

B. (Acute pancreatitis) Epigastric pain radiating to the back, vomiting and fever are typical features of pancreatitis which can occur after alcohol excess. Management is with fluids, analgesia and nutritional support.

Question 9

D. (Sigmoid volvulus) Severe abdominal pain and vomiting are the typical features of acute bowel obstruction. Volvulus often presents with preceding episodes of abdominal pain which resolve after passing stool or gas. Sigmoid is the most common type. Adhesions relating to prior abdominal surgery are the most common cause.

Question 10

C. (Oesophagitis) Frank small volume haematemesis suggests UGIB. GORD increases the risk of oesophagitis, irritation of the oesophageal lining due to chronic acid reflux, which can cause minor bleeding.

Question 11

B. (Pregnancy test) Migratory abdominal pain which becomes localized to the right iliac fossa, nausea and vomiting and peritonitic features on examination are the typical features of appendicitis. Appendicitis is a clinical diagnosis, however in females of childbearing age, it is essential to exclude ectopic pregnancy with a pregnancy test before appendectomy.

Question 12

C. (Ascending cholangitis) RUQ pain, jaundice and fever are Charcot's triad of ascending cholangitis. Cholangitis develops following impaction of gallstone in the common bile duct and local inflammation and infection. Cholecystitis presents with abdominal pain and fever, but no jaundice, as there is no biliary tract obstruction.

Question 13

E. (Nasogastric tube insertion and IV fluids) Acute bowel obstruction presents with abdominal pain, distension, vomiting and obstipation. Bowel sounds are initially high pitched, and later absent. Management is with bowel decompression, with NG tube insertion with free drainage, and intravenous fluid resuscitation.

Question 14

C. (Intravenous fluids) UGIB is indicated by coffee-ground vomit and melaena. Chronic NSAID use makes a bleeding peptic ulcer the likely aetiology. Management is with resuscitation and urgent endoscopic haemostasis. Fluids should be used initially, with transfusion restricted to those with Hb <80 g/dL. The role of IV PPIs prior to endoscopy in peptic ulcer bleeding is controversial, but not currently recommended.

Question 15

E. (Ultrasound of abdomen) RUQ pain, nausea and flatulent dyspepsia after eating, suggest biliary colic, best investigated with US. Middle-aged women are at particular risk for gallstones.

Question 16

A. (Direct inguinal hernia) A reducible groin lump superomedial to the pubic tubercle, which does not transilluminate, suggests inguinal hernia. Reappearance of the lump on coughing while being reduced suggests direct protrusion of the abdominal contents through the inguinal canal.

Question 17

C. (Endoscopic retrograde cholangiopancreatography) Ascending cholangitis presents with RUQ pain, jaundice and fever. Following resuscitation and antibiotics, definitive management is with gallbladder drainage and removal of the obstructing stone. ERCP is used first line, with EUS and biliary drainage if ERCP is unsuccessful.

Question 18

D. (Nasogastric tube insertion and IV fluids) A coffee-bean sign on abdominal film with symptoms of acute bowel obstruction suggests sigmoid volvulus. Immediate management is with NG tube insertion to decompress the bowel and intravenous fluids. Definitive management is with endoscopic decompression, typically by flexible sigmoidoscopy.

Question 19

B. (Colonoscopy) Patients >60 with a new anaemia should have an urgent colonoscopy to exclude colorectal carcinoma. Smoking is a risk factor. If there were respiratory symptoms or weight loss, investigation for lung cancer with CXR would be advised.

Question 20

B. (Emergency colectomy) A peritonitic abdomen with guarding and abdominal rigidity and sepsis suggests acute diverticular perforation. Emergency colectomy is required in these cases. CT-guided drainage can be used for abscesses associated with diverticula.

Question 21

A. (Barrett's oesophagus) Barrett oesophagus is a premalignant metaplasia of the oesophageal epithelium from squamous to columnar cells. Poorly controlled GORD, male sex, older age and obesity increase the risk. Management is with PPIs and endoscopic surveillance, to detect dysplastic change to carcinoma.

Question 22

E. (Ultrasound of abdomen) Acute cholecystitis presents with abdominal pain, fever and Murphy sign, with worsening pain on inspiration during palpation. The history of diabetes, hormonal contraceptives and obesity, and being middle aged and female place her at increased risk. Diagnosis is with abdominal ultrasound. LFTs will typically be normal, as there is no biliary obstruction.

Question 23

E. (Small bowel obstruction) Bowel obstruction presents with abdominal pain, vomiting, constipation and abdominal distention. Hyperactive bowel sounds are typical in the early stages. The abdominal film demonstrates dilated central bowel loops, with valvulae conniventes traversing the full width of the bowel, suggesting SBO.

Question 24

A. (Appendicitis) Appendicitis presents with migratory abdominal pain, nausea and anorexia, with a low-grade fever. A positive urinalysis is a common feature, but in the absence of urinary symptoms, appendicitis is the more likely diagnosis.

Question 25

B. (Left hemicolectomy) Patients with localized colorectal carcinoma who are otherwise fit and well are candidates for curative surgery. A left hemicolectomy with regional lymph node dissection is appropriate for the location of the lesion.

Question 26

C. (Elective mesh repair) A reducible groin lump inferomedial to the pubic tubercle suggests femoral hernia. Femoral hernias are more common in women, and are at increased risk of strangulation, hence all must be repaired. Emergency surgery is indicated in complicated cases of incarceration, strangulation and bowel obstruction.

Question 27

C.(Glasgow-Blatchford score) UGIBs with frank haematemesis, a history of alcoholic excess and signs of chronic liver disease suggest oesophageal varices. The Glasgow-Blatchford score is used to risk stratify prior to endoscopy, and Rockall score to calculate the risk of rebleeding following endoscopy.

Question 28

A. (Endoscopic mucosal resection) Haematochezia can occur with colorectal polyps. Risk factors include obesity, smoking, alcohol and poor diet. Management is with endoscopic resection, to reduce the risk of progression to colorectal carcinoma.

Question 29

A. (ECG) GORD presents with chest pain and dyspepsia. It is very common in pregnancy due to increased intraabdominal pressure. GORD is a clinical diagnosis – once cardiac causes of chest pain are excluded, empiric therapy with a proton pump inhibitor can be initiated. Further investigations can be considered if symptoms fail to resolve after delivery.

Question 30

D. (Endoscopy) Gastric cancer presents with epigastric pain, nausea and weight loss. Heavy drinking is a significant risk factor. Presence of Virchow node is highly suggestive of gastric cancer. Endoscopy and biopsy will provide the diagnosis.

Question 31

C. (Watchful waiting) A reducible groin lump superomedial to the pubic tubercle which appeared after heavy lifting is the typical feature of an inguinal hernia. Management in symptomatic patients is open or laparoscopic mesh repair – however in patients without pain or complications, watchful waiting initially is appropriate. If symptoms worsen or complications develop, repair can be performed.

Question 32

A. (Colonoscopy) Colorectal carcinoma presents with abdominal pain, change in bowel habit, fatigue, weight loss and anaemia. The diagnosis should be confirmed with colonoscopy, which will allow biopsy for staging.

Question 33

B. (Dietary modifications) Abdominal pain, bloating and change in bowel habit suggest IBS, an important but benign differential for IBD. Management is with dietary modifications, exercise, stress management and psychobehavioural therapies.

Question 34

D. (Peritoneal carcinomatosis) New fatigue, abdominal pain and distention, with a history of colorectal cancer, suggest metastatic disease, which can occur via peritoneal seeding in up to 10% of patients. This is often a terminal feature.

Question 35

C. (Liver transplant) Acute liver failure presents with abdominal distention, asterixis, hepatic encephalopathy and coagulopathy, and can occur after an overdose of hepatotoxic medications. The King's College risk stratification criteria indicate that patients between 10 and 40 years old, with an INR >3.5 and bilirubin >17.5 are candidates for early transplant where available, which is the only cure.

Question 36

C. (CT of abdomen) Pancreatic cancer presents with weight loss and painless jaundice. Relevant risk factors include type 2 diabetes and chronic high alcohol use. The most appropriate investigation is CT abdomen. Biopsy and tissue samples for histopathology will then confirm the diagnosis.

Question 37

C. (Colonoscopy) Diverticulosis presents with colicky abdominal pain and constipation. Relevant risk factors include chronic constipation, smoking and hypothyroidism. Diagnosis is with colonoscopy, to visualize outpouchings of colonic mucosa. Management is with conservative lifestyle modifications to reduce constipation, and laxatives.

Question 38

D. (Perforated peptic ulcer) Perforated peptic ulcers present with peritonitic abdominal symptoms and risk factors including NSAID use, alcohol and cigarette smoking. Shoulder tip pain results from irritation of the phrenic nerve by intraabdominal free fluid. Treatment is with bowel rest and surgical repair.

Question 39

E. (Emergency laparotomy) Acute abdominal pain, bloody diarrhoea and atrial fibrillation, is the classic triad of acute mesenteric ischaemia. There is evidence of sepsis and haemodynamic instability, meaning emergency laparotomy with resection of necrotic bowel is the appropriate management. For stable patients, anticoagulation and endovascular intervention can be considered in the first instance.

Question 40

E. (Pneumatic dilation) Achalasia presents with dysphagia and effortless regurgitation of food, and weight loss. For patients at low surgical risk, endoscopy-guided pneumatic dilation is appropriate. Botox and medical therapies are indicated in frail patients at increased surgical risk, but there is a high likelihood of recurrence.

Question 41

D. (Diverticular bleed) Diverticular bleeding presents with left iliac fossa pain and bright red rectal bleeding. A history of alternating constipation and diarrhoea suggests diverticular disease. Acute mesenteric ischaemia is typically found in those with AF. Angiodysplasia is painless, and haemorrhoids present with minimal blood upon wiping and a perianal mass. Patients with colorectal cancer will likely have constitutional features in addition to gastrointestinal symptoms.

Question 42

D. (Intravenous cyclizine) Mallory-Weiss tears are small oesophageal tears which result from profuse vomiting and present with minimal haematemesis. Management is with fluids and antiemetics to stop the vomiting and promote mucosal recovery.

Question 43

B. (Emergency colectomy) An acute ulcerative colitis flares presents with profuse bloody diarrhoea and abdominal pain. He is haemodynamically unstable, with a metabolic acidosis with raised lactate suggesting perforation, peritonitis and sepsis – hence emergency surgery is appropriate. In less severe cases, intravenous steroids are used to induce remission.

Question 44

C. (Diclofenac) Biliary colic presents with RUQ pain, nausea and dyspepsia. The history suggests gallstones. Management is with NSAID analgesia, and surgical consult for elective cholecystectomy once the acute episode has resolved

Question 45

D. (Intravenous antibiotics) Acute cholecystitis presents with RUQ pain and fever. The history suggests biliary colic, placing him at risk of acute obstruction of the cystic duct and gallbladder inflammation. Initial management is with empirical antibiotic therapy. Cholecystectomy is subsequently performed as soon as possible.

Question 46

E. (Urgent 2-week wait referral) Change in bowel habit for over 6 weeks and rectal bleeding is a red flag for colorectal cancer, regardless of age. A 2-week wait referral for colonoscopy is appropriate.

Question 47

A. (Acute mesenteric ischaemia) Sudden acute abdominal pain, bloody diarrhoea and AF suggest acute mesenteric ischaemia. Management is with lifelong anticoagulation and resection of necrotic bowel, if present.

Question 48

D. (Faecal elastase) Chronic pancreatitis presents with chronic abdominal pain, malabsorptive symptoms and a history of alcohol excess. Initial screening is with faecal elastase, which will demonstrate pancreatic insufficiency. Amylase and lipase are often normal in chronic pancreatitis, even in acute exacerbations.

Question 49

D. (Endoscopy) Oesophageal carcinoma presents with progressive dysphagia, weight loss and a history of self-treated reflux symptoms. Smokers are at significantly increased risk of head and neck malignancy. First-line investigation is endoscopy, which will allow biopsy of suspicious lesions.

Question 50

A. (Alcohol abstinence therapies) Chronic pancreatitis presents with chronic abdominal pain and malabsorptive symptoms. The history suggests repeat episodes of acute pancreatitis. Ongoing excess alcohol use is the biggest risk factor. Management includes nutritional support, pain management and enzyme replacement, and cessation of aggravating factors. Enzyme replacement may be appropriate, but it would be more useful to attempt psychological therapies to support alcohol cessation and engagement with health services in the long term.

Question 51

D. (Perianal fistula) A perianal fistula presents with perianal discharge and pain during defecation. Crohn disease is a risk factor.

Question 52

C. (Intravenous fluids) Severe infectious colitis presents with profuse watery, bloody diarrhoea, abdominal pain, fever and dehydration. Resuscitation is the most important first step.

Question 53

D. (Pancreatic cancer) Pancreatic cancer presents with nausea and anorexia, weight loss and steatorrhoea. Painless jaundice and palpable gallbladder (Courvoisier's sign) are the hallmark features and indicate late-stage disease. Management is typically palliative in such cases. Diabetes and smoking are significant risk factors.

Question 54

B. (Oesophageal adenocarcinoma) Dysphagia and retrosternal discomfort, with a history of GORD, suggests oesophageal malignancy. Oesophageal adenocarcinoma is often asymptomatic or presents with mild symptoms in early stages. Smokers are at significantly increased risk.

Question 55

D. (Liver function tests) Cholestasis presents with pale urine and dark stools, as well as pruritus and jaundice. The history of ulcerative colitis places him at risk of primary sclerosing cholangitis, an autoimmune inflammatory condition of the intra and extrahepatic bile ducts. Initial screening is with LFTs, which will demonstrate a cholestatic picture (↑ALP/GGT) with subsequent abdominal imaging (initial by ultrasound, then MRCP) to evaluate for biliary strictures.

Question 56

E. (Choledocholithiasis) Biliary colic presents with postprandial RUQ pain. Jaundice suggests obstruction of biliary flow, which can occur secondary to gallstones in the extrahepatic bile ducts, known as choledocholithiasis. The pain in choledocholithiasis is often prolonged and more severe than in biliary colic. There is no evidence of acute infection at present.

Question 57

A. (Femoral hernia) Femoral hernias are common in older women, and present with a groin lump inferolateral to the pubic tubercle. Risk factors include increased intraabdominal pressure (obesity, multiparity, chronic cough). Management is with operative repair, due to the increased risk of strangulation.

Question 58

D. (Peritoneal fluid analysis) Patients with chronic ascites are at risk of spontaneous bacterial infection of ascitic fluid. Symptoms of SBP include worsening ascites, abdominal pain and fever. Peritoneal fluid analysis with a neutrophil count of $\geq 250/mm^3$ is diagnostic.

Question 59

B. (Chest X-ray) Oesophageal perforation presents following significant vomiting with chest pain and subcutaneous emphysema. CXR will show a widened mediastinum, pneumomediastinum and air-fluid levels. The diagnosis is then confirmed on CT thorax or contrast oesophagography.

Question 60

E. (Ultrasound of abdomen) Hepatocellular carcinoma presents with RUQ pain, hepatomegaly, jaundice and weight loss. Chronic hepatitis B infection is a significant risk factor. Initial investigation is with abdominal US. Serum AFP can support the diagnosis, but US is more specific.

Question 61

D. (Oral antibiotics) Acute diverticulitis presents with fever, left lower abdominal pain and a palpable mass. Risk factors for chronic constipation include codeine use and hypothyroidism, which can predispose to diverticular disease. There is no haemodynamic instability, suggesting mild diverticulitis, which can be managed with oral antibiotics.

Question 62

A. (Gastric cancer) Gastric cancer is often only mildly symptomatic in early stages. Later stages present with abdominal pain, early satiety and weight loss. Risk factors include poorly managed GORD and smoking.

Question 63

E. (Rectopexy) A full-thickness rectal prolapse is indicated by concentric mucosal folds on rectal examination. Management of full-thickness prolapse is with rectopexy, and management of underlying risk factors (constipation, chronic cough). Mucosal prolapse can be managed with digital reduction and injection sclerotherapy.

Question 64

A. (Intramuscular hydroxocobalamin) Vitamin B_{12} deficiency presents with anaemia and peripheral neuropathy. A history of Crohn's disease places her at risk of malabsorption at the terminal ileum, where the majority of B_{12} is absorbed. Management is with intramuscular B_{12} replacement. Folate deficiency should be tested for and replaced, after B_{12} is corrected, to avoid precipitating subacute combined degeneration of the spinal cord.

Question 65

B. (Increase dietary fibre) Haemorrhoids present with minimal fresh rectal bleeding. Pregnancy is a risk factor. Management of internal, non–thrombosed haemorrhoids is conservative, with increased dietary fibre to reduce constipation and straining. This patient has no pain, so local anaesthetic and steroid creams are not indicated in the first instance.

Question 66

E. (Oesophageal manometry) Achalasia presents with dysphagia and painless regurgitation when lying flat. Weight loss is common. The gold standard confirmatory test is oesophageal manometry.

Question 67

E. (Thrombosed haemorrhoid) Thrombosed haemorrhoids present with sudden anorectal pain and painful vascular anorectal mass. Anal fissures and fistulas are associated with IBD.

Question 68

D. (Duplex ultrasound abdomen) Chronic mesenteric ischaemia presents with postprandial pain and weight loss due to food aversion. Diagnosis is with duplex US, which will show stenosis of the mesenteric arteries. Management is with reduction of vascular risk (smoking cessation, weight loss, management of blood pressure and antiplatelet agents) and endovascular interventions if severe.

Question 69

A. (Analgesia, fluids and bowel rest) In patients with atherosclerotic disease, hypovolaemia risks ischaemia of the watershed areas of the colon, presenting with abdominal pain and bloody diarrhoea. Mild cases (without haemodynamic compromise or signs of sepsis) are likely to resolve within several days without specific medical or surgical intervention. Long-term management involves reduction of vascular risk.

Question 70

A. (Acute respiratory distress syndrome) Acute pancreatitis presents with epigastric pain radiating to the back, vomiting and fever, following an alcoholic binge. New chest pain, dyspnoea and oxygen requirement suggest development of acute respiratory distress syndrome, which is a significant complication of acute pancreatitis and other systemic inflammatory syndromes. Management is with ventilatory support and ICU consult.

Question 71

C. (Incision and drainage) Perianal abscess present with a warm, subcutaneous mass on the anal margin. Abscesses can progress to sepsis or chronic perianal tissue damage without early incision and drainage. Antibiotics may be used postoperatively for immunocompromised patients, including those with IBD.

Question 72

B. (Hiatus hernia) Hiatal hernia present with retrosternal pain worse during meals and at night, nausea and flatulence. Obesity and a chronic cough are risk factors for hernia formation.

Question 73

C. (Ischaemic colitis) Ischaemic colitis can occur with intercurrent illness or dehydration and hypoperfusion of the watershed areas of the colon (splenic flexure and rectosigmoid junction), presenting with abdominal pain and dark red rectal bleeding. A history of atherosclerotic disease is typical.

Question 74

C. (Hepatocellular carcinoma) Unintentional weight loss with a history of chronic liver disease is suggestive of malignancy. Symptoms of abdominal pain jaundice and ascites may only occur late in the disease process.

Question 75

E. (Topical glyceryl trinitrate ointment) Anal fissures present with sharp defecatory pain and rectal bleeding. He is not constipated, so laxatives are unlikely to help, although they are preferred first line in those with fissures relating to chronic constipation. Topical vasodilators, including GTN, are used first line. Surgery is reserved for refractory cases.

Question 76

E. (Radiochemotherapy) The majority of anal cancers are managed with radiochemotherapy. Resection is performed for tumours involving the anal margin. Remission may be achieved with radiochemotherapy alone. Recurrent cancers are treated surgically.

Question 77

B. (Endoscopic dilation) Oesophageal strictures present with dysphagia and regurgitation, with the risk factor of GORD. The barium swallow findings suggest stricture formation. There are no red flags to suggest malignancy at this point. Management is with endoscopic dilation.

Question 78

E. (Total gastrectomy) Localized gastric cancer without nodal or distant metastases is appropriate for surgical resection; however prognosis remains poor, with high recurrence rates. Proximal lesions are managed with total gastrectomy, and distal lesions subtotal gastrectomy. Chemotherapy may be used as an adjunct, but radiation is rarely used.

Question 79

E. (Enterolithotomy) Acute bowel obstruction presents with abdominal pain, vomiting and obstipation. The history suggests gallstones, suggesting a gallstone ileus as the underlying aetiology. Enterolithotomy is performed to remove the obstructing stone. Following this, cholecystectomy can be performed to prevent recurrence or other gallstone-related complications.

Question 80

B. (Anal fissure) Anal fissures present with sharp defecatory pain, perianal blood and itch. Constipation and IBD increases the risk of fissure formation, which commonly occur in the posterior anal commissure.

Cardiothoracics and vascular 27

Question 1

C. (Smoking cessation) Intermittent claudication presents with cramping calf pain on exercise, relieved by rest. Cardiovascular comorbidities and smoking increase the risk of PAD. Smoking cessation is the most important step. Antiplatelets and statins should be prescribed if not already.

Question 2

A. (Carotid duplex ultrasound) Carotid artery disease presents with transient amaurosis fugax and an audible carotid bruit. Risk factors include diabetes, hypertension and smoking. Initial screening is with carotid ultrasound, following which stenosis can be further assessed on CT or MRI.

Question 3

C. (Deep vein thrombosis) DVTs present with calf swelling, pain, redness and warmth. IBD and smoking are VTE risk factors.

Question 4

A. (Apixaban) PEs present with chest pain, dyspnoea, low-grade fever, tachycardia and hypoxia, with risk factors including recent surgery and immobility. Management is with anticoagulation – in a provoked, low-risk VTE, a DOAC can be started immediately and continued for 3–6 months.

Question 5

D. (Ultrasound of abdomen) AAA's present with lower back pain and an expansile abdominal mass with a bruit. Risk factors include high cholesterol, hypertension and cigarette smoking. The first-line investigation is abdominal US.

Question 6

B. (CT angiogram) Aortic dissection presents with central tearing chest pain, presyncope and nausea, with hypertension, a wide pulse pressure, and pulse differences between arms. Risk factors include hypertension, high cholesterol and smoking. Urgent CT angiogram will confirm the diagnosis.

Question 7

A. (Chest drain) A spontaneous pneumothorax presents with chest pain and respiratory distress. Young, thin, tall males who smoke are at risk. He is stable, and hence does not require needle decompression, but the pneumothorax is over 2 cm, so definitive management with chest drain placement is required.

Question 8

C. (Diabetic neuropathy) Diabetic neuropathy presents with bilateral sensory loss, neuropathic pain and a diabetic ulcer. Chronic poor glycaemic control risks neuropathic injury, leading to sensory loss and chronic repetitive microtrauma, leading to ulcer formation. ABPI >1.4 suggests calcified, stenotic vessels, associated with diabetes.

Question 9

A. (Amputation) Wet gangrene is suggested by black discolouration of the foot, oedema and blistering, and sepsis. Once infection has set in, the likelihood of limb salvage is exceedingly low. Management is with broad-spectrum antibiotics and amputation.

Question 10

A. (Ankle brachial pressure index) Intermittent claudication presents with cramping muscular pain on exertion, relieved by rest, suggesting underlying PAD. Risk factors including age, renal disease, AF and smoking. Initial investigation is with ABPI, with a ratio of 0.5–0.8 diagnosing PAD.

Question 11

A. (Acute limb ischaemia) The 6Ps of ALI are pain, pallor, pulselessness, paralysis, paraesthesia and poikilothermia (coldness). AF places him at risk of acute embolic occlusion of the lower limb arteries. Urgent revascularization is essential.

Question 12

A. (Compression stockings) Varicose veins present with leg swelling and pain, worse in the heat. Compression stockings are first line with other conservative measures including leg elevation, weight loss and smoking cessation if appropriate. If conservative measures fail, surgical intervention includes ablation, sclerotherapy and vein stripping.

Question 13

D. (Repeat ultrasound at 12 months) Males age 65 are offered one-off abdominal aortic aneurysm screening with abdominal US. If the aortic diameter is 3–5.5 cm, repeat US screening is required with the frequency depending on the size of the aneurysm to determine growth rates and assess the need for intervention. For aneurysms 4.2 cm, repeat US at 12-month interval is appropriate.

Question 14

E. (Transthoracic echocardiogram) Mitral regurgitation presents with dyspnoea, palpitations and fatigue. A pan systolic murmur radiating to the axilla is classical. Transthoracic echocardiogram is required to assess the mitral valve function.

Question 15

C. (Intravenous labetalol) Aortic dissection presents with chest pain and presyncope. Risk factors include hypertension and smoking. Management of Stanford B dissections involving the descending aorta is with tight blood pressure control (target 100–120 systolic). Patients who remain stable can be discharged on oral medications with outpatient surveillance.

Question 16

A. (Cardiac tamponade) Cardiac tamponade presents with hypotension, muffled heart sounds and distended neck veins with a raised JVP. This case likely relates to malignant pericardial effusion. Management is with urgent pericardiocentesis to prevent cardiac arrest.

Question 17

C. (Revascularization) CLI presents with rest pain, ulceration and gangrene, indicating limb-threatening arterial occlusion. In cases of dry gangrene, the limb may be salvageable with revascularization.

Question 18

E. (Venous ulcer) A painless, itchy, ulcer that is shallow, sloughy, with an irregular border, over the medial malleolus, suggests venous ulceration. There is evidence of chronic venous eczema, placing her at risk of ulceration if poorly controlled.

Question 19

E. (Echocardiogram) Pericardial effusions present with aching chest pain, dyspnoea and orthopnoea. Autoimmune diseases can cause spontaneous pericardial effusions. The best confirmatory test is an echocardiogram.

Question 20

C. (CT angiogram) Thoracic aortic aneurysms present with upper back pain and compressive symptoms of cough and dysphagia. Risk factors include smoking and hypertension. CT angiogram will show dilation of the thoracic aorta.

Question 21

A. (Aspirin) TIAs present with focal neurological symptoms lasting less than 24 hours, and can develop secondary to stenosis of the carotid arteries. 50%–69% stenosis is deemed moderate, and an indication for surgery in young, fit patients. A 94-year-old woman with significant medical comorbidities is unlikely to be an appropriate surgical candidate.

Question 22

E. (Transcatheter aortic valve replacement) Syncope, angina and dyspnoea suggest aortic stenosis, confirmed by echocardiography findings. Symptomatic patients should undergo surgery. Management for younger patients is with open surgery; however for older patients, TAVR is appropriate.

Question 23

C. (Endovascular aneurysm repair) Ruptured AAAs present with severe tearing abdominal pain, hypotension and presyncope. Unstable patients should have urgent aneurysm repair. Endovascular routes are preferred, particularly in high surgical risk.

Question 24

E. (Venous duplex ultrasound) Chronic venous insufficiency presents with bilateral leg aching and swelling, worse after standing, relieved by elevation. Obesity and smoking are risk factors. First-line assessment is with venous ultrasound.

Question 25

E. (Trigger avoidance) Raynaud phenomenon presents with intermittent vasospastic attacks in the fingers, causing ischaemic, hypoxia and reactive hyperaemia upon trigger exposure, which are commonly the cold and stress. The mainstay of treatment is trigger avoidance.

Question 26

A. (Aortoiliac occlusive disease) Leriche syndrome presents with bilateral buttock and calf pain and absent femoral pulses. Leriche syndrome results from aortoiliac occlusive disease. In men, erectile dysfunction is common.

Question 27

C. (Lung cancer) Pleural effusion presents with dyspnoea, chest pain and total whiteout with meniscus level on CXR. Pleural fluid analysis can help to determine the likely cause. Light's criteria can be applied: acidic fluid with a high protein, glucose, LDH, and cholesterol suggests an exudative effusion, relating to infection or malignancy. In this case, a three-week history with preceding fatigue and weight loss is more likely to represent cancer than infection.

Question 28

E. (Lymphoedema) Pelvic surgery and radiation risks lymphatic vessel damage and lymphedema, which presents with nonpitting leg oedema. Management is with compression bandages and manual lymphatic drainage to prevent irreversible skin fibrosis.

Question 29

B. (Lobectomy) Surgical intervention is appropriate for localized lung adenocarcinoma, with lobectomy the most common procedure.

Question 30

B. (Endovascular venography and stenting) SVC syndrome presents with hypotension, facial plethora, raised JVP and distended neck veins. For unstable patients, management is with urgent endovascular stenting, following which definitive treatment relating to the underlying condition is performed. Dexamethasone, radiotherapy, and loop diuretics can all be considered, but in acutely unstable patients urgent stenting is required.

Orthopaedics 28

Question 1

B. (Intravenous flucloxacillin) Cellulitis presents with a tender, warm, red swollen leg and fever. Pathogen entry is typically via small skin breaks. Patients with diabetes are at particular risk. Management is with intravenous antibiotics.

Question 2

A. (Aspiration of left knee joint for microscopy and culture) Septic arthritis presents with a warm, tender joint with reduced range of motion and fever. Diabetics are at increased risk. Investigation is with knee joint aspirate and MC&S, which will show a turbid fluid sample with raised white blood cells and neutrophil dominance. Culture and sensitivity will guide antibiotic therapy.

Question 3

B. (Cast removal) Acute compartment syndrome presents with severe pain, swelling and neurovascular impairment. Immediate management should be with cast removal, to reduce limb compartment pressures, then fasciotomy.

Question 4

B. (Osteoarthritis) Osteoarthritis presents with bilateral pain and stiffness, worsens on exertion and relieved by rest. Crepitus and reduced range of motion are typical. Management is with exercise, weight loss, analgesia and physiotherapy. Surgery is reserved for refractory, severe cases.

Question 5

A. (Intravenous antibiotic therapy) Bone marrow oedema on MRI is the earliest and most sensitive feature of osteomyelitis. Treatment is with intravenous antibiotic therapy, and surgery in refractory cases.

Question 6

B. (Empirical antibiotic therapy) Septic arthritis presents with a warm, red, swollen knee with reduced range of motion, and fever, and aspirate indicating joint infection. Patients with existing joint disease are at increased risk. Management is with empirical antibiotics, tailored to culture results.

Question 7

E. (Total hip replacement) Fractured NOF present with a shortened and externally rotated leg following trauma. In younger adults with minimal comorbidities, THR is preferred over hemiarthroplasty for intracapsular fractures as the prosthesis will last longer and may avoid repeat surgery.

Question 8

B. (Fasciotomy) Compartment syndrome presents with severe pain, swelling and neurovascular impairment. Crush injuries are a common cause. Management is with urgent fasciotomy to reduce compartmental pressures and salvage the limb.

Question 9

E. (Surgical exploration and debridement) Necrotizing fasciitis presents with severe pain, erythema and skin necrosis, tissue induration and subcutaneous crepitus. Fever, rigors and altered mental status are common. Definitive management is with surgical debridement.

Question 10

E. (Therapeutic arthrocentesis) Septic arthritis presents with a warm, red tender and swollen joint, with reduced range of motion. Intravenous drug users are at risk of introduction of bacteria at injection sites and haematogenous spread to regional and distant joints. Diagnostic and therapeutic arthrocentesis with MC&S should be performed in all patients first. Patients at high risk of atypical organisms (i.e. intravenous drug users) should be discussed with microbiology first to identify the most appropriate antibiotic regime before antibiotics are prescribed.

Question 11

D. (MR of foot) Osteomyelitis is suggested by a warm, painful, tender foot with a deep local ulcer and fever. Diabetics are at risk of deep tissue infection without effective foot to care and blood sugar management. The most appropriate investigation is MRI of the foot which will show cortical destruction and soft tissue inflammation.

Question 12
E. (Septic arthritis) Septic arthritis presents with a hot red swollen joint, with reduced range of motion. The synovial fluid sample suggests bacterial infection, most commonly related to Staphylococcus aureus, as suggested by the gram stain. Prosthetic joints are at particular risk of infection. Management is with empirical antibiotic therapy and orthopaedic consult for potential debridement and joint replacement if severe.

Question 13
A. (Cauda equina syndrome) CES presents with lower back pain and lower motor neuron signs (reduced tone and power) in the lower limbs, with saddle anaesthesia. Urgent lumbosacral MRI and neurosurgical consultation is required. Bowel and bladder impairment are late signs in CES.

Question 14
B. (Arthroplasty) Refractory osteoarthritic knee pain can be managed with arthroplasty, which has excellent outcomes for younger patients with minimal comorbidities. Arthroscopy is used for meniscus or cartilage damage, osteotomy for malalignment deformity and arthrodesis for wrist or ankle disease.

Question 15
E. (Necrotizing fasciitis) Necrotizing fasciitis presents with systemic features of confusion, fever and haemodynamic instability, and severe leg pain, black skin discolouration, blistering and skin shearing. Urgent deep tissue biopsies and surgical debridement is required.

Question 16
C. (Deep tissue biopsy) Necrotizing fasciitis affecting the perineum is known as Fournier gangrene. Alcohol excess, intravenous drug use and poor nutrition are risk factors. Infection can enter locally if groin vessels are used to inject drugs. Definitive diagnosis is with deep tissue biopsy during surgical debridement.

Question 17
A. (Compartmental pressures) Acute compartment syndrome presents with severe pain, swelling, paralysis, paraesthesia and sensory loss. Excessively constrictive bandaging is a risk. Compartment syndrome is primarily a clinical diagnosis, but intracompartmental pressure measures >30 mmHg confirms the diagnosis, following which urgent fasciotomy should be performed.

Question 18
C. (Debridement and external fixation) Management of a displaced open fracture of a long bone with significant tissue loss involves debridement of devitalized tissue and definitive skeletal stabilization. Antibiotics should be given to all patients as a prophylactic adjunctive measure.

Question 19
C. (MR of lumbosacral spine) Spinal cord compression presents with back pain, lower limb sensorimotor weakness and brisk reflexes. A history of breast cancer suggests bony metastasis compressing the spinal cord.

Question 20
C. (Neck of femur fracture) Groin pain and shortened externally rotated hip suggest NOF fracture. The X-ray demonstrates an intracapsular fracture of the femoral neck.

Question 21
E. (Wrist splinting) Carpal tunnel syndrome presents with pain and tingling in the distribution of the median nerve, worse at night and with prolonged use. Positive Phalen test is highly suggestive. Diabetes and hypothyroidism are common risk factors. Initial management is conservative, with wrist splinting. Steroid injections can then be trailed.

Question 22
B. (No investigation required) Osteoarthritis presents with joint pain and reduced range of motion, morning stiffness and joint crepitus. No specific investigations are required, as findings typically do not correlate well with symptoms, and should only be used if the diagnosis is in doubt.

Question 23
B. (Alendronic acid) Atraumatic vertebral fractures are typically related to osteoporosis, termed fragility fractures. Long-term therapy with levothyroxine and PPIs are risk factors. Management of stable fractures is conservative, with optimization of bone health, typically with bisphosphonates first line. Vitamin D and calcium deficiency should be treated if present. Smoking cessation is also essential.

Question 24
B. (Ibuprofen gel) Osteoarthritis is suggested by pain and stiffness in the hands, worse on exertion. Heberdens

(DIPJs) and Bouchard (PIPJs) nodes are evident on examination. Management is with topical analgesia. Capsaicin is typically recommended for OA of the knee.

Question 25

C. (MR of knee) An acute ACL tear presents with knee swelling and pain. A positive anterior draw test suggests ACL instability. MRI of knee will delineate the soft tissue injury and identify associated bony contusions.

Question 26

B. (MR of cervical spine) C6/C7 radiculopathy is suggested by neck pain, neuropathic pain and sensorimotor weakness in the left C6/C7 dermatomes and myotomes. Cervical spine MR will delineate any disk degeneration or spinal stenosis resulting in impingement or compression of a spinal nerve root.

Question 27

A. (Carpal tunnel syndrome) Carpal tunnel syndrome presents with neuropathic pain and sensorimotor weakness in the area of the median nerve distribution, reproducible with Tinel's test. Pregnancy is a risk, with generalized peripheral oedema resulting in compression of the median nerve in the carpal tunnel.

Question 28

C. (Chronic osteomyelitis) Chronic osteomyelitis presents with a subacute history of pain and reduced mobility, and local inflammation and sinus formation. Diabetics are at particular risk. X-ray findings suggest chronic inflammation leading to bony destruction. Septic arthritis presents much more acutely.

Question 29

A. (Open reduction and internal fixation) A displaced bimalleolar fracture is inherently unstable, hence ORIF is required. Casting can be used for stable, isolated fractures.

Question 30

D. (Ultrasound of ankle) Achilles tendon rupture presents with a sudden loud popping, severe pain and difficulty mobilizing. Simmonds test (absent plantar flexion on calf compression) is pathognomonic. The US will show swelling and separation of the Achilles tendon.

Question 31

E. (Physiotherapy) Adhesive capsulitis presents with pain and stiffness in the shoulder joint affecting external rotation and abduction. Following rotator cuff injury and surgical repair, adhesive capsulitis is a risk without early physiotherapy and joint mobilization. Symptoms will gradually resolve over one to two years, with physiotherapy the mainstay of treatment.

Question 32

B. (Hemiarthroplasty) Avascular necrosis of the femoral head can develop secondary to steroid use. Conservative measures are indicated first line, but in significant necrosis with compromised bone structure, surgery is required.

Question 33

A. (Functional brace and physiotherapy) MCL injuries present with swelling, bruising and tenderness and medial laxity of the knee with valgus force application. There is no evidence of cruciate ligament injury or meniscus injury, hence conservative treatment with a functional brace and physiotherapy is appropriate.

Question 34

C. (Meniscal tear) Meniscal tears present with sharp knee pain, swelling and locking of the knee with popping and clicking of the knee on movement. They commonly relate to twisting injuries. Management is typically conservative, with arthroscopic meniscal repair used for complex or nonhealing injuries.

Question 35

D. (Intramedullary nail) A NOF fracture presents with pain, inability to weight bear and a shortened and externally rotated leg. Extracapsular fractures are unstable, and mostly treated with surgery, unless the surgical risk is unacceptably high. A long intramedullary nail is used.

Question 36

B. (Closed reduction) Shoulder dislocation presents with pain and reduced mobility following a fall on an outstretched hand. The X-ray findings suggest anterior dislocation. Numbness over the deltoid bulk and weakness to abduct suggest axillary nerve injury, a common finding in anterior dislocations. Most can be managed with closed reduction.

Question 37

B. (Osteonecrosis) Nontraumatic hip pain and reduced range of motion, with a history of steroid use, suggest avascular necrosis of the femoral head. Hip MRI will show cystic and sclerotic changes and bone marrow oedema. Management is with bone protective measures (avoid steroids, smoking cessation, bisphosphonates and statins), and surgery if conservative measures fail.

Question 38

B. (DEXA scan) A hip fracture after a fall from a standing height suggests underlying osteoporosis. Long-term steroid use and smoking are risk factors. A DEXA scan will assess her bone mineral density and confirm the diagnosis.

Question 39

A. (Adhesive capsulitis) Adhesive capsulitis presents with pain and severe shoulder stiffness, worse in external rotation and abduction. Management is with physiotherapy and analgesia. Symptoms will gradually resolve over several years. Diabetes and hypothyroidism are risk factors.

Question 40

E. (Weber B fracture) Ankle fractures are common after pronation injuries, and present with pain, swelling and inability to weight bear. A fibular fracture at the level of the syndesmosis is classified as a Weber B fracture.

Question 41

A. (MR of hip) Hip pain and a shortened, externally rotated hip are suggestive of a NOF fracture. Those with risk factors for osteoporosis (smoking, steroid use) are at increased risk. If there is high clinical suspicion, MR of hip should be performed to detect occult injuries.

Question 42

A. (Disc herniation) Sciatica and sensorimotor weakness in the L4/5 dermatomes suggest L4 radiculopathy, which commonly relates to intervertebral disc herniation. Management is with physiotherapy and analgesia, with surgery reserved for refractory pain.

Question 43

D. (Rotator cuff repair) Rotator cuff tears present with sudden severe shoulder pain on abduction, weak external rotation and tenderness over the acromioclavicular joint and deltoid. Management in the young with traumatic injuries is typically rotator cuff repair.

Question 44

C. (No investigation required) Ankle sprains present with pain and swelling, but preserved weight bearing. According to the Ottawa ankle rules an X-ray is not required.

Question 45

D. (Physiotherapy) C4/5 radiculopathy presents with bilateral pain and sensorimotor weakness in the C4/5 dermatomes and myotomes, with reduced biceps reflexes, commonly relating to intervertebral disc protrusion. Management is with physiotherapy and analgesia, with discectomy reserved for refractory symptoms.

Question 46

E. (Posterior shoulder dislocation) Seizures are a common cause of posterior shoulder dislocation, which present with inability to externally rotate the arm with the arm held in adduction and internal rotation. The X-ray shows the ‘light bulb’ sign, with abnormal vertical positioning of the humeral head, suggesting posterior dislocation.

Question 47

C. (Fracture nonunion) Pain, swelling and reduced range of motion following closed fracture reduction suggest nonunion. Management is with ORIF to realign the bones and allow effective healing.

Question 48

B. (Anti-CCP antibodies) Rheumatoid arthritis presents with symmetrical pain and swelling of the MCP and PIP joints. Young women are the most common demographic. The most specific blood test is anti-CCP antibodies. Rheumatoid factor is sensitive, but not specific, and can be raised in many autoimmune conditions.

Question 49

B. (Osteonecrosis of the jaw) Jaw pain and gum inflammation following dental work while on bisphosphonates suggest osteonecrosis. Bisphosphonates can impair healing following dental procedures, resulting in exposed bone, pain, inflammation and infection. It is typically recommended to stop bisphosphonates for 2–3 months before dental work.

Question 50

B. (Lateral epicondylitis) Lateral epicondylitis presents with lateral elbow and forearm pain, worse on movements involving the extensor tendons. Epicondylitis results from repetitive supination, pronation and extension of the wrist. Management is conservative, with rest and topical analgesia.

Question 51

D. (Spinal osteotomy) Ankylosing spondylitis can result in vertebral body fusion and fixed flexion spinal deformities if poorly controlled. For axial disease, with severe pain and disabling symptoms, spinal osteotomy can correct the deformity.

Question 52

C. (De Quervain tenosynovitis) De Quervain tenosynovitis results from swelling and inflammation of the abductor pollicis long and extensor pollicis brevis tendon sheaths. It is a repetitive strain injury common in new mothers due to repetitive lifting of newborns. Management is with rest, wrist splinting and analgesia, with physiotherapy and steroid injections if refractory.

Question 53

A. (Escharotomy) Circumferential burns risk formation of a constrictive eschar which can result in acute compartment syndrome without early surgical debridement. Escharotomy is appropriate in the first instance. Fasciotomy can be performed if there is ongoing neurovascular impairment.

Question 54

C. (Ewing sarcoma) Constitutional features of malignancy with atraumatic shoulder pain, swelling, erythema and warmth, with lytic bone lesions and an onion skin reaction of the periosteum on X-ray suggest Ewing sarcoma.

Question 55

B. (Iliotibial band syndrome) Iliotibial band syndrome presents with lateral knee pain worse after exercise and hip abductor weakness. This is common in runners due to overtraining and underlying weakness of the hip abductors. Management is with activity modification, icing and NSAIDs, with physiotherapy to increase hip abductor strength.

Question 56

E. (Trochanteric bursitis) Trochanteric bursitis presents with neuropathic hip pain worse on exertion, extended sitting, and at night, and a positive Trendelenburg test. Trochanteric bursitis in older adults may relate to trauma, friction from repetitive movements or inflammatory arthritis. Management is with conservative measures and intraarticular steroid injections.

Question 57

C. (Denosumab) Osteoporosis is suggested by an atraumatic fragility fracture and a T score <-2.5. Management is with optimization of bone health, typically with bisphosphonates first line – however PUD and CKD mean bisphosphonates should be avoided. Denosumab is a monoclonal antibody used as second-line prophylaxis.

Question 58

A. (Intraarticular steroid injections) Trochanteric bursitis can develop as a complication of inflammatory arthritis and presents with greater trochanter pain, pain on internal and external rotation of the hip and hip abduction, and a positive Trendelenburg test. Management options include NSAID analgesia, physiotherapy and steroid injections. Given uncontrolled pain with ibuprofen, a trial of intraarticular steroid injections is appropriate in this case.

Question 59

C. (Physiotherapy) Shoulder impingement presents with pain on abduction and external rotation, and palpable superomedial tenderness of the shoulder joint. Management is with physiotherapy, with steroid injections and surgical decompression if physiotherapy fails to control symptoms.

Question 60

B. (Chronic compartment syndrome) Muscular swelling during exercise can result in recurrent reversible increase in compartmental pressures, compromising limb perfusion and causing pain. Management is with avoidance of triggers, with elective fasciotomy if conservative measures fail.

Urology 29

Question 1

E. (Ultrasound of testes) Testicular cancer presents with a painless, firm testicular mass and is diagnosed with US. Seminomas are homogenous, hypoechoic with sharp margins, and nonseminomas associated with variable echogenicity, calcifications and cystic lesions. Alpha-fetoprotein and human chorionic gonadotropin can support the diagnosis, but US is more specific.

Question 2

C. (Oral antibiotics) Simple UTIs present with dysuria and urinary frequency, and should be managed with empirical antibiotics, typically nitrofurantoin for 5 days. There is no evidence of flank pain or fever to suggest pyelonephritis.

Question 3

E. (Transurethral catheterization) Acute urinary retention is common in older males with BPH. Management is with immediate catheterization to relieve the pain relating to bladder distention.

Question 4

D. (Urinalysis and microscopy, culture and sensitivity) Pyelonephritis presents with flank pain, fever and rigors. Urinalysis and MC&S will confirm the diagnosis and allow tailoring of antibiotics.

Question 5

A. (Benign prostatic hyperplasia) BPH presents with LUTS and a smooth enlarged prostate on DRE. There are no red flag features of malignancy or fever to suggest infection.

Question 6

E. (Surgical reduction and orchiopexy) Testicular torsion presents with lower abdominal and testicular pain and swelling, with a high riding testis with transverse lie. Management is with urgent scrotal exploration and orchiopexy. There is a 6-hour window to save the testis.

Question 7

A. (Ceftriaxone and doxycycline) Acute epididymo-orchitis presents with testicular pain, redness and swelling following UPSI. Management in patients with a likely STI cause is antibiotic therapy, with ceftriaxone and doxycycline an appropriate option to cover the likely organisms. Scrotal packs, icing and NSAIDs can be used as adjunctive measures.

Question 8

C. (Ultrasound of testicles) Testicular torsion presents with sudden onset severe abdominal and testicular pain and vomiting, a high riding testis with a transverse line and a negative Prehn sign (no relief of pain on elevation of the scrotum). Torsion is a clinical diagnosis, but US can be used to confirm the diagnosis if it does not delay scrotal exploration.

Question 9

C. (Cystoscopy and biopsy) Painless haematuria is the hallmark of bladder cancer. Cystoscopy and biopsy will allow direct visualization and confirmation of the diagnosis.

Question 10

D. (Transurethral resection of the prostate) In BPH with a failure of dual medical therapy to control symptoms, surgical management with TURP is appropriate.

Question 11

B. (Nucleic acid amplification test) Testicular pain, swelling, erythema and low-grade fever suggest acute epididymo-orchitis. In sexually active males, the most common cause is Chlamydia trachomatis or Neisseria gonorrhoeae; hence, NAAT testing will confirm the diagnosis and guide antibiotic treatment.

Question 12

A. (Bladder cancer) Bladder cancer presents with gross haematuria. Suprapubic discomfort is common. Smokers are at particular risk.

Question 13

A. (Active surveillance) Early-stage prostate cancer is often managed with active surveillance in patients with life expectancy >5 years, with regular monitoring with DRE, PSA and multiparametric MRI screening.

Question 14

C. (Radical cystectomy) For TCC involving the detrusor muscle wall without regional or distant metastasis, radical cystectomy (with or without neoadjuvant chemoradiotherapy) is indicated.

Question 15

A. (Intravenous antibiotics) Pyelonephritis presents with flank pain, fevers and urinary symptoms. Tachycardia and hypotension suggest sepsis, hence intravenous antibiotics are appropriate. Percutaneous nephrostomy is used if there is a perinephric abscess.

Question 16

A. (Multiparametric MR of prostate) Prostate cancer can present with LUTS and constitutional features including unintentional weight loss, and is diagnosed with multiparametric MRI. PSA would be elevated regardless due to BPH. DRE may be unremarkable in cancer as tumours are commonly peripherally located.

Question 17

A. (Bladder scan) Acute urinary retention presents as an acute inability to pass urine. Bedside bladder US will demonstrate residual bladder volume. Parkinson disease can impair detrusor muscle contraction and result in acute retention. Urgent urinary catheterization is required.

Question 18

A. (*Chlamydia trachomatis*) In young males the most common cause of epididymo-orchitis are STIs. In older males, enteric organisms including E. coli are more common.

Question 19

D. (Radical inguinal orchiectomy) A solid testicular mass likely represents testicular malignancy. The US findings suggest nonseminoma. Management is with orchiectomy and radical inguinal lymph node dissection. Following staging, adjuvant radiochemotherapy can be considered.

Question 20

D. (Tamsulosin) BPH presents with urinary frequency and urgency, nocturia and difficulties with the urinary stream. Conservative management involves bladder retraining and moderating fluid intake. Most patients require medical management, with alpha-blockers (tamsulosin) for symptom control or 5-alpha reductase inhibitors (finasteride) to reduce the size of the prostate.

Question 21

D. (Testicular torsion) In patients with cryptorchidism (undescended testes), sudden lower abdominal pain and vomiting is a red flag for testicular torsion. In all cases of young males with abdominal pain, scrotal examination should be considered, as pain can radiate to the lower abdomen from a torted testis.

Question 22

A. (Epididymal cyst) A painless, soft, fluctuant groin lump not tethered to the testes suggests epididymal cyst. Hydroceles transilluminate and varicoceles feel like a 'bag of worms'. If you could not palpate above the lump, this would suggest inguinal hernia.

Question 23

E. (PR diclofenac) Renal colic presents with severe, 'colicky' loin-to-groin pain, nausea and vomiting, dysuria and haematuria. NSAIDs reduce ureteric peristalsis and oedema, and the PR route is known to be highly effective.

Question 24

B. (CT of abdomen) Renal carcinoma presents with flank pain, haematuria and a palpable mass. CT abdomen will most effectively delineate the lesion.

Question 25

E. (Watchful waiting) Hydroceles can develop following an acute scrotal infection, and typically spontaneously resolve without specific treatment. If symptoms fail to improve, aspiration or surgical correction can be performed.

Question 26

C. (Manual foreskin reduction) Paraphimosis presents with pain and swelling of the glans, and a band of constricting tissue at the coronal sulcus. Initially, manual reduction is attempted, with dorsal slit reduction surgery if manual reduction fails. There is a risk of penile necrosis.

Question 27

A. (CT of kidneys, ureters, bladder) Renal colic presents with intermittent severe loin-the-groin pain, nausea, vomiting, urinary symptoms and haematuria. CT KUB will demonstrate the obstruction stone and guide management.

Question 28

C. (Chronic urinary retention) Chronic urinary retention presents with nocturnal incontinence and painless abdominal distention. Management is with urinary catheterization and management of the underlying cause.

Question 29

B. (Medication review) Stress incontinence presents with involuntary leakage of urine when increasing intra-abdominal pressure. Conservative measures targeting risk factors are appropriate in the first instance – she is on a diuretic, which could be modified to reduce her symptoms, and her asthma management is optimized to reduce coughing which is triggering her symptoms.

Question 30

D. (Tamsulosin) Renal colic presents with intermittent, 'colicky' loin-to-groin pain, restlessness and costovertebral angle tenderness. The investigations confirm an 8 mm stone, which can be managed conservatively with medical expulsive therapy (alpha-blockers) in the first instance.

Question 31

E. (Urinalysis) BPH presents with storage (frequency and nocturia) and voiding (hesitancy and terminal dribbling) LUTS. BPH is a clinical diagnosis; however urinalysis to exclude urinary tract infection is essential.

Question 32

E. (Urge incontinence) Urge incontinence presents with sudden urinary urgency and incontinence. Constipation is a risk factor.

Question 33

D. (Testicular seminoma) Painless scrotal swelling with negative transillumination suggests testicular cancer. Males 20–35 are at particular risk. Seminomas are associated with hypoechoic, homogenous, well-defined lesions on US and nonseminomas cystic lesions and calcifications.

Question 34

C. (Suprapubic catheterization) A sudden, painful inability to void and residual bladder volume indicates acute urinary retention. BPH is a common cause in older men. A history of urethral strictures and surgery means suprapubic catheterization is the preferred approach.

Question 35

B. (Balanoposthitis) Balanoposthitis presents with pain and swelling of the glans and foreskin, with penile discharge, ulcerations and dysuria. Balanitis refers to irritation of the glans penis only. The most common aetiology is poor genital hygiene or contact irritation. Yeast infections are also common.

Question 36

C. (Cystolith) The US demonstrates a cystolith (bladder stone), which may be asymptomatic but can cause irritation to the bladder wall or neck, causing LUTS. BPH may be an aggravating factor.

Question 37

E. (Neurogenic bladder) CES can occur after intervertebral disc prolapse. Acute urinary retention suggests compression of the spinal nerve roots supplying the pudendal nerve, which controls voluntary micturition. Management is with urgent catheterization and investigation and treatment of the underlying cause.

Question 38

D. (PSA) Widespread sclerotic lesions of the lumbosacral spine and hips suggest advanced metastatic malignancy. In an older man, sclerotic bony lesions suggest prostate cancer; hence DRE, PSA and multiparametric MRI should be performed as a comprehensive screen for prostate cancer.

Question 39

C. (Indapamide) Recurrent renal stones are an indication for chemoprophylaxis alongside lifestyle measures. For calcium stones (which are radiopaque), thiazide diuretics such as indapamide can be used. Low-calcium diets should be avoided as they increase the osteoporosis risk.

Question 40

B. (Foreskin reaction and bathing) Balanitis presents with pain, swelling and erythema of the glans penis. Most cases relate to poor genital hygiene; hence management involves daily foreskin retraction and bathing. If there is evidence of underlying fungal or bacterial infection, antimicrobials can be prescribed. Steroids are used for contact dermatitis.

Question 41

C. (Reassurance and discharge) Screening for prostate cancer is not recommended, as investigations such as

PSA are nonspecific and may lead to further unnecessary or invasive tests. There are no LUTS or constitutional features to warrant investigation in this case. PSA would be raised regardless in BPH.

Question 42

D. (Uric acid) Uric acid stones are radiolucent and associated with conditions of high cell turnover (i.e. myelodysplastic syndrome). Management is with increased fluid intake and uric acid-lowering agents including allopurinol.

Question 43

D. (Urinalysis and microscopy, culture and sensitivity) While UTIs are typically a clinical diagnosis, in complicated cases (in males, or those with risk factors for severe infection including CKD and immunosuppression), urine culture should be sent to guide effective antibiotic therapy.

Question 44

D. (Radical nephrectomy) Renal malignancy presents with flank pain, a palpable mass and haematuria, and is managed with radical nephrectomy. Immunotherapy is used if there is evidence of distant metastatic disease.

Question 45

C. (Prostatitis) Acute bacterial prostatitis presents with LUTS, abdominal and back pain, fever and prostatic swelling and tenderness. Management is with antibiotic therapy.

Question 46

A. (Leydig cell tumour) Leydig cell tumours arise from hormone-producing stromal cells, and are associated with features of androgen excess, including gynaecomastia and breast tenderness.

Question 47

D. (Oral antibiotics) Chronic bacterial prostatitis presents with an extended history of LUTS following incompletely treated acute bacterial prostatitis. Erectile dysfunction, ejaculatory pain and haematospermia are common. Management is with extended antibiotic therapy (up to 12 weeks).

Question 48

C. (Intravenous hydrocortisone) Graft versus host disease can develop due to a systemic inflammatory response to a transplanted organ and presents with abdominal pain, rash and hepatosplenomegaly. It is associated with HLA mismatching and typically manifests within 100 days following transplant. If there is evidence of liver involvement, steroids are required. If not, optimization of prophylaxis (ciclosporin) is sufficient.

Question 49

E. (Hyponatraemia) Post-TURP syndrome results from systemic absorption of irrigation fluids used during TURP, resulting in plasma dilution, hyponatraemia and hypothermia. Hyponatremia can lead to seizures.

Question 50

C. (Percutaneous drainage) Obstructing renal stones can lead to stagnation and infection of urine, resulting in perinephric abscesses, presenting with flank pain, fever and a palpable mass. Management is with percutaneous drainage. Antibiotics should be started following urinalysis and MC&S.

Question 51

B. (CT of abdomen) Perinephric abscesses present with fever, flank pain, dysuria and a palpable flank mass. Diabetics are at increased risk. Abdominal CT will demonstrate the abscess extending from the renal pelvis into the perinephric space.

Question 52

B. (Interstitial cystitis) UTIs with a sterile culture suggest interstitial cystitis, an intrinsic renal injury commonly caused by medication toxicity (in this case, valproate combined with NSAIDs).

Question 53

A. (Bladder retraining) Overactive bladder presents with urinary frequency and urgency, in the absence of infective symptoms or incontinence. Conservative measures including bladder retraining (progress increase in voiding intervals) and modifying caffeine and alcohol intake are appropriate in the first instance.

Question 54

A. (Chronic epididymitis) Over 6 weeks of scrotal pain and swelling, with a thickened epididymis, and multiple episodes of acute epididymo-orchitis suggests chronic epididymitis. Management involves symptomatic treatment with scrotal support, warm baths and analgesia.

Question 55

E. (Urethral stricture) Chronic bladder outflow obstruction presents with hesitancy and poor urinary stream. Urethral strictures can occur following repeated urinary infections and traumatic catheterizations. Management is with urethrotomy (resection of fibrotic urethral tissue) or urethral stents.

Question 56

D. (Testicular cancer) A first seizure and multiple 'cannonball' lung lesions suggest disseminated malignancy. Cannonball metastases are commonly associated with testicular and renal cell carcinoma. In this demographic, testicular cancer is the most likely aetiology. Renal cell carcinoma presents in older adults and pulmonary and bone metastasis are most common.

Question 57

E. (Oxybutynin) Neurogenic bladder dysfunction presents with intermittent involuntary leakage of small volumes without associated urgency or symptoms of stress incontinence. Management is with conservative measures (regular voiding, avoidance of diuretics and appropriate fluid intake and timing) and muscarinic antagonists initially. If patients are severely frail, long-term catheterization may be appropriate.

Question 58

C. (Transrectal ultrasound of prostate) Prostatic abscesses present with LUTS, fevers and a tender, fluctuant prostate. Abscesses are a complication of acute bacterial prostatitis and should be managed with transrectal US and drainage, and antibiotics.

Question 59

B. (CT of abdomen) A right-sided renal malignancy may obstruct the spermatic vein and lead to a unilateral varicocele. Abdominal imaging is required to investigate for malignancy.

Question 60

C. (Reassurance and safety netting) Phimosis can develop following balanitis. In relative phimosis (difficult retracting the foreskin) conservative management is used initially, as symptoms will likely spontaneously resolve. Surgical management is used for full phimosis (inability to retract the foreskin) or if conservative measures fail to resolve symptoms.

Breast surgery 30

Question 1

B. (Cerebral metastasis) In patients with a history of breast cancer, cerebral metastasis can occur and provoke seizures. A first presentation of epilepsy at 78 is uncommon, and there are no meningitic features.

Question 2

D. (No investigations required) Mastitis presents with pain, erythema, swelling and tenderness in the breast. Pain and difficulty breastfeeding is common. Mastitis is a clinical diagnosis. Investigations are only required if there are atypical symptoms or a poor response to initial antibiotic therapy

Question 3

C. (Oral antibiotics) Mastitis presents with pain and swelling of the breast, with pain and difficulty breastfeeding. An erythematous breast lump is common due to inflammation of the lactiferous ducts. Empirical treatment with oral antibiotics is appropriate. Continued breastfeeding should be encouraged to reduce the risk of a breast abscess.

Question 4

B. (Double mastectomy) The personal and family history significantly increases the breast cancer risk. In such cases, annual mammography or prophylactic surgery can be offered depending on patient preferences. In this case, double mastectomy is the most effective way to reduce her risk.

Question 5

E. (Ultrasound of breast) An unexplained breast lump should be assessed with clinical examination, breast imaging and biopsy. The initial investigation of a breast lump in younger patients (<30) is with breast US, as dense breast tissue in younger patients makes lesions more difficult to characterize on mammography. Following US, appropriate biopsy is performed depending on the features of the lesion and risk of malignancy.

Question 6

B. (Herceptin) All HER2+ve breast cancers are treated with targeted monoclonal antibiotics to HER2 receptors, to inhibit tumour growth, reducing the risk of recurrence. There is a risk of cardiomyopathy.

Question 7

C. (Mammography every 3 years) There are no red flag features of breast cancer, or history increasing the risk of cancer development. In such cases, mammography every 3 years between the ages 50 and 70 is appropriate. While hormone replacement therapy may increase the risk of breast cancer, it is not an indication for enhanced screening in the absence of symptoms or other risk factors.

Question 8

C. (Incision and drainage) There are features of a severe breast abscess with skin necrosis, which should be managed surgically with incision and drainage. Percutaneous drainage is used when there is no associated skin necrosis.

Question 9

B. (Mammogram) Breast cancer presents with a firm, fixed lump in the breast, often with associated nipple changes. Older patients (>30) with a breast lump should undergo mammography, then biopsy to confirm the underlying aetiology.

Question 10

E. (Total mastectomy with axillary dissection) Stage two breast cancers with local lymphatic spread can be managed with breast-conserving surgery or mastectomy. Breast-conserving surgery is contraindicated if there is nipple involvement. Radical mastectomy is less common in recent years in preference for less invasive procedures.

Question 11

B. (Reassurance) Gynaecomastia is common in pubertal boys, relating to oestrogen and androgen imbalance, and typically spontaneously resolves by late teenage years. Pharmacotherapy with selective oestrogen modulators (i.e., tamoxifen) or surgical intervention can be considered if there is persistence past puberty or severe psychological distress.

Question 12

E. (Fibroadenoma) Fibroadenomas are benign tumours of stromal and epithelial tissue which present with small, very mobile lumps within the breast tissue. They are the most common benign breast tumours in women under 35, and are managed conservatively, unless large or distort the appearance of the breast.

Question 13

C. (Prolactin level) Galactorrhoea is painless milky nipple discharge not associated with lactation. Typical antipsychotics such as risperidone are common causes of hyperprolactinaemia, which can result in galactorrhoea. Alternative medications can be considered if symptoms are troubling, but should be undertaken under specialist supervision due to the risk of psychiatric disturbances.

Question 14

A. (Excisional biopsy) Complex breast cysts have a high risk of malignant transformation and should be managed with a core needle or excisional biopsy, to confirm the diagnosis and detect malignancy.

Question 15

E. (Reassurance) Simple breast cysts are benign fluid collections common in premenopausal women. Most resolve spontaneously.

Question 16

D. (Periductal mastitis) Periductal mastitis is noninfectious mastitis common in smokers and diabetic patients. It is rare. There are no skin changes to suggest inflammatory breast cancer or Paget disease of the nipple. Breast abscesses are associated with severe systemic illness.

Question 17

A. (Ductal carcinoma in situ) A nontender, poorly defined, fixed breast lump suggests cancer. Triple assessment should be performed, involving clinical examination, age-appropriate imaging (in this case mammography) and biopsy to confirm the diagnosis. Ductal carcinoma in situ is a noninvasive carcinoma that can precede invasive carcinoma, and appears as grouped microcalcifications on mammography.

Question 18

C. (Inflammatory breast cancer) Inflammatory breast cancer is a rare form of invasive breast cancer that presents with rapid onset of oedema, erythema, skin changes and blood-stained nipple discharge. There is often no palpable mass. Inflammatory breast cancer is treated with radical mastectomy and chemoradiotherapy but has a poor prognosis.

Question 19

B. (Manual lymphatic drainage) Lymphoedema can develop in limbs following surgical intervention or radiotherapy to regional lymph nodes. Management is with manual lymphatic drainage and compression garments. Exercise and elevation of the affected limb can help but will likely be insufficient in isolation to control symptoms.

Question 20

E. (Paget disease of the nipple) Paget disease of the nipple presents with a scaly erythematous nipple rash with nipple retraction, ulceration and blood-stained discharge. This suggests an underlying ductal carcinoma in situ or invasive ductal carcinoma. A complete triple assessment should be performed and managed appropriately for the underlying aetiology.

Question 21

E. (Ultrasound of breast) Breast abscesses present with breast pain, swelling and erythema, with a fluctuant mass and purulent nipple discharge. US will confirm the diagnosis, which can be treated with fine needle aspiration.

Question 22

E. (Ultrasound of breast) Fibrocystic breast changes are nonspecific cystic changes associated with hormone fluctuations, presenting with bilateral pain and lumpiness around menstruation. They are very common. Breast imaging is indicated for all breast lumps to detect concerning features of malignancy. In this age group, breast US should be performed, which will demonstrate scattered microcysts and calcifications. Complex cystic lesions should be further excised to detect atypia.

Question 23

D. (Radical mastectomy) Paget disease of the breast is an external lesion commonly associated with underlying ductal carcinoma in situ or invasive ductal carcinoma. Management involves assessment of the underlying cause and surgical tumour removal. Breast-conserving surgery is used in localized, small lesions, but is contraindicated with skin or nipple involvement.

Question 24

A. (Breast abscess) Breast abscesses can complicate mastitis, and present with breast pain, erythema and oedema, with a fluctuant mass. High fever and nausea are common.

Question 25

C. (Nipple swabs) Nipple thrush presents with pain and itch while breastfeeding. It is common in breastfeeding mothers and associated with diabetes. Swabs will confirm the diagnosis and antifungal agents can be prescribed.

Question 26

A. (Core needle biopsy) Intraductal papillomas are benign breast lesions that commonly cause bloody nipple discharge. Core needle biopsy will confirm the diagnosis and detect atypia. Intraductal papillomas with atypia should be excused due to the risk of malignant transformation.

Question 27

E. (Topical NSAIDs) Cyclical mastalgia presents with breast pain associated with the menstrual cycle. Oral contraceptive use can trigger or worsen the pain. Topical NSAIDs are the most effective treatment, alongside a supportive, well-fitting bra. In unexplained, noncyclical mastalgia, age-appropriate imaging should be performed to determine the underlying aetiology.

Question 28

C. (Fat necrosis) Fat necrosis occurs when trauma leads to fibrosis and calcification of breast tissue. It is relatively common following surgery, and may be difficult to distinguish from breast cancer. Imaging and biopsy should be performed; however recurrence of malignancy in this time frame following surgery would be uncommon.

Question 29

B. (Duct ectasia) Duct ectasia results from periductal inflammation and fibrosis of the breast tissue, resulting in nipple retraction and green, grey or bloody nipple discharge. Smoking and obesity increase the risk. Breast imaging and biopsy should be performed to confirm the diagnosis and exclude malignancy.

Question 30

E. (Phyllodes tumour) Phyllodes tumours are fast-growing benign tumours common in older women just prior to menopause. Stromal cellularity and leaf-like architecture are the classical histology findings. Fibroadenomas are smaller lesions which typically affect younger women.

Section 5

UKMLA DIAGNOSTIC AND FULL MOCKS – QUESTIONS

UKMLA diagnostic mock – medicine 31

CARDIOVASCULAR

1. A 52-year-old woman has severe chest pain radiating to her left shoulder for 2 hours. Her pulse is 114 bpm and BP 123/87 mmHg. She is pale and clammy to the touch.

Investigations:
ECG: ST elevation in leads I, V5 and V6.

Which is the most likely diagnosis?
   A. Anterior STEMI
   B. Anterolateral STEMI
   C. Inferior STEMI
   D. Lateral STEMI
   E. Posterior STEMI

2. A 59-year-old man has recurrent exertional chest tightness for 5 minutes, relieved by rest for 3 months. He has hypercholesterolaemia, managed with atorvastatin.

Investigations:
ECG: ST depression in the inferior leads.
Troponin: normal

Which is the most likely diagnosis?
   A. Non-ST-elevated myocardial infarction
   B. Prinzmetal angina
   C. Stable angina
   D. ST-elevated myocardial infarction
   E. Unstable angina

3. A 33-year-old woman has left-sided chest pain worsened by deep inspiration, relieved by leaning forward. She has systemic lupus erythematosus, managed with hydroxychloroquine. A scratchy sound is heard on the chest auscultation, accentuated when she leans forward.

Investigations:
ECG: concave ST elevation in the precordial leads

Which is the most likely diagnosis?
   A. Acute pericarditis
   B. Constrictive pericarditis
   C. Pulmonary embolism
   D. ST-elevated myocardial infarction
   E. Unstable angina

4. A 64-year-old woman has shortness of breath and chest pain worsened by deep inspiration for 2 hours. She had surgery for a hip fracture 3 weeks ago. Her BP is 120 bpm and respiratory rate 27 breaths per minute. She has leg swelling and dilated, swollen, tender lower leg veins bilaterally.

Which is the most likely diagnosis?
   A. Acute pericarditis
   B. Aortic dissection
   C. Congestive heart failure
   D. Pulmonary embolism
   E. ST-elevated myocardial infarction

5. A 61-year-old man has a sudden loss of consciousness and a collapse. He arrives at the emergency department pulseless and unresponsive.

Investigations:
ECG: irregular deflections of varying amplitude, with no discernible p waves and QRS complexes.

Which is the most likely diagnosis?
   A. Atrial fibrillation
   B. Cardiac arrest
   C. Hypertrophic obstructive cardiomyopathy
   D. ST-elevated myocardial infarction
   E. Stroke

6. A 74-year-old woman has had increasing fatigue and shortness of breath for a month. She has hypertension and type 2 diabetes mellitus, managed with ramipril and metformin. She has bilateral pitting oedema, an S3 heart sound and bibasal crepitations on chest auscultation.

Which is the most likely diagnosis?

A. Aortic stenosis
B. Heart failure
C. Pulmonary embolism
D. Stable angina
E. ST-elevated myocardial infarction

7. A 40-year-old man has chest pain and progressively worsening shortness of breath for 2 days. His pulse is 130 bpm and BP 87/58 mmHg. He has elevated jugular venous pressure, with an absent y descent and softened heart sounds on chest auscultation.

Investigations:
ECG: alternation of QRS complex amplitude between beats

Which is the most likely diagnosis?

A. Cardiac tamponade
B. Constrictive pericarditis
C. Pulmonary embolism
D. Simple pneumothorax
E. Tension pneumothorax

8. A 25-year-old man has chest pain and shortness of breath for 2 weeks. He uses recreational IV heroin once a month. His temperature is 38.7°C. He has small, painless red spots on his palms and soles and a pansystolic murmur best heard on inspiration.

Which is the most likely diagnosis?

A. Aortic dissection
B. Atrial myxoma
C. Infective endocarditis
D. Rheumatic fever
E. Pulmonary embolism

9. A 74-year-old woman has intermittent palpitations and shortness of breath for 4 months. She has hypertension, managed with amlodipine. Her pulse is 120 bpm and BP 165/102 mmHg.

Investigations:
ECG: irregularly irregular R-R intervals and absent p waves.

Which is the most likely diagnosis?

A. Atrial fibrillation
B. Torsades de pointes
C. Ventricular tachycardia
D. Ventricular fibrillation
E. Wolff–Parkinson–White syndrome

10. An 80-year-old man has shortness of breath and chest pain on exertion. He has hypertension, managed with amlodipine. He has an ejection systolic murmur loudest at the second right intercostal space, radiating to the carotids. His lungs are clear on auscultation.

Which is the most likely diagnosis?

A. Aortic regurgitation
B. Aortic stenosis
C. Atrial septal defect
D. Hypertrophic cardiomyopathy
E. Mitral valve prolapse

GASTROENTEROLOGY

1. A 31-year-old woman has had recurrent bloody diarrhoea, abdominal cramping and incomplete evacuation three times a day for 6 months. She has left lower quadrant abdominal pain and painful, red eyes bilaterally.

Investigations:
Colonoscopy: regenerating mucosa.

Which is the most likely diagnosis?

A. Coeliac disease
B. Crohn disease
C. Gastric cancer
D. Irritable bowel syndrome
E. Ulcerative colitis

2. A 27-year-old man has right lower quadrant pain and nonbloody diarrhoea five times a day for 3 months. She has perianal skin tags, mouth ulcers and joint pain bilaterally in the hands and wrists.

Investigations:
Colonoscopy: skip lesions.

Which is the most likely diagnosis?

A. Coeliac disease
B. Colorectal cancer
C. Crohn disease
D. Irritable bowel syndrome
E. Ulcerative colitis

3. A 25-year-old man has had stomach cramps and pale diarrhoea for 3 months. He has type 1 diabetes mellitus, managed with a basal-bolus insulin regime. He has abdominal bloating and itchy, vesicular skin lesions on the elbows and knees.

Investigations:
IgA tissue transglutaminase: 17.1 U/mL (<15).
Duodenal biopsy: 1:1 villous to crypt ratio.

Which is the most likely diagnosis?
   A. Coeliac disease
   B. Crohn disease
   C. Duodenal ulcer
   D. Irritable bowel syndrome
   E. Small bowel overgrowth syndrome

4. A 63-year-old woman has had fatigue and a loss of appetite for 4 months. She has chronic alcohol abuse, drinking 30 units of alcohol per week for 30 years. He has yellowing of his skin, a distended abdomen with visible veins and tenderness in the right upper quadrant.

Which is the most likely diagnosis?
   A. Acute cholecystitis
   B. Hepatitis B
   C. Hepatitis C
   D. Liver abscess
   E. Liver cirrhosis

5. A 31-year-old man has had a fever and right upper quadrant pain for 3 weeks. He returned from Thailand a month ago, where most of his meals were from street food vendors. He has scleral icterus, tender liver enlargement and right upper quadrant tenderness.

Which is the most likely diagnosis?
   A. Hepatitis A
   B. Hepatitis B
   C. Hepatitis C
   D. Hepatitis D
   E. Hepatitis E

6. A 27-year-old woman has crampy abdominal pain relieved by passing gas and bowel movements alternating between diarrhoea and constipation for 8 months. Her symptoms are worsened by stress and eating meals.

Which is the most likely diagnosis?
   A. Coeliac disease
   B. Crohn disease
   C. Diverticulitis
   D. Irritable bowel syndrome
   E. Ulcerative colitis

7. A 48-year-old man has had right upper quadrant pain and confusion for 4 days. He has chronic alcohol misuse, consuming 25 units of alcohol per week. His abdomen is tender in the right upper quadrant and has scleral icterus.

Investigations:
Prothrombin time: 24 seconds (11.5–15.5).

Which is the most likely diagnosis?
   A. Acute cholecystitis
   B. Acute pancreatitis
   C. Gastric ulcer
   D. Hepatitis B
   E. Liver failure

8. An 18-year-old woman has had a declining academic performance at university and increased irritability for 5 months. She has a resting tremor bilaterally, yellowing of the skin and brownish-green discolouration of the corneas.

Which is the most likely diagnosis?
   A. Autoimmune hepatitis
   B. Haemochromatosis
   C. Huntington disease
   D. Parkinson disease
   E. Wilson disease

9. A 46-year-old man has difficulty swallowing solids and liquids progressively worsening for 7 months, causing central chest pain, and he has also lost 4 kg unintentionally.

Investigations:
Barium swallow: dilated distal oesophagus with tapering at the gastroesophageal junction.

Which is the most likely diagnosis?
   A. Achalasia
   B. Gastroesophageal reflux disease
   C. Hiatus hernia
   D. Oesophageal cancer
   E. Oesophageal stricture

10. A 33-year-old woman has had bilateral joint pain in the hands and right upper quadrant pain for 3 months. She has hepatomegaly and skin hyperpigmentation.

Investigations:
Serum iron: 45 g/L (12–30).

Which is the most likely diagnosis?
A. Acute liver failure
B. Haemochromatosis
C. Hepatocellular carcinoma
D. Liver cirrhosis
E. Wilson disease

RESPIRATORY

1. A 30-year-old woman has had shortness of breath and a cough, worse at night for a month. She has eczema, managed with topical betamethasone. She has a bilateral expiratory wheeze.

Investigations:
Forced expiratory volume (FEV1)/forced vital capacity (FVC) ratio: 0.63.

Which is the most likely diagnosis?
A. Asthma
B. Chronic bronchitis
C. Chronic obstructive pulmonary disease (COPD)
D. Pneumonia
E. Pulmonary embolism

2. A 62-year-old man has had progressive shortness of breath and cough for 5 years. The cough has been producing more sputum for 6 months. He has smoked 20 cigarettes for 30 years. He has decreased breath sounds and scattered bilateral expiratory wheezes.

Investigations:
Forced expiratory volume (FEV1)/forced vital capacity (FVC) ratio: 0.61.

Which is the most likely diagnosis?
A. Alpha-1 antitrypsin deficiencny
B. Asthma
C. Bronchiectasis
D. Chronic obstructive pulmonary disease (COPD)
E. Pneumonia

3. A 47-year-old woman has a chronic cough, producing thick yellow sputum for 3 months, with occasional blood in the sputum. She has frequent respiratory infections. She has coarse crepitations bilaterally on chest auscultation.

Which is the most likely diagnosis?
A. Bronchiectasis
B. Chronic obstructive pulmonary disease (COPD)
C. Chronic sinusitis
D. Pulmonary fibrosis
E. Tuberculosis

4. A 69-year-old man has had a productive cough and progressive shortness of breath for 5 days. He has hypertension, managed with amlodipine. She has crepitations and bronchial breath sounds in the left lower lobe on chest auscultation.

Which is the most likely diagnosis?
A. Acute exacerbation of COPD
B. Pneumonia
C. Pulmonary embolism
D. Sarcoidosis
E. Tuberculosis

5. A 24-year-old woman has had a persistent cough producing yellowish sputum for 3 weeks. He is a healthcare assistant and was recently exposed to a patient with a chronic cough. He has decreased breath sounds and fine crepitations in the right upper lobe on chest auscultation.

Which is the most likely diagnosis?
A. Bronchitis
B. Lung cancer
C. Pneumonia
D. Sarcoidosis
E. Tuberculosis

6. A 29-year-old man has had shortness of breath and left-sided chest pain worsened by deep breathing for an hour. He has Marfan syndrome. He has left-sided decreased breath sounds and hyperresonant percussion.

Investigations:
CXR: absence of lung markings on the left chest.

Which is the most likely diagnosis?

A. Mallory-Weiss tear
B. Pneumonia
C. Pulmonary embolism
D. Simple pneumothorax
E. Tension pneumothorax

7. A 56-year-old woman has a persistent cough, occasional blood in her sputum and unintentional weight loss of 6 kg for 5 months. She has smoked 20 cigarettes a day for 35 years. She has decreased breath sounds in the left upper lobe on chest auscultation.

Which is the most likely diagnosis?

A. Amyloidosis
B. Lung cancer
C. Pneumonia
D. Sarcoidosis
E. Tuberculosis

RENAL

1. A 41-year-old woman has right flank pain and decreased urine output. She had a urinary tract infection, managed with nitrofurantoin. She has a diffuse maculopapular rash over her back and right costovertebral angle tenderness.

Investigations:
Serum urea: 7.6 mmol/L (2.5–7.0).
Serum creatinine: 127 μmol/L (60–110).
Eosinophils: 0.49×10^9/L (0–0.40).

Which is the most likely diagnosis?

A. Acute glomerulonephritis
B. Acute interstitial nephritis
C. Acute tubular necrosis
D. Eosinophilic granulomatosis with polyangiitis
E. Renal cell carcinoma

2. A 58-year-old woman has fatigue and increased urination during the night. She has hypertension and type 2 diabetes mellitus, managed with amlodipine and metformin. Her BP is 165/113 mmHg. She has oedema to the knees bilaterally.

Investigations:
Serum urea: 7.5 mmol/L (2.5–7.0).
Serum creatinine: 137 μmol/L (60–110).
Estimated glomerular filtration rate (eGFR): 53 mL/min/ 1.73 m^2 (>90).

Which is the most likely diagnosis?

A. Acute kidney injury
B. Chronic kidney disease
C. Nephrotic syndrome
D. Renal artery stenosis
E. Urinary tract infection

3. A 6-year-old boy has had facial and leg swelling, frothy urine and decreased appetite for a week. He has mild pallor, periorbital oedema and pitting oedema to the knees bilaterally.

Investigations:
Urinalysis: protein ++, blood -, glucose -, leucocytes –
24-h urinary albumin: 23 mg (<30)

Which is the most likely diagnosis?

A. Alport syndrome
B. Focal segmental glomerulosclerosis
C. IgA nephropathy
D. Minimal change disease
E. Post-streptococcal glomerulonephritis

4. A 23-year-old man has painless blood in his urine and intermittent flank pain for 24 hours. He had an upper respiratory infection that resolved 2 days ago. He has pitting oedema in his legs.

Investigations:
Urinalysis: protein ++, blood ++, glucose -, leucocytes -
Renal biopsy: mesangial hypercellularity.

Which is the most likely diagnosis?

A. Antiglomerular basement membrane disease
B. Henoch–Schönlein purpura
C. IgA nephropathy
D. Minimal change disease
E. Poststreptococcal glomerulonephritis

5. A 47-year-old man has had recurrent abdominal pain and intermittent blood in his urine for 4 months. Both his father and paternal grandmother had renal transplants in their fifties. He has bilateral palpable flank masses.

Which is the most likely diagnosis?
A. Acute tubular necrosis
B. IgA nephropathy
C. Polycystic kidney disease
D. Tuberous sclerosis
E. Urinary tract calculi

NEUROLOGY

1. A 42-year-old woman has a severe occipital headache for an hour. She has polycystic kidney disease. She has photophobia and neck stiffness.

Investigations:
CT head: hyperdensities in the basal cisterns.

Which is the most likely diagnosis?
A. Cluster headache
B. Extradural haematoma
C. Meningitis
D. Subarachnoid haemorrhage
E. Subdural haematoma

2. A 67-year-old man has weakness in his right arm and leg and has inarticulate speech for 2 hours. His BP is 165/102 mmHg. He has right-sided facial droop and homonymous hemianopia, and his speech is not fluent, but his comprehension is intact.

Investigations:
CT head: hypodense area in the left middle cerebral artery territory.

Which is the most likely diagnosis?
A. Lacunar infarct
B. Lateral medullary syndrome
C. Partial anterior circulation infarct
D. Posterior circulation infarct
E. Total anterior circulation infarct

3. A 23-year-old man has a severe headache and low-grade fever for a day. He has neck stiffness, photophobia and pain with passive extension of his knees bilaterally.

Investigations:
Lumbar puncture: low glucose, high protein, neutrophil predominance

Which is the most likely diagnosis?
A. Bacterial meningitis
B. Encephalitis
C. Fungal meningitis
D. Subarachnoid haemorrhage
E. Viral meningitis

4. A 32-year-old woman has severe headaches localized around her right temple lasting several hours, preceded by zigzag lines in her vision. The headaches are more frequent when she menstruates and are improved by entering a dark, quiet room.

Which is the most likely diagnosis?
A. Cluster headache
B. Migraine
C. Sinusitis
D. Temporal arteritis
E. Tension headache

5. A 45-year-old man has had a severe headache and confusion for 2 days. His temperature is 39.1°C, and he is not orientated to person, place or time.

Investigations:
MRI head: increased signal intensity in the mediotemporal lobes bilaterally.

Which is the most likely diagnosis?
A. Brain tumour
B. Encephalitis
C. Meningitis
D. Stroke
E. Subarachnoid haemorrhage

6. A 63-year-old woman has had a gradual decline in her memory and difficulty performing formerly routine tasks for 9 months. Her husband says that she forgets important events and frequently misplaces her belongings. Her mother suffered similar symptoms in her seventies. She is disoriented to time and place.

Investigations:
Mini-mental state examination (MMSE): 17 out of 30.

Which is the most likely diagnosis?
A. Alzheimer disease
B. Frontotemporal dementia
C. Lewy body dementia
D. Parkinson disease
E. Vascular dementia

7. A 31-year-old man has a sudden loss of consciousness, causing a fall. During this episode, his family says that his whole body stiffened for 30 seconds before the rhythmic jerking of his arms and legs for 2 minutes; however, he has no recollection of this occurring.

Which is the most likely diagnosis?
   A. Absence seizure
   B. Atonic seizure
   C. Focal seizure
   D. Generalized tonic-clonic seizure
   E. Myoclonic seizure

8. A 64-year-old woman has a resting tremor in her right hand, progressively worsening for a year. She has increased muscle tone in both arms and a shuffling gait with a decreased arm swing while walking.

Which is the most likely diagnosis?
   A. Essential tremor
   B. Huntington disease
   C. Multiple sclerosis
   D. Myasthenia gravis
   E. Parkinson disease

9. A 33-year-old man has had severe stabbing pain around his left eye for about 45 minutes for 2 months. He has smoked 20 cigarettes a year for 10 years. He has nasal stuffiness and drooping of his left eyelid.

Which is the most likely diagnosis?
   A. Cluster headache
   B. Migraine
   C. Subarachnoid haemorrhage
   D. Temporal arteritis
   E. Trigeminal neuralgia

10. A 29-year-old woman has had recurrent double vision in her right eye for 6 months. She also has numbness and tingling in her legs, with weakness in her left leg. She had similar symptoms 18 months ago. She has paraesthesia bilaterally in the limbs on neck flexion.

Which is the most likely diagnosis?
   A. Guillain-Barré syndrome
   B. Migraine
   C. Motor neuron disease
   D. Multiple sclerosis
   E. Myasthenia gravis

RHEUMATOLOGY

1. A 32-year-old man has had bilateral pain and stiffness in his wrists and hands for 4 months, with his stiffness improving as the day progresses. He has bilateral swelling and tenderness in the wrists, with pain on the metacarpal squeeze.

Which is the most likely diagnosis?
   A. Ankylosing spondylitis
   B. Osteoarthritis
   C. Osteoporosis
   D. Rheumatoid arthritis
   E. Septic arthritis

2. A 67-year-old woman has had gradually worsening pain and stiffness in her right hand for 2 years. Her stiffness is worse after long periods of immobility. She has hypertension, managed with amlodipine. She has bone growths on the distal interphalangeal joint of her right hand.

Which is the most likely diagnosis?
   A. Ankylosing spondylitis
   B. Bursitis
   C. Osteoarthritis
   D. Rheumatoid arthritis
   E. Septic arthritis

3. A 54-year-old man has sudden pain and swelling in his left big toe, causing difficulty walking. He has Conn syndrome, managed with spironolactone. He has erythema and tenderness of his left first metatarsophalangeal joint.

Investigations:
Synovial fluid analysis: negatively birefringent, needle-shaped crystals

Which is the most likely diagnosis?
   A. Gout
   B. Osteoarthritis
   C. Pseudogout
   D. Rheumatoid arthritis
   E. Septic arthritis

4. A 31-year-old woman has had joint pain in her hands and wrists and fatigue for 4 months. She has a butterfly-shaped rash over her cheeks and the bridge of her nose. She also has metacarpophalangeal joint tenderness.

Investigations:
Antibody testing: antinuclear antibody (ANA) positive.

Which is the most likely diagnosis?
- A. Ankylosing spondylitis
- B. Psoriatic arthritis
- C. Rheumatoid arthritis
- D. Sjögren syndrome
- E. Systemic lupus erythematosus

5. A 65-year-old man has shoulder and hip pain and stiffness, affecting his ability to perform daily activities. He also has appetite loss and fatigue. He has a limited range of motion and tenderness in his shoulders and hips.

Investigations:
Erythrocyte sedimentation rate (ESR): 47 mm/h (<20).
C-reactive protein (CRP): 36 mg/L (<10).
Temporal artery biopsy: negative.

Which is the most likely diagnosis?
- A. Giant cell arteritis
- B. Fibromyalgia
- C. Osteoarthritis
- D. Polymyalgia rheumatica
- E. Polymyositis

6. A 43-year-old woman has had dryness in her eyes and mouth for 3 months, frequently drinking water while eating. She has rheumatoid arthritis, managed with methotrexate. She has swollen and tender joints in the hands bilaterally.

Investigations:
Antibody testing: anti-Ro and anti-La antibody positive.

Which is the most likely diagnosis?
- A. Ankylosing spondylitis
- B. Limited cutaneous systemic sclerosis
- C. Psoriatic arthritis
- D. Sjögren syndrome
- E. Systemic lupus erythematosus

ENDOCRINOLOGY

1. A 45-year-old man has had rapid weight gain despite no changes to his diet or exercise regime, muscle weakness and easy bruising for 4 months. His BP is 163/108 mmHg. He has purple stretch marks on his abdomen, and his arms and legs have significant muscular atrophy.

Which is the most likely diagnosis?
- A. Acromegaly
- B. Addison disease
- C. Cushing syndrome
- D. Phaeochromocytoma
- E. Polycystic ovarian syndrome

2. A 61-year-old man has extreme weakness and unintentional weight loss of 4 kg for 3 months. He had tuberculosis 5 months ago, managed with the RIPE regimen. He has a darkening of his palmar creases and proximal muscle weakness.

Investigations:
Serum sodium: 133 mmol/L (137–144).
Serum potassium: 5.6 mmol/L (3.5–4.9).

Which is the most likely diagnosis?
- A. Addison disease
- B. Acute kidney injury
- C. Cushing disease
- D. Phaeochromocytoma
- E. Primary hyperaldosteronism

3. A 33-year-old woman has an unintentional weight loss of 5 kg and palpitation for 3 months. Her mother has type 1 diabetes mellitus. She has an abnormal protrusion of her eyeballs bilaterally, waxy discolouration of her shins and clubbing in both hands.

Which is the most likely diagnosis?
- A. De Quervain thyroiditis
- B. Graves disease
- C. Hashimoto thyroiditis
- D. Subacute thyroiditis
- E. Thyroid adenoma

4. A 51-year-old man has had fatigue and increased thirst for 4 months. His mother had renal stones 20 years ago. Her BP is 172/104 mmHg. There is a loss of sensation in her hands and feet bilaterally, and she has generalized bone pain.

Investigations:
Serum-corrected calcium: 2.93 mmol/L (2.20–2.60).
Serum phosphate: 0.75 mmol/L (0.8–1.4).

Which is the most likely diagnosis?

A. Cushing syndrome
B. Hyperthyroidism
C. Hypoparathyroidism
D. Primary hyperparathyroidism
E. Secondary hyperparathyroidism

5. A 57-year-old woman has increased thirst and blurry vision for 3 months. She has hypertension, managed with amlodipine. She has a BMI of 32 kg/m^2.

Investigations:
HbA1c: 54 mmol/mol (<48 mmol/mol).

Which is the most likely diagnosis?

A. Latent autoimmune diabetes mellitus of adults
B. Nephrogenic diabetes mellitus insipidus
C. Prediabetes
D. Type 1 diabetes mellitus
E. Type 2 diabetes mellitus

6. A 44-year-old man has noticed his hands and feet have become more prominent, and knee pain for 3 years. He has hypertension, managed with ramipril. He has coarse facial features, a prominent jaw and an enlarged nose.

Investigations:
Insulin-like growth factor 1 (IGF-1): elevated.

Which is the most likely diagnosis?

A. Acromegaly
B. Cushing syndrome
C. Gigantism
D. Hyperparathyroidism
E. Hypothyroidism

7. A 26-year-old woman has had irregular menstrual periods for 6 months, with heavy bleeding and severe cramping. She has a BMI of 33 kg/m^2, acne and excess hair growth on her face, back and chest.

Investigations:
Plasma follicle-stimulating hormone: 8.3 U/L (1.0–7.0).
Serum luteinizing hormone: 11.5 U/L (1.0–10.0).
Serum testosterone: 46 nmol/L (9–35).

Which is the most likely diagnosis?

A. Addison disease
B. Hypogonadotropic hypogonadism
C. Hypothyroidism
D. Premature ovarian failure
E. Polycystic ovarian syndrome

HAEMATOLOGY

1. An 11-year-old boy has sudden severe joint pain in his arms and legs, shortness of breath and fatigue. He has pale conjunctivae and swelling of the fingers bilaterally.

Investigations:
Haemoglobin: 105 g/L (130–180).
Reticulocytes: 2.9% (0.5–2.4).

Which is the most likely diagnosis?

A. Aplastic anaemia
B. G6PD deficiency
C. Haemophilia
D. Sickle cell disease
E. Thalassaemia

2. A 29-year-old woman has painless swelling of her cervical lymph nodes and unintentional weight loss of 4 kg for 3 months. She has enlarged and firm lymph nodes in the axilla.

Investigations:
Haemoglobin: 106 g/L (115–165).
MCV: 83 fL (80–96).
Eosinophils: 0.69 × 10^9/L (0.0–0.6).
Lymph node biopsy: Reed-Sternberg cells.

Which is the most likely diagnosis?

A. Acute myeloid leukaemia
B. Chronic myeloid leukaemia
C. Hodgkin lymphoma
D. Non-Hodgkin lymphoma
E. Multiple myeloma

3. A 62-year-old man has night sweats and unintentional weight loss of 5 kg for 4 months. He has hypercholesterolaemia, managed with atorvastatin. He has enlarged lymph nodes in the neck and axillae.

Investigations:
Haemoglobin: 111 g/L (130–180).
Platelets: 135 × 10^9/L (150–400).
Blood film: smear cells.

Which is the most likely diagnosis?

A. Acute lymphoblastic leukaemia
B. Acute myeloid leukaemia
C. Chronic lymphocytic leukaemia
D. Chronic myeloid leukaemia
E. Multiple myeloma

4. A 75-year-old man has had bone pain worse in his lower back and the ribs and unintentional weight loss of 5 kg for 3 months. He has mild pallor and tenderness over the lower back.

Investigations:
Haemoglobin: 112 g/L (130–180).
Serum calcium: 2.73 mmol/L (2.20–2.60).
Blood film: RBC's stacked like coins.

Which is the most likely diagnosis?

A. Acute myeloid leukaemia
B. Chronic lymphocytic leukaemia
C. Chronic myeloid leukaemia
D. Hodgkin lymphoma
E. Multiple myeloma

5. A 7-year-old girl has persistent bleeding from a laceration in her left knee after falling in the playground 3 hours ago. The knee has been swollen and painful since the fall. Her left knee is warm with limited ROM due to pain.

Investigations:
Prothrombin time: 13.3 s (11.5–15.5)
Activated partial thromboplastin time: 45.6 s (30–40)

Which is the most likely diagnosis?

A. Haemophilia
B. Idiopathic thrombocytopenic purpura
C. Sickle cell disease
D. Thalassaemia
E. von Willebrand disease

UKMLA diagnostic mock – surgery 32

GENERAL SURGERY

1. A 54-year-old man has central burning chest discomfort worse after meals and at night, with nausea and occasional regurgitation. He has type 2 diabetes mellitus and hypercholesterolaemia, managed with metformin and atorvastatin. He has smoked 20 cigarettes a day for 20 years.

Which is the most likely diagnosis?

A. Cholecystitis
B. Duodenal ulcer
C. Gastroesophageal reflux disease
D. Hiatus hernia
E. Pancreatitis

2. A 42-year-old man has 2 months of gnawing upper abdominal pain and nausea, worse at night, relieved by eating, with 3 kg of weight gain. He has osteoarthritis, managed with naproxen. He drinks 30 units of alcohol a week. He has mild epigastric discomfort.

Which is the most likely diagnosis?

A. Biliary colic
B. Chronic pancreatitis
C. Duodenal ulcer
D. Gastric ulcer
E. Gastroesophageal reflux disease

3. A 48-year-old woman has 2 days of worsening right upper quadrant pain, nausea and fever, after 3 months of intermittent upper abdominal pain after meals. Her temperature is 38.1°C, pulse 112 bpm and BP 132/92 mmHg. She has severe right upper quadrant tenderness, with worsening pain on inspiration during abdominal palpation.

Which is the most likely diagnosis?

A. Biliary colic
B. Cholangitis
C. Cholecystitis
D. Choledocholithiasis
E. Pancreatitis

4. A 38-year-old woman has sudden severe right upper quadrant pain, nausea and fevers. She has Crohn disease and gallstones, managed with azathioprine and naproxen. Her temperature is 38.3°C, pulse 128 bpm and BP 95/71 mmHg. She has severe pain and guarding in the right upper quadrant and yellowing of the sclera.

Which is the most likely diagnosis?

A. Biliary colic
B. Cholecystitis
C. Cholangitis
D. Hepatitis
E. Pancreatitis

5. A 32-year-old man has 12 hours of severe abdominal pain radiating to the back and vomiting following an alcoholic binge. His temperature is 37.8°C, pulse 102 bpm and BP 103/88 mmHg. He has severe epigastric pain and guarding, marked abdominal distension and reduced bowel sounds.

Which is the most likely diagnosis?

A. Acute mesenteric ischaemia
B. Acute pancreatitis
C. Chronic pancreatitis
D. Peritonitis
E. Perforated peptic ulcer

6. A 62-year-old man has 4 months of nausea, poor appetite and intermittent foul, loose stools with 6 kg of unintentional weight loss. He has type 2 diabetes mellitus and high cholesterol, managed with metformin and atorvastatin, and has smoked 30 cigarettes a day for 30 years. He has a scleral icterus and a painless upper abdominal mass.

Investigations:
CT pancreas: heterogenous mass in the pancreatic head

Which is the most likely diagnosis?

A. Cholangiocarcinoma
B. Cholangitis
C. Chronic pancreatitis
D. Crohn disease
E. Pancreatic cancer

7. A 65-year-old man has 3 months of intermittent abdominal discomfort with increased frequency of loose stool, fatigue and 3 kg of weight loss. He has type 2 diabetes mellitus and high cholesterol, managed with metformin and atorvastatin, and has smoked 20 cigarettes a day for 40 years. He has mild right lower abdominal tenderness.

Which is the most likely diagnosis?
   A. Acute diverticulitis
   B. Colorectal carcinoma
   C. Crohn disease
   D. Irritable bowel syndrome
   E. Ulcerative colitis

8. A 21-year-old girl has 3 days of abdominal pain, which began as mild central discomfort and is now sharp and localized to the right lower quadrant, with nausea and loss of appetite. Her temperature is 37.8°C, pulse 109 bpm and BP 113/94 mmHg. She has severe tenderness in the right lower quadrant, worse on palpation of the left lower quadrant, with abdominal guarding and rigidity.

Which is the most likely diagnosis?
   A. Appendicitis
   B. Diverticulitis
   C. Ectopic pregnancy
   D. Ovarian torsion
   E. Pyelonephritis

9. A 74-year-old woman has sudden severe abdominal pain, nausea and profuse bloody diarrhoea. Her temperature is 38.1°C, pulse 122 bpm and BP 98/71 mmHg. She has atrial fibrillation and hypertension, managed with bisoprolol and amlodipine. She has severe generalized abdominal tenderness and guarding, with fresh red blood per rectum.

Which is the most likely diagnosis?
   A. Acute mesenteric ischemia
   B. Angiodysplasia
   C. Colonic ischaemia
   D. Colorectal carcinoma
   E. Diverticulitis

10. A 28-year-old man has a left groin lump, which appeared suddenly when moving some boxes at work. There is a soft, painless, lump superomedial to the pubic tubercle, which does not transilluminate, which is reducible.

Which is the most likely diagnosis?
   A. Direct inguinal hernia
   B. Epididymo-orchitis
   C. Femoral hernia
   D. Hydrocele
   E. Indirect inguinal hernia

11. A 43-year-old woman has intermittent upper abdominal discomfort after meals, nausea, bloating and indigestion, lasting up to 6 hours. She has type 2 diabetes mellitus and high cholesterol, managed with empagliflozin and atorvastatin. Her abdomen is soft and nontender.

Which is the most likely diagnosis?
   A. Acute pancreatitis
   B. Biliary colic
   C. Cholecystitis
   D. Gastroesophageal reflux disease
   E. Peptic ulcer disease

TRAUMA

1. A 23-year-old man has severe abdominal pain after being tackled in a rugby match. His pulse is 131 bpm, BP 88/54, respiratory rate 32 breaths per minute and oxygen saturation 98% on breathing air. He has diffuse abdominal pain radiating to the shoulder, guarding and rigidity, with dull percussion on the left.

Which is the most likely diagnosis?
   A. Diaphragmatic rupture
   B. Liver laceration
   C. Pneumothorax
   D. Rib fracture
   E. Splenic rupture

2. An 18-year-old boy had a 5-minute episode of loss of consciousness after a blow to the head, which has now resolved. He has since become drowsy and confused with a severe left-sided headache, nausea and two vomiting episodes. His GCS is 12 (E3V4M5). He has a large bruise over the left temporal area and a fixed, dilated left pupil.

Which is the most likely diagnosis?
A. Basal skull fracture
B. Extradural haematoma
C. Intracerebral haemorrhage
D. Subarachnoid haemorrhage
E. Subdural haematoma

3. A 28-year-old man has severe chest pain after being stabbed. His pulse is 128 bpm, BP 112/97, respiratory rate 35 breaths per minute and oxygen ssaturation 91% on breathing air. He has a 2 cm laceration on the right lateral chest wall, reduced breath sounds and hyperresonance to percussion on the right, with tracheal deviation to the left.

Which is the most likely diagnosis?
A. Aortic dissection
B. Diaphragmatic rupture
C. Flail chest
D. Pulmonary embolism
E. Tension pneumothorax

CARDIOTHORACIC AND VASCULAR SURGERY

1. A 54-year-old man has 1 month of cramping pain in his left calf, worse on exertion, relieved by rest. He has hypertension and high cholesterol, managed with losartan and atorvastatin. His left calf is cool and pale, and his pain is reproducible on walking.

Which is the most likely diagnosis?
A. Acute limb ischaemia
B. Critical limb ischaemia
C. Deep vein thrombosis
D. Intermittent claudication
E. Neurogenic claudication

2. A 62-year-old man has sudden severe pain in his right calf and burning in his foot with difficulty walking. He has hypertension and peripheral arterial disease, managed with amlodipine, clopidogrel and atorvastatin. His right leg is pale, and cold, with absent pedal pulses, and he is unable to weight bear.

Which is the most likely diagnosis?
A. Acute limb ischaemia
B. Compartment syndrome
C. Deep vein thrombosis
D. Intermittent claudication
E. Peroneal nerve palsy

3. A 57-year-old man has 2 months of dull lower back pain. He has hypertension, type 2 diabetes mellitus and high cholesterol, managed with ramipril, metformin, gliclazide and atorvastatin. There is no focal spinal tenderness or lower limb sensorimotor loss. He has an expansile mass in his umbilical area, with an audible bruit.

Which is the most likely diagnosis?
A. Abdominal aortic aneurysm
B. Aortic dissection
C. Fibromuscular dysplasia
D. Mesenteric ischaemia
E. Renal artery stenosis

4. A 72-year-old man has sudden tearing chest pain radiating to the back, nausea and lightheadedness. He has hypertension and ischaemic heart disease, managed with ramipril, bisoprolol, atorvastatin and GTN spray. His heart rate is 123 beats per minute, blood pressure 137/102 mmHg in the right arm and 95/67 mmHg in the left.

Which is the most likely diagnosis?
A. Acute coronary syndrome
B. Aortic dissection
C. Oesophageal perforation
D. Pulmonary embolism
E. Thoracic aortic aneurysms

5. A 42-year-old woman has left calf pain and swelling since returning from holiday. She has type 2 diabetes mellitus, managed with metformin, takes the oral contraceptive pill and has smoked 20 cigarettes a day for 20 years. Her left calf is swollen 3 cm larger than the right, with diffuse, warm skin erythema.

Which is the most likely diagnosis?
A. Cellulitis
B. Compartment syndrome
C. Deep vein thrombosis
D. Intermittent claudication
E. Superficial thrombophlebitis

6. A 68-year-old man has 2 months of a painless, itchy left ankle ulcer. He has type 2 diabetes mellitus, hypertension high cholesterol and a previous deep vein thrombosis in the left leg. He has a 6 cm shallow irregular ulcer on the left medial malleolus, with an erythematous, sloughy base.

Which is the most likely diagnosis?
A. Arterial ulcer
B. Diabetic ulcer
C. Marjorlin's ulcer
D. Pressure ulcer
E. Venous ulcer

ORTHOPAEDICS

1. A 72-year-old woman has right groin pain following a fall. She has hypothyroidism, managed with levothyroxine, and has smoked 20 cigarettes a day for 40 years. She has right groin tenderness and a shortened and externally rotated right leg, and is unable to weight bear.

Which is the most likely diagnosis?
A. Neck of femur fracture
B. Osteoarthritis
C. Posterior hip dislocation
D. Pubic rami fracture
E. Sacroiliitis

2. A 54-year-old man has 3 days of worsening pain, redness and swelling of the right lower leg, with fevers and confusion. He has type 2 diabetes mellitus and peripheral arterial disease, managed with metformin, gliclazide, clopidogrel and atorvastatin. His temperature is 38.4°C, pulse 129 bpm and BP 113/94 mmHg. He has pain, diffuse erythema and violaceous discolouration of the right calf, with palpable subcutaneous crepitus and bullae formation.

Which is the most likely diagnosis?
A. Cellulitis
B. Compartment syndrome
C. Deep vein thrombosis
D. Necrotizing fasciitis
E. Superficial thrombophlebitis

3. A 74-year-old woman has 2 days of left hip pain and difficulty mobilizing. She has osteoarthritis and type 2 diabetes mellitus managed with metformin, naproxen and recent left hip steroid injection. Her temperature is 38.2°C, pulse 103 bpm and BP 123/88 mmHg. She has a tender warm, swollen, right hip, with reduced range of motion and pain on weight bearing.
A. Gout
B. Osteoarthritis
C. Osteomyelitis
D. Septic arthritis
E. Trochanteric bursitis

4. A 28-year-old man has severe pain and swelling in the right lower leg and the inability to weight bear following a motorcycle accident. He has an exquisitely tender right calf, worse on leg extension, with marked swelling and sensory loss to the mid-shin. His foot is cold, and pedal pulses are absent.

Which is the most likely diagnosis?
A. Acute limb ischaemia
B. Compartment syndrome
C. Critical limb ischaemia
D. Deep vein thrombosis
E. Peroneal nerve palsy

5. A 57-year-old woman has right knee pain, worse on exertion, and relieved by rest, with morning stiffness. She takes over-the-counter paracetamol and ibuprofen for the pain. She has a reduced range of flexion and extension in the right knee and palpable joint crepitus.

Which is the most likely diagnosis?
A. Gout
B. Osteoarthritis
C. Pseudogout
D. Reactive arthritis
E. Rheumatoid arthritis

6. A 32-year-old woman has right ankle pain after everting her ankle. There is swelling, bruising and tenderness over the right lateral malleolus, with a reduced range of motion in all planes. She was unable to weight bear immediately after the injury and could not walk more than two steps in the emergency department.

Which is the most likely diagnosis?
A. Achilles tendon rupture
B. Distal fibular fracture
C. Lateral malleolar fracture
D. Lateral ligament sprain
E. Peroneal tendonitis

7. A 22-year-old man has severe right shoulder pain and an inability to weight bear following a fall on an outstretched hand. His right arm is externally rotated and slightly abducted, with tenderness around the glenohumeral joint. The humeral head is palpable below the coracoid process.

Which is the most likely diagnosis?
A. Adhesive capsulitis
B. Anterior shoulder dislocation
C. Posterior shoulder dislocation
D. Proximal humeral fracture
E. Rotator cuff tear

8. A 23-year-old man has left knee pain and an inability to weight bear after a direct blow to the knee and loud popping sound while playing football. He has a marked left knee effusion and severe pain on palpation, with a positive Lachman test.

Which is the most likely diagnosis?
A. Anterior cruciate ligament injury
B. Medial collateral ligament injury
C. Medial meniscus tear
D. Patellar dislocation
E. Posterior cruciate ligament injury

UROLOGY

1. A 28-year-old man has 6 hours of sudden, severe pain in the left flank radiating to the groin, nausea and vomiting, and pain and visible blood when he passes urine. His temperature is 37.2°C, pulse 114 bpm and BP 134/91 mmHg. He is sweaty and restless, with left-sided costovertebral angle tenderness.

Which is the most likely diagnosis?
A. Epididymo-orchitis
B. Prostatitis
C. Pyelonephritis
D. Renal stones
E. Urethritis

2. A 72-year-old man has 6 months of urinary frequency, urgency and nocturia, difficulty initiating the urinary stream, with poor flow and terminal dribbling. His abdomen is soft and non-tender. Digital rectal examination reveals a symmetrically enlarged, smooth, firm, nontender prostate.

Which is the most likely diagnosis?
A. Benign prostatic hyperplasia
B. Prostate cancer
C. Prostatitis
D. Urethral stricture
E. Urinary tract infection

3. A 78-year-old man has 3 months of difficulty initiating the urinary stream, weak urinary flow and nocturia, fatigue, a poor appetite and 5 kg of weight loss. His abdomen is soft and nontender. Digital rectal examination reveals a hard, nontender, indurated nodule on the right lobe of the prostate, with obliteration of the central sulcus.

Which is the most likely diagnosis?
A. Benign prostatic hyperplasia
B. Bladder cancer
C. Prostate cancer
D. Prostatitis
E. Prostatic abscess

4. A 23-year-old woman has 3 days of frequency and pain when passing urine, right back pain, nausea and fevers. Her temperature is 38.3°C, pulse 123 bpm and BP 112/81 mmHg. She is shivery, with right flank pain and costovertebral angle tenderness.

Which is the most likely diagnosis?
A. Appendicitis
B. Pelvic inflammatory disease
C. Pyelonephritis
D. Renal colic
E. Urinary tract infection

5. A 63-year-old man has 1 week of visible blood in his urine. He feels otherwise well. He has hypertension, managed with ramipril, and has smoked 30 cigarettes a day for 30 years. He has mild suprapubic tenderness.

Which is the most likely diagnosis?
A. Bladder cancer
B. Interstitial cystitis
C. Prostatitis
D. Renal stones
E. Urinary tract infection

6. A 16-year-old boy has sudden, severe, lower abdominal and right groin pain, nausea and vomiting. His temperature is 37.1°C, pulse 102 bpm and BP 123/91 mmHg. He has lower abdominal tenderness and a swollen, tender right testis, with right hemiscrotal elevation and a transverse lie. The cremasteric reflex is absent. Elevation of the right hemiscrotum does not relieve the pain.

Which is the most likely diagnosis?

A. Epididymo-orchitis
B. Hydrocele
C. Testicular torsion
D. Urinary tract infection
E. Varicocele

7. A 23-year-old man has 3 days of left groin pain, urinary frequency and pain when passing urine. His temperature is 38.3°C, pulse 92 bpm and BP 119/83 mmHg. He has a tender, swollen, erythematous left hemiscrotum, with relief of pain on scrotal elevation.

Which is the most likely diagnosis?

A. Epididymo-orchitis
B. Hydrocele
C. Testicular cancer
D. Testicular torsion
E. Urinary tract infection

8. A 72-year-old man has sudden severe lower abdominal pain and an inability to pass urine. He has benign prostatic hyperplasia and hypertension, managed with tamsulosin and amlodipine. His temperature is 36.8°C, pulse 108 bpm and BP 134/93 mmHg. He is agitated, with significant lower abdominal pain and distention and a palpable bladder.

Which is the most likely diagnosis?

A. Bladder outlet obstruction
B. Detrusor-sphincter dyssynergia
C. Neurogenic bladder
D. Prostatitis
E. Urethral stricture

BREAST SURGERY

1. A 32-year-old woman 3 weeks postpartum has 3 days of increasing left breast tenderness and difficulty breastfeeding. Her temperature is 37.9°C, pulse 68 bpm and BP 128/81 mmHg. She has a tender, firm, swollen and erythematous left breast, with milky discharge expressible from the nipple.

Which is the most likely diagnosis?

A. Breast abscess
B. Breast cancer
C. Breast cyst
D. Duct ectasia
E. Mastitis

2. A 38-year-old woman 2 weeks postpartum has worsening right breast pain, reduced breast milk supply, nausea and vomiting. Her temperature is 38.6°C, pulse 102 bpm and BP 106/69 mmHg. She has an exquisitely tender, swollen and erythematous right breast, with a fluctuant mass in the medial inferior quadrant, and purulent discharge from the nipple.

Which is the most likely diagnosis?

A. Breast abscess
B. Duct ectasia
C. Galactocele
D. Inflammatory breast cancer
E. Mastitis

3. A 48-year-old woman has 3 weeks of a painless left breast lump. She takes the combined oral contraceptive pill, has smoked 20 cigarettes a day for 30 years and drinks two bottles of wine a week. She has a nontender 2 cm irregular lesion in the upper outer quadrant of the left breast, with dimpling of the overlying skin and axillary lymphadenopathy.

Which is the most likely diagnosis?

A. Breast abscess
B. Breast cancer
C. Fat necrosis
D. Fibroadenoma
E. Mastitis.

POSTOPERATIVE SURGERY

1. A 64-year-old man 1 day post cholecystectomy has right chest pain, shortness of breath and fever. His temperature is 38.1°C, pulse 102 bpm, BP 134/97 mmHg, respiratory rate 28 breaths per minute and oxygen saturations 92% on breathing air. He has dullness to percussion and reduced breath sounds in the right lung base.

Which is the most likely diagnosis?

A. Aspiration pneumonia
B. Atelectasis
C. Community-acquired pneumonia
D. Pneumothorax
E. Pulmonary embolism

UKMLA mixed topics mock – medicine and surgery 100 Qs

33

1. A 38-year-old woman has sharp central chest pain worsened by deep inspiration. She has Hashimoto thyroiditis, managed by levothyroxine. Her temperature is 38.5°C. She has a pericardial friction rub on her chest auscultation.

Investigations:
ECG: concave ST elevation and PR depression in the precordial leads.

Which is the most appropriate management?
   A. IV antibiotics
   B. NSAID + colchicine
   C. Pericardiocentesis
   D. Percutaneous coronary intervention
   E. Rivaroxaban

2. A 32-year-old man has sudden abdominal pain and dark urine after consuming broad beans. He has mild pallor and scleral icterus, with generalized abdominal tenderness.

Investigations:
Haemoglobin: 102 g/L (130–180).
Blood film: small, round cytoplasmic inclusions

Which is the most appropriate management?
   A. Fresh frozen plasma
   B. IV iron infusion
   C. Packed red blood cells
   D. Splenectomy
   E. Supportive care and avoiding triggers

3. A 72-year-old man has 2 months of fatigue, weakness and poor appetite, with 5 kg of unintentional weight loss. He has type 2 diabetes mellitus, managed with metformin, and has smoked 30 cigarettes a day for 40 years. He has a marked scleral icterus and a palpable, painless mass in the right upper quadrant.

Which is the most appropriate diagnostic investigation?
   A. Abdominal US
   B. CT abdomen
   C. Liver function tests
   D. Oesophagogastroduodenoscopy
   E. Serum amylase

4. A 26-year-old woman has chronic diarrhoea and abdominal bloating for 5 months, worse when eating foods containing wheat. Her mother has type 1 diabetes mellitus. She has itchy papulovesicular lesions bilaterally over the extensor surfaces of the arms.

Which is the most appropriate investigation?
   A. Abdominal US
   B. Antigliadin antibodies
   C. Serum amylase
   D. Serum IgA tissue transglutaminase (tTG) antibodies
   E. Upper gastrointestinal endoscopy

5. A 39-year-old woman has had daily, dull right-sided headaches increasing in intensity throughout the day for a month. She had an elective right hip replacement two weeks prior to the onset of the headache.

Which is the most likely diagnosis?
   A. Cluster headache
   B. Medication overuse headache
   C. Migraine
   D. Temporal arteritis
   E. Tension-type headache

6. A 23-year-old man has right-sided chest pain after a road traffic accident. His pulse is 131 bpm, BP 125/97 mmHg, respiratory rate 35 breaths per minute and oxygen saturation 90% on breathing air. He has absent breath sounds and dull percussion on the right.

Investigations:
Haemoglobin: 78 g/L (115–165).
Platelet count: 54 × 10^9/L (150–400).
Haematocrit: 17% (36–48).
PT: 26 seconds (11.5–15.5).
APTT: 84 seconds (30–40).
Fibrinogen: 78 mg/dL (200–400).
D-dimer: 1.98 (<0.50).

Which is the most likely explanation for the blood results?
   A. Acute liver failure
   B. Disseminated intravascular coagulation
   C. Haemolytic uraemic syndrome
   D. Massive haemorrhage
   E. Splenic sequestration crisis

7. A 31-year-old woman has had a racing heartbeat and heat intolerance for a month. She is currently 9 weeks pregnant. She has a diffusely enlarged thyroid gland and waxy discolouration of the shins.

Investigations:
Serum TSH: 0.3 mU/L (0.4–5.0).
Serum-free T4: 25.8 pmol/L (10.0–22.0).

Which is the most appropriate management?
   A. Amiodarone
   B. Carbimazole
   C. Levothyroxine
   D. Propylthiouracil
   E. Radioactive iodine

8. A 64-year-old man has 2 months of cramping calf pain on exertion, improved by rest, with painful left leg ulceration. He has hypertension and high cholesterol, managed with amlodipine, ramipril and atorvastatin. His pain is reproducible on walking 50 metres.

Figure 33.1 (see Chapter 37).

Which test is most likely to confirm the diagnosis?
   A. Arterial brachial pressure index
   B. Capillary blood glucose
   C. D-dimer
   D. Deep tissue biopsy
   E. Duplex ultrasound

9. A 58-year-old man has 1 month of increasing difficulty swallowing, with mild retrosternal discomfort. He has Barrett's oesophagus, managed with omeprazole, and has smoked 20 cigarettes a day for 25 years. He has conjunctival pallor and bilateral cervical lymphadenopathy.

Which is the most appropriate investigation?
   A. Barium swallow
   B. Chest X-ray
   C. CT chest
   D. Endoscopy
   E. Oesophageal manometry

10. A 61-year-old woman has sudden left-sided chest pain radiating to the left arm. She has hypertension, managed with amlodipine. Her pulse is 120 bpm and BP 165/100 mmHg.

Investigations:
Troponin: elevated.
ECG: ST elevation in leads I, V5 and V6.

Which is the most likely diagnosis?
   A. Anterior STEMI
   B. Anterolateral STEMI
   C. Inferior STEMI
   D. Lateral STEMI
   E. Posterior STEMI

11. A 33-year-old man has had bloody diarrhoea and an increased urge to defecate urgently for 4 months. He has rheumatoid arthritis, managed with methotrexate. He has left lower quadrant abdominal pain and tender, red bumps on his shins bilaterally.

Which biopsy findings are most likely to be observed in this man?
   A. Crypt abscesses
   B. Crypt elongation
   C. Eosinophil accumulation in the lamina propria
   D. Transmural inflammation
   E. Villous atrophy

12. A 54-year-old woman has 2 weeks of left shoulder pain and stiffness. She has type 2 diabetes mellitus managed with metformin. She has tenderness over the left glenohumeral joint and significant restriction of active and passive external rotation and abduction of the left shoulder.

Which is the most appropriate management option?
   A. Ibuprofen
   B. Intraarticular steroid injections
   C. Morphine
   D. Physiotherapy
   E. Prednisolone

13. A 62-year-old woman has had bone pain and fatigue for 4 months. She has chronic kidney disease, managed with ramipril. Her BP is 153/97 mmHg. She has twitching of her facial muscles when her facial nerve is tapped and generalized bone tenderness.

Investigations:
Serum-corrected calcium: 2.17 mmol/L (2.20–2.60).
Serum phosphate: 1.54 mmol/L (0.8–1.4).
Plasma parathyroid hormone: 8.03 pmol/L (0.9–5.4).

Which is the most likely diagnosis?
- A. Hypercalcaemia of malignancy
- B. Hypoparathyroidism
- C. Primary hyperparathyroidism
- D. Secondary hyperparathyroidism
- E. Tertiary hyperparathyroidism

14. A 54-year-old woman has 6 months of daily involuntary urine leakage when she sneezes or coughs. There is no dysuria, frequency or urgency and only a small urine volume is passed each time.

Which is the most appropriate initial management?
- A. Bladder retraining
- B. Duloxetine
- C. Oxybutynin
- D. Pelvic floor exercises
- E. Urethral sling

15. A 54-year-old man has sudden, severe chest pain radiating to his back. He has hypertension, managed with ramipril. His BP is 183/112 mmHg in his right arm and 157/96 mmHg in his left arm. He has an early diastolic murmur over the left sternal border on chest auscultation.

Which of the following would be most likely seen on CXR?
- A. Bibasilar consolidation
- B. Bilateral pleural effusions
- C. Flattening of the diaphragm
- D. Normal X-ray
- E. Widening of the mediastinum

16. A 27-year-old woman has recurrent cough and shortness of breath, worse at night. She frequently has to wake up during the night due to difficulty breathing. She is currently on salbutamol and beclomethasone inhalers. She has a bilateral expiratory wheeze on chest auscultation.

Which is the most appropriate management?
- A. Ipratropium
- B. Montelukast
- C. Prednisolone
- D. Salmeterol
- E. Theophylline

17. A 45-year-old woman has excrutiating perianal pain and bleeding when opening her bowels for 5 hours. She typically opens her bowels once a week and takes over-the-counter laxatives. She has a tender, purple mass on the anal verge that bleeds on palpation and hard stool in the rectum.

Which is the most appropriate management?
- A. Hydrocortisone and lidocaine cream
- B. Laxatives
- C. Sphincterotomy
- D. Surgical excision
- E. Topical calcium channel blockers

18. A 39-year-old man has had severe right orbital pain for 2 weeks, lasting 45 minutes to an hour. He also has nasal congestion and a runny nose during these episodes. He has a red, teary right eye with a drooping right eyelid.

Which is the most appropriate prophylaxis?
- A. High-flow oxygen
- B. Naproxen
- C. Sumatriptan
- D. Topiramate
- E. Verapamil

19. A 62-year-old woman has left hip pain radiating to the knee and an inability to bear weight following a fall. Her left leg is shortened and internally rotated, with tenderness over the left greater trochanter.

Figure 33.2 (see Chapter 37).

Which is the most appropriate management option?
- A. Dynamic hip screw
- B. Hemiarthroplasty
- C. Manual reduction
- D. Open reduction
- E. Total hip replacement

20. A 45-year-old woman has had worsening weakness and visual problems for a month. She has myasthenia gravis, managed with pyridostigmine and was diagnosed with hypertension 3 months ago and started on medication. She has drooping of her eyelids bilaterally and double vision that worsens when attempting to gaze upwards.

Which of the following antihypertensives can exacerbate her symptoms?
- A. Amlodipine
- B. Bisoprolol
- C. Hydrochlorothiazide
- D. Losartan
- E. Ramipril

21. A 31-year-old man has swelling in his legs and ankles and foamy urine for a week. His BP is 172/103 mmHg. He has a rash on his nose and cheeks, worsened by exposure to sunlight and generalized joint pain and stiffness.

Investigations:
Urinalysis: protein ++, blood ++, glucose -, leucocytes -

Which is the most likely diagnosis?
   A. Acute pyelonephritis
   B. Diabetic nephropathy
   C. IgA nephropathy
   D. Lupus nephritis
   E. Polycystic kidney disease

22. A 38-year-old woman 2 weeks postpartum has 3 days of left breast pain and difficulty breastfeeding. Her temperature is 38.2°C, pulse 109 bpm and BP 114/87 mmHg. She has a tender, swollen, warm, erythematous left breast, a fluctuant 2 cm mass in the subareolar area and a purulent nipple discharge.

Which is the most appropriate management?
   A. Continue breastfeeding
   B. Intravenous flucloxacillin
   C. Oral analgesia
   D. Percutaneous drainage
   E. Warm and cold compresses

23. A 43-year-old woman has had intermittent pain and stiffness of the hand joints bilaterally for 3 months. She has type 1 diabetes mellitus, managed with a basal-bolus insulin regime. She has swelling and tenderness in the proximal interphalangeal joints and wrists bilaterally and pain when squeezing across the metacarpal joints.

Which is the most sensitive investigation?
   A. Anti-CCP antibodies
   B. Antinuclear antibodies
   C. HLA-B27 levels
   D. Rheumatoid Factor
   E. Synovial fluid analysis

24. A 33-year-old woman has severe abdominal pain following a road traffic accident.

Investigations:
Haemoglobin: 64 g/L (115–165).
Platelet count: 102 × 10^9/L (150–400).
Reticulocytes: 8.5% (0.5–2.5).
PT: 14 (11.5–15.5).
APTT: 47 (30–40).
Fibrinogen: 378 mg/dL (200–400).
Bilirubin: 34 µmol/L (1–22).
FAST scan: splenic laceration.
During blood transfusion, her temperature was 37.9°C, pulse 121 bpm, BP 89/64 mmHg, respiratory rate 33 breaths per minute and oxygen saturation 91% on breathing air. She has marked scleral icterus, bilateral flank pain and burning pain at the cannula site.

Which is the most important initial management step?
   A. Cessation of transfusion
   B. High-flow oxygen therapy
   C. Intravenous fluid resuscitation
   D. Intravenous furosemide
   E. IM adrenaline 1:1000

25. A 54-year-old woman has sudden abdominal pain and three episodes of frank haematemesis. She drinks 3 L of vodka a week. Her temperature is 36.7°C, pulse 128 bpm and BP 91/63 mmHg. She has excoriations over her arms and abdomen and dilated superficial veins over the abdominal wall.

Which is the most appropriate next step in management?
   A. Blood transfusion
   B. Intravenous antibiotics
   C. Intravenous fluids
   D. Sengstaken-Blakemore tube
   E. Terlipressin

26. A 47-year-old man has shortness of breath after a car accident. His pulse is 126 bpm, BP 89/58 mmHg and respiratory rate 29 breaths per minute. He has an absent y descent in JVP, decreased heart sounds and decreased breath sounds on chest auscultation.

Which is the most likely diagnosis?
   A. Aortic dissection
   B. Cardiac tamponade
   C. Constrictive pericarditis
   D. Pulmonary embolism
   E. ST-elevated myocardial infarction

27. A 45-year-old woman has had irregular, jerky movements involving her arms and legs for 4 months. Her father and paternal grandfather had similar symptoms in their fifties and sixties. She has an unsteady gait on tandem walking and slurred speech.

Which is the most likely method of inheritance?
   A. Autosomal dominant
   B. Autosomal recessive
   C. Mitochondrial
   D. X-linked dominant
   E. X-linked recessive

28. A 59-year-old woman has had fatigue and leg swelling for a month. She has hypertension, managed with ramipril and indapamide. Her BP is 172/104 mmHg. She has mild pitting oedema to the knees bilaterally and multiple excoriations on her shins.

Investigations:
Serum urea: 7.4 mmol/L (2.5–7.0).
Serum creatinine: 119 μmol/L (60–110).
Estimated glomerular filtration rate (eGFR): 56 mL/min/ 1.73 m^2 (>90).

What stage of disease does this woman have?
   A. Stage 2
   B. Stage 3a
   C. Stage 3b
   D. Stage 4
   E. Stage 5

29. A 72-year-old man has 2 weeks of severe right foot pain. He has hypertension and type 2 diabetes mellitus, managed with ramipril and metformin. He has grey-black discolouration to the midfoot, with oedema, blistering and discharge of the overlying skin. The second toe is absent.

Which is the most appropriate initial treatment?
   A. Amputation
   B. Analgesia
   C. Debridement
   D. Intravenous antibiotics
   E. Revascularization

30. A 62-year-old woman has 2 weeks of aching lower back pain. She has polymyalgia rheumatica, managed with prednisolone and omeprazole. She has focal L4 tenderness.

Investigations:

Figure 33.3 (see Chapter 37).

Which is the most appropriate diagnostic investigation?
   A. Bone profile
   B. DEXA scan
   C. Parathyroid hormone level
   D. Serum-free light chains
   E. Vitamin D level

31. A 29-year-old woman has had a swollen, painful right knee for 24 hours. She is sexually active with multiple partners. Her temperature is 38.8°C. Her right knee is erythematous, tender to palpation and has a limited range of motion.

Investigations:
Erythrocyte sedimentation rate (ESR): 51 mm/h (<20).

Which is the most likely diagnosis?
   A. Polymyalgia rheumatica
   B. Psoriatic arthritis
   C. Reactive arthritis
   D. Septic arthritis
   E. Transient synovitis

32. A 56-year-old man has had weakness and dizziness for 2 months. He also has an itch, especially worse after a hot bath. His BP is 167/102 mmHg. He has a palpable spleen and has engorged veins on his face and neck.

Investigations:
Neutrophils: 8.2×10^9/L (1.5–7.0)
Platelets: 436×10^9/L (150–400).

Which is the most likely diagnosis?
   A. Acute myeloid leukaemia
   B. Chronic lymphocytic leukaemia
   C. Essential thrombocytosis
   D. Hereditary spherocytosis
   E. Polycythaemia rubra vera

33. A 23-year-old man has severe retrosternal pain radiating to the back following profuse episodes of vomiting after an alcoholic binge. His temperature is 37.8°C, pulse 133 bpm, BP 127/93 mmHg, respiratory rate 32 breaths per minute and oxygen saturation 91% on breathing air. He has palpable subcutaneous crepitus in the suprasternal notch.

Which is the most appropriate diagnostic investigation?
- A. Barium swallow
- B. Chest X-ray
- C. CT chest
- D. Endoscopy
- E. Oesophageal manometry

34. A 54-year-old woman has 2 months of a painless left breast lump. She takes combined, continuous hormonal replacement therapy and has smoked 20 cigarettes a day for 30 years. She has a 3 cm, firm nodule in the upper outer quadrant of the left breast, with skin dimpling and retraction.

Which is the most appropriate investigation?
- A. Breast milk MC&S
- B. Breast MRI
- C. Breast ultrasound
- D. Core needle biopsy
- E. Mammogram

35. A 19-year-old man has had difficulty writing and slurred speech for 3 months. He is very irritable and has a resting tremor bilaterally.

Investigations:
Serum caeruloplasmin: 185 mg/L (200–350).
24-hour urinary copper: 0.73 μmol (0.2–0.6).

Which is the most appropriate management?
- A. Cholestyramine
- B. Desferrioxamine
- C. Levodopa
- D. Penicillamine
- E. Ursodeoxycholic acid

36. A 28-year-old man has 3 days of right scrotal pain, urinary frequency and pain when passing urine after unprotected sexual intercourse with a new partner. His temperature is 37.8°C. He has a swollen, erythematous and tender right hemiscrotum, with pain relief upon elevation of the hemiscrotum.

Which is the most appropriate investigation?
- A. CT KUB
- B. Nucleic acid antigen testing of the urine
- C. Scrotal ultrasound
- D. Urinalysis and MC&S
- E. VDRL screening

37. A 74-year-old man has intermittent headaches and confusion after a slip in the bathroom 2 months ago, after which there were no visible injuries or significant symptoms. He has atrial fibrillation, managed with warfarin. He has left-sided limb weakness and pronator drift.

Investigations:
CT head: right-sided crescent-shaped hypodense area.

Which is the most likely vessel affected?
- A. Basilar artery
- B. Bridging vein
- C. Circle of Willis
- D. Middle meningeal artery
- E. Posterior inferior cerebellar artery

38. A 48-year-old man is admitted for elective cholecystectomy. He has type 1 diabetes mellitus, managed with once-daily Lantus and three times a day Novorapid insulin injections.

Which is the most appropriate intraoperative blood sugar management option?
- A. Fixed-rate insulin infusion
- B. Omit morning Lantus
- C. Omit morning Novorapid
- D. Reduce Lantus dose to 80%
- E. Variable rate insulin infusion

39. A 62-year-old woman has right upper quadrant pain and fever for 3 hours. She has COPD, managed with salbutamol. Her temperature is 38.8°C. She has yellowing of her sclera and tenderness in the right upper quadrant.

Investigations:
Abdominal US: stones in the bile duct.

Which is the most appropriate initial management?
- A. Endoscopic retrograde cholangiopancreatography
- B. IV antibiotics
- C. Laparoscopic cholecystectomy
- D. Simple enterolithotomy
- E. Ursodeoxycholic acid

40. An 18-year-old man has had progressive unsteadiness and frequent stumbling for 3 years. His older sister had similar symptoms 10 years ago. He has absent ankle jerks, faded colour vision and curvature of the spine in the coronal and sagittal planes.

Which of the following is a complication of the likely diagnosis?

A. Aortic regurgitation
B. Aortic stenosis
C. Dilated cardiomyopathy
D. Hypertrophic obstructive cardiomyopathy
E. Takotsubo cardiomyopathy

41. A 46-year-old woman has 3 days of worsening abdominal pain and fevers after 2 months of intermittent crampy upper abdominal pain after meals lasting for several hours. Her temperature is 38.1°C, pulse 127 bpm and BP 114/83 mmHg. She has scleral icterus and severe right upper quadrant tenderness.

Investigations
Haemoglobin: 123 g/L (115–165).
WBC: 18 × 109/L (4.0–11.0)
CRP: 102 (<1)
Bilirubin: 37 μmol/L (1–22)
Alanine aminotransferase: 2 U/L (5–35).
Alkaline phosphatase: 195 U/L (45–105).
Amylase: 160 U/L (30–110).

Which is the most likely complication of the diagnosis?

A. Acute cholecystitis
B. Acute pancreatitis
C. Gallstone ileus
D. Hepatitis
E. Liver abscess

42. A 33-year-old woman has a sudden loss of consciousness, which causes her to fall to the ground. Her body stiffened for 20 seconds before the limbs started rhythmically jerking. She has since regained consciousness, but she is confused and fatigued.

Which is the most appropriate management?

A. Carbamazepine
B. Ethosuximide
C. Lamotrigine
D. Sodium valproate
E. Zonisamide

43. A 47-year-old woman has sudden severe epigastric pain on the background of recurrent peptic ulcers; however, the pain usually is not this bad. Her BP is 86/55 mmHg. She has guarding and rebound tenderness of the epigastric region.

Which is the most appropriate investigation?

A. Chest X-ray
B. CT abdomen
C. Jejunal biopsy
D. Urea breath tests
E. US abdomen

44. A 63-year-old man has sudden chest pain worse on inspiration and shortness of breath. He has a metallic aortic valve. He has smoked 20 cigarettes a day for 38 years. He has not had recent surgery or trauma. His pulse is 110 bpm and respiratory rate 29 breaths per minute. He has decreased breath sounds at the right base.

Investigations:
CT pulmonary angiogram: thrombus in pulmonary artery.

Which is the most appropriate management?

A. IV alteplase
B. Rivaroxaban for 6 months
C. Rivaroxaban for 3 months
D. Warfarin for 6 months
E. Warfarin for 3 months

45. A 28-year-old woman has 12 hours of a severe headache affecting the entire head, radiating to the neck, with nausea, confusion and photophobia. Her temperature is 37.2°C, pulse 117 bpm and BP 108/73 mmHg,

Which test is most likely to confirm the diagnosis?

A. CT angiography
B. Digital subtraction angiography
C. Lumbar puncture
D. MRI head
E. Non-contrast CT head

46. A 69-year-old woman has had a cognitive decline for 3 years. Initially, she had forgetfulness and difficulty finding words before suddenly getting lost in familiar places and having difficulty following conversations. She has hypertension and hypercholesterolaemia, managed with amlodipine and atorvastatin.

Investigations:
MMSE: 16 out of 30.

Which is the most likely diagnosis?

A. Alzheimer disease
B. Frontotemporal dementia
C. Huntington disease
D. Lewy body dementia
E. Vascular dementia

47. A 65-year-old man has had recurrent central chest pain and a metallic taste in his mouth for 1 year, particularly after meals. He has hypercholesterolaemia, managed with atorvastatin. His BMI of 37kg/m^2.

Investigations:
Barium swallow: gastroesophageal junction is above the diaphragm.

Which is the most likely diagnosis?
   A. Achalasia
   B. Boeerhaave syndrome
   C. Hiatus hernia
   D. Mallory-Weiss tear
   E. Oesophageal cancer

48. A 61-year-old man has had a dry cough and progressive exertional shortness of breath for a year. He has clubbing of his fingers bilaterally and bibasal end-inspiratory fine crepitations on chest auscultation.

Investigations:
Forced expiratory volume 1 second (FEV1)/forced vital capacity (FVC): 0.89.

Which of the following findings would most likely be seen on CXR?
   A. Bilateral hilar lymphadenopathy
   B. Bilateral reticular opacities
   C. Egg-shell calcification of the hilar lymph nodes
   D. Lower zone fibrosis
   E. Signet ring sign

49. A 54-year-old woman has 1 week of right calf pain after 6 months of ankle swelling and tenderness, worse in the heat, relieved by elevation. There is pain, erythema and induration of the right lower leg, with a palpable cord in the medial aspect of the calf.

Which is the most appropriate management?
   A. Apixaban
   B. Heparinoid
   C. Oral flucloxacillin
   D. Structured exercise therapy
   E. Treatment dose enoxaparin

50. A 67-year-old woman has left upper and lower limb weakness and speech problems. She has hypertension, managed by amlodipine. She struggles to understand what is asked and cannot form a meaningful sentence, but her speech is fluent.

Which type of aphasia is this man displaying?
   A. Anomic aphasia
   B. Broca aphasia
   C. Conduction aphasia
   D. Global aphasia
   E. Wernicke aphasia

51. A 48-year-old man has watery, foul-smelling diarrhoea with unintentional weight loss of 3 kg over 3 months. She has joint pain, swelling in her knees and skin hyperpigmentation.

Investigations:
Jejunal biopsy: macrophage deposition containing Periodic acid-Schiff granules.

Which is the most likely diagnosis?
   A. Coeliac disease
   B. Colon cancer
   C. Liver abscess
   D. Ulcerative colitis
   E. Whipple disease

52. A 23-year-old woman has left wrist pain following a fall on an outstretched hand. She has pain and swelling of the left wrist joint, with a reduced range of motion in all planes. There is no sensory loss, and radial and ulnar pulses are palpable.

Investigations:

Figure 33.4 (see Chapter 37).

Which is the most appropriate management?
   A. Closed reduction
   B. Intramedullary nail
   C. K-wire fixation
   D. Open reduction and internal fixation
   E. Spica cast

53. A 27-year-old woman has a severe headache, worse in the morning. She takes the combined oral contraceptive pill. Her BMI is 36 kg/m^2. She has an enlargement of her blind spot bilaterally, and both her eyes are deviated inwards.

Investigations:
Fundoscopy: bilateral papilloedema.

Which is the most appropriate initial management?
A. Acetalozamide
B. Naproxen
C. Topiramate
D. Sumatriptan
E. Weight loss

54. A 72-year-old man has 6 months of difficulty initiating the urinary stream, a feeling of incomplete bladder emptying and occasional nocturnal incontinence. He has benign prostatic hyperplasia, managed with tamsulosin. He has mild lower abdominal distention and a palpable bladder.

Which is the most appropriate investigation?
A. Multiparametric MRI
B. Postvoid residual bladder scan
C. Prostate-specific antigen
D. Urinalysis and MC&S
E. Urodynamic studies

55. A 68-year-old man has a sudden high-grade fever and increased shortness of breath. His temperature is 38.9°C, pulse 114 bpm and respiratory rate 25 breaths per minute. He has decreased breath sounds and crepitations at the right lower lung base.

Which is the most likely causative organism?
A. *Haemophilus influenzae*
B. *Klebsiella pneumoniae*
C. *Legionella pneumophila*
D. *Mycoplasma pneumoniae*
E. *Streptococcus pneumoniae*

56. A 56-year-old man has had recurrent central chest pain and a metallic taste in his mouth for 4 months. His symptoms worsen when lying down and are improved by over-the-counter antacids. He has a BMI of 36 kg/m^2.

Investigations:
Barium swallow: gastroesophageal junction above the diaphragm.

Which is the most appropriate management?
A. Endoscopic diverticulectomy
B. Heller cardiomyotomy
C. Ivor-Lewis oesophagectomy
D. Omeprazole
E. Pneumatic dilation

57. A 72-year-old man has 3 days of colicky central abdominal pain, nausea and vomiting. He last opened his bowels 5 days ago and cannot remember passing gas. He has marked abdominal distension and a tympanic abdomen, with high-pitched bowel sounds.

Which is the most appropriate initial management?
A. Flexible sigmoidoscopic decompression
B. Intravenous antibiotics
C. Laparotomy
D. Nasogastric tube insertion and intravenous fluids
E. Phosphate enema

58. A 29-year-old man has lower back pain and stiffness, progressively worsening for 6 months. The pain is worse in the morning and is improved by exercise. He has had anterior uveitis, managed by atropine. He has hip discomfort, limited lumbar spinal mobility and spinal tenderness.

Which would be most likely seen on imaging, given the likely diagnosis?
A. Intervertebral disc herniation
B. Lumbar lordosis
C. Osteopenia
D. Periarticular erosions
E. Sacroiliitis

59. A 4-year-old boy has a chronic cough and difficulty breathing during exertion. He has had recurrent sinus infections and steatorrhoea. He has mild clubbing and coarse crepitations bilaterally on chest auscultation.

Investigations:
Sweat test: sweat chloride level of 69 mmol/L.
Gene analysis: homozygous for delta F508 mutation

Which is the most appropriate initial management?
A. Chest physiotherapy and postural drainage
B. Doxycycline
C. Lumacaftor/Ivacaftor
D. Lung transplantation
E. Salbutamol

60. A 65-year-old man has a one-off abdominal aortic aneurysm screening. He has hypertension and peripheral arterial disease, managed with ramipril, clopidogrel and atorvastatin, drinks a bottle of rum a week and has smoked 20 cigarettes a day for 40 years.

Investigations:
US abdomen: 4.5 cm dilation of the abdominal aorta.
12-month aneurysm surveillance is arranged.

Which is the most important additional management step?

A. Alcohol reduction
B. Dietician referral
C. Smoking cessation
D. Stress reduction
E. Structured exercise therapy

61. A 77-year-old woman has difficulty moving around the house, often falling when getting out of bed. She has a pill-rolling right-sided tremor and cogwheel rigidity in the right arm. She can also not look upwards, even though her pupils are equal and reactive to light.

Which is the most likely diagnosis?

A. Drug-induced parkinsonism
B. Essential tremor
C. Idiopathic Parkinson disease
D. Multiple-system atrophy
E. Progressive supranuclear palsy

62. A 16-year-old boy has 1 hour of sudden, severe left groin pain radiating to the lower abdomen, with nausea and vomiting. He has lower abdominal tenderness, a swollen, tender left scrotum and a high-riding left testis with a transverse lie. The cremasteric reflex is absent.

Which is the most appropriate management?

A. Analgesia
B. Antiemetics
C. Manual testicular detorsion
D. Scrotal exploration and bilateral orchidopexy
E. Scrotal exploration and orchiectomy

63. A 45-year-old man has had a chronic cough and decreased exercise tolerance for 5 years. He had recurrent childhood ear infections. He has bilateral finger clubbing and coarse crepitations on chest auscultation.

Imaging:
CXR: thick-walled dilated bronchi.

Which is the most likely causative organism?

A. *Haemophilus influenzae*
B. *Legionella pneumophilia*
C. *Mycobacterium tuberculosis*
D. *Pseudomonas aeruginosa*
E. *Streptococcus pneumoniae*

64. A 63-year-old woman has had fatigue and bone pain in her ribs for 4 months. She has had recurrent sinus infections. She has mild pallor and multiple bruises all over her body.

Investigations:
Haemoglobin: 105 g/L (115–165).
Serum calcium: 2.87 mmol/L (2.20–2.60).

Which of the following would most likely be seen on blood film?

A. Howell-Jolly bodies
B. Hypersegmented neutrophils
C. Rouleaux formation
D. Schistocytes
E. Tear-drop poikilocytes

65. A 68-year-old man has sudden, severe abdominal pain and bloody diarrhoea. He has atrial fibrillation, managed with bisoprolol and apixaban. His temperature is 37.8°C, pulse 119 bpm and BP 98/61 mmHg. He has severe periumbilical pain and fresh red blood per rectum.

Which is the most appropriate investigation?

A. Abdominal X-ray
B. Colonoscopy
C. CT angiogram
D. Laparotomy
E. US abdomen

66. A 68-year-old man has right upper quadrant pain and yellowing of his eyes for a week after having epididymo-orchitis 3 weeks ago. He has scleral icterus, right upper quadrant tenderness and hepatomegaly.

Investigations:
Liver US: fluid-filled cavity in the right lobe of the liver.

Which is the most likely diagnosis?

A. Liver abscess
B. Peptic ulcer perforation
C. Small bowel obstruction
D. Ulcerative colitis
E. Whipple disease

67. A 23-year-old man has painless swelling of her lymph nodes, night sweats and unintentional weight loss of 5 kg for 4 months. He had infectious mononucleosis 5 months ago. He has a palpable, rubbery, nontender mass in the right cervical area.

Investigations:
Haemoglobin: 112 g/L (130–180).
MCV: 89 fL (80–96).
Eosinophils: 0.71×10^9/L (0.0–0.6).
Lymph node biopsy: Reed-Sternberg cells.

What is the name for the staging criteria for the likely diagnosis?

A. Ann Arbor staging
B. Breslow staging
C. FAB staging
D. Ranson criteria
E. TNM staging

68. A 54-year-old man has 3 months of bilateral knee pain and stiffness, which worsens throughout the day and is relieved by rest. He is a healthy weight, though not regularly active, and has smoked 20 cigarettes a day for 30 years. He has a reduced range of knee flexion and extension bilaterally, with crepitus and pain on joint movement.

Which is the most appropriate additional management option?

A. Increase weight-bearing exercise
B. Hot and cold packs
C. Physiotherapy
D. Smoking cessation
E. Weight loss

69. A 47-year-old man has loss of consciousness without associated palpitations or shortness of breath. His father died suddenly from cardiac issues at age 50.

Investigations:
ECG: convex ST-segment elevation of 3 mm in leads V1–V3 followed by a negative T wave.

Which is the most appropriate management?

A. Ajmaline
B. Implantable cardioverter-defibrillator
C. Percutaneous coronary intervention
D. Pericardiocentesis
E. Radiofrequency catheter ablation

70. A 54-year-old man has 3 hours of sudden central chest pain, radiating to the back and abdomen, with nausea and lightheadedness. He has hypertension and type 2 diabetes mellitus, managed with ramipril, amlodipine and metformin, and has smoked 30 cigarettes a day for 25 years. His pulse is 107 bpm and BP 167/85 mmHg.

Which test is most likely to confirm the diagnosis?

A. Chest X-ray
B. CT angiography
C. D-dimer
D. Transthoracic echocardiogram
E. US Chest

71. A 54-year-old woman has sudden severe pain and swelling in her right knee. She has Wilson disease, managed with penicillamine. Her right knee is warm, she cannot bear weight on her right leg and has a limited range of motion due to pain.

Investigations:
Synovial fluid analysis: rhomboid-shaped, weakly positively birefringent crystals.

Which is the most likely diagnosis?

A. Gout
B. Osteoarthritis
C. Pseudogout
D. Rheumatoid arthritis
E. Septic arthritis

72. A 67-year-old woman has had confusion and extreme thirst for 4 days. She has type 2 diabetes mellitus, managed with metformin. Her pulse is 120 bpm and BP 156/97 mmHg. She has dry mucous membranes and is not oriented to time or place.

Investigations:
Random blood glucose: 34.1 mmol/L (4.0–7.0).
Blood ketones: 1.3 mmol/L (<0.6).
Serum osmolality: 326 mOsmol/kg (278–300).

Which is the most appropriate management?

A. IV 5% dextrose
B. IV insulin
C. IV potassium chloride
D. IV saline
E. IV sodium bicarbonate

73. A 72-year-old man has 2 months of bilateral hip and lower back pain, with fatigue and 5 kg of weight loss. He has L4/5 tenderness and tenderness over the sacroiliac joints and greater trochanters bilaterally.

Investigations:

Figure 33.5 (see Chapter 37).

Which is the most likely underlying aetiology?
A. Lung adenocarcinoma
B. Medullary thyroid carcinoma
C. Multiple myeloma
D. Prostate adenocarcinoma
E. Renal cell carcinoma

74. A 54-year-old woman has 2 months of constant, cramping abdominal pain, nausea, bloating, and increased frequency of foul stools, with 3 kg of weight loss. She drinks four bottles of wine a week and has smoked 20 cigarettes a day for 30 years.

Which test is most likely to confirm the diagnosis?
A. Amylase
B. Faecal calprotectin
C. Faecal elastase
D. Lipase
E. Stool MC&S

75. A 42-year-old man has swelling in his legs and decreased urine output for a month. He is a known recreational IV drug user. His BP is 157/98 mmHg,

Investigations:
Urinalysis: protein ++++, blood ++, glucose -, leucocytes -_
CD4 cell count: 243 × 10^6/L (430–1690).

Which is the most likely diagnosis?
A. Diabetic nephropathy
B. Focal segmental glomerulosclerosis
C. HIV-associated nephropathy
D. IgA nephropathy
E. Minimal change disease

76. A 33-year-old woman has excessive thirst and has to wake up multiple times during the night to urinate despite no changes in fluid intake. She has haemochromatosis, managed with regular venesection.

Investigations:
Blood glucose: normal.
Water deprivation test: low urine osmolality originally; after desmopressin, the urine osmolality increases.

Which is the most likely diagnosis?
A. Cranial diabetes insipidus
B. Nephrogenic diabetes insipidus
C. Psychogenic polydipsia
D. Syndrome of inappropriate antidiuretic hormone secretion
E. Type 2 diabetes mellitus

77. A 57-year-old man has shortness of breath and an irregular heartbeat. He has hypertension, managed with ramipril. He has a pansystolic murmur heard best heard on expiration at the apex radiating to the axilla on chest auscultation.

Which is the most likely diagnosis?
A. Aortic regurgitation
B. Aortic stenosis
C. Mitral regurgitation
D. Pulmonary regurgitation
E. Tricuspid regurgitation

78. A 54-year-old man has pain and weakness in his right lower leg following right anterior tibial artery angioplasty. His right calf is swollen and exquisitely tender, with paraesthesia and sensory loss to the knee and weak pedal pulses.

Which test is most likely to confirm the diagnosis?
A. ABPI
B. Compartmental pressures
C. CT angiography
D. D-dimer
E. Duplex ultrasound

79. A 24-year-old man has had blood in his urine for a week. He has had similar episodes since childhood, but they resolve after a day. His abdomen is soft and non-tender, while his Rinne test was positive in both ears, and his Weber's test was equally heard in both ears.

Investigations:
Serum urea: 8.5 mmol/L (2.5–7.0).
Serum creatinine: 123 µmol/L (60–110).

Which type of collagen is primarily affected in the likely diagnosis?
A. Collagen type I
B. Collagen type II
C. Collagen type III
D. Collagen type IV
E. Collagen type V

80. A 23-year-old woman has had a constant headache for 3 months. Her BP is 172/104 mmHg. She has a mid-systolic murmur, maximal over the back on chest auscultation and radio-femoral delay bilaterally.

Which congenital condition is associated with the likely diagnosis?

A. Brugada syndrome
B. Down's syndrome
C. Marfan's syndrome
D. Noonan's syndrome
E. Turner's syndrome

81. A 54-year-old woman has 1 month of central lower back pain and cramping calf pain, worse on walking and prolonged standing, relieved by sitting down. She has an unsteady broad-based gait, reduced knee and ankle jerk reflexes, and postural instability when closing her eyes while standing.

Which is the most appropriate investigation?

A. ABPI
B. CT myelogram
C. Lumbar spine X-ray
D. Lumbosacral MRI
E. Ultrasound lower limbs

82. A 43-year-old woman has had sudden abdominal pain and bilious vomiting for 48 hours. She had a caesarean section 8 years ago. Her abdomen is distended and she has high-pitched bowel sounds.

Investigations:
Abdominal X-ray: small bowel diameter of 6 cm.

Which is the most likely diagnosis?

A. Liver abscess
B. Peptic ulcer perforation
C. Small bowel obstruction
D. Ulcerative colitis
E. Whipple disease

83. A 59-year-old man has 3 months of increasing difficulty acquiring and maintaining an erection. He has hypertension, high cholesterol and angina, managed with ramipril, atorvastatin and nicorandil.

Which is the most appropriate management?

A. Penile prosthesis
B. Phosphodiesterase-5 inhibitors
C. Psychological therapy
D. Testosterone replacement therapy
E. Vacuum-assisted erectile device

84. A 50-year-old woman has had weight gain and fatigue for 4 months. She has also been bruising more easily and noticed thinning of her skin. Her BP is 172/107 mmHg. She has proximal muscle weakness and purple abdominal striae.

Investigations:
Abdominal CT: well-defined, nonenhancing mass in the right adrenal cortex.

What result would be expected in a high-dose dexamethasone suppression test?

A. High cortisol and high ACTH
B. High cortisol and low ACTH
C. Low cortisol and high ACTH
D. Low cortisol and low ACTH
E. Low cortisol and normal ACTH

85. A 68-year-old man has 3 days of left calf pain and fevers. He has type 2 diabetes mellitus managed with metformin. His temperature is 38.1°C, pulse 97 bpm and BP 147/102 mmHg. He has a tender, swollen, erythematous left calf.

Which is the most appropriate management?

A. Apixaban
B. Compression stockings
C. Intravenous flucloxacillin
D. Oral flucloxacillin
E. Surgical debridement

86. A 34-year-old man has had a cough and night sweats for 3 weeks. He has decreased breath sounds and crepitations on right upper lobe auscultation.

Investigations:
CXR: right upper lobe cavitary lesion.

Which is the most appropriate investigation?

A. Chest X-ray
B. CT chest
C. Mantoux test
D. Spirometry
E. Sputum culture

87. A 40-year-old man has had progressively worsening joint pain and fatigue for 3 months. He has mottled skin and palpable nodules on his shins.

Investigations:
pANCA: elevated.
Serum urea: 8.8 mmol/L (2.5–7.0).
Serum creatinine: 172 µmol/L (60–110).

Which is the most likely diagnosis?
A. Behcet disease
B. Polyarteritis nodosa
C. Polymyositis
D. Rheumatoid arthritis
E. Systemic lupus erythematosus

88. A 72-year-old woman has 2 days of severe lower abdominal pain and fevers. She has not opened her bowels for a week and describes intermittent diarrhoea and constipation for the past year. Her temperature is 38.2°C, pulse 124 bpm and BP 102/84 mmHg. She has severe generalized abdominal pain, guarding and rigidity.

Which is the most appropriate immediate treatment?
A. Emergency colectomy
B. Intravenous antibiotics
C. Intravenous fluids
D. Laxatives
E. Percutaneous abscess drainage

89. A 31-year-old woman has had shortness of breath and fatigue for 6 months. She had multiple childhood respiratory infections. She has a fixed, widely split S2 heart sound and an ejection systolic murmur heard loudest at the left sternal border on chest auscultation.

Investigations:
Echocardiogram: left-to-right shunt.

Which is the most likely diagnosis?
A. Atrial septal defect
B. Patent ductus arteriosus
C. Tetralogy of Fallot
D. Transposition of the great arteries
E. Ventricular septal defect

90. A 68-year-old man has 2 weeks of visible blood when he passes urine. There is no urinary frequency or pain when passing urine. He has benign prostatic hyperplasia, managed with finasteride, and has smoked 30 cigarettes a day for 30 years.

Which test is most likely to confirm the diagnosis?
A. CT KUB
B. Cystoscopy and biopsy
C. Multiparametric MRI
D. Urinalysis and MC&S
E. Urinary tract ultrasound

91. A 45-year-old man is brought to the emergency department after falling unconscious at work after feeling weak and shaky. He has type 2 diabetes mellitus, managed with metformin and empagliflozin. He is unresponsive, diaphoretic and has mild pallor.

Investigations:
Blood sugar level: 1.7 mmol/L (4.0–7.0).

Which is the most appropriate management?
A. IM glucagon
B. IV insulin
C. IV metformin
D. Oral GlucoGel
E. Oral glucose

92. A 24-year-old man has 6 hours of intermittent, severe right back pain radiating to his groin, with nausea, urinary frequency, pain and visible blood when passing urine.

Investigations:
CT KUB: 12 mm stone in the right proximal ureter.

Which is the most appropriate management?
A. Extracorporeal shock wave lithotripsy
B. Percutaneous nephrostomy
C. PR diclofenac
D. Tamsulosin
E. Ureterolithotomy

93. A 42-year-old woman has 2 weeks of a painless right breast lump. She has a nontender, mobile, fluctuant mass in the subareolar area with no skin or nipple changes.

Investigations:
Breast ultrasound: simple breast cyst.

Which is the most appropriate management?
A. Analgesia
B. Excisional biopsy
C. Fine needle aspiration
D. Oral flucloxacillin
E. Reassurance

94. A 7-year-old boy has concerns over his growth as he has a small head size and is in the 20th percentile for height for his age. His older brother died aged 10 due to acute lymphoblastic leukaemia. He has tan patches of skin throughout the body.

Investigations:
Haemoglobin: 99 g/L (130–180).
White cell count: 2.1 × 10^9/L (3.0–10.0).
Platelets: 116 × 10^9/L (150–400).
Bone marrow biopsy: hypocellular marrow with fatty infiltrates.

Which is the most likely diagnosis?
A. Beta thalassaemia
B. Disseminated intravascular coagulation
C. Fanconi anaemia
D. Haemophilia A
E. Thrombotic thrombocytopenic purpura

95. A 56-year-old woman has had nausea and decreased urine output for 3 days. She had otitis externa a week ago, treated with gentamicin. Her pulse is 98 bpm and BP 173/104 mmHg. She has mild pallor.

Investigations:
Serum urea: 8.3 mmol/L (2.5–7.0).
Serum creatinine: 149 μmol/L (60–110).
Urinalysis: urinary casts.

Which of the following urinary casts would most likely be seen?
A. Brown granular casts
B. Fatty casts
C. Hyaline casts
D. Red cell casts
E. White cell casts

96. A 54-year-old man has 2 months of gnawing upper abdominal pain, worse at night and relieved by meals, with nausea and indigestion. He has osteoarthritis managed with ibuprofen and drinks a crate of beers weekly. He has epigastric tenderness.

Which is the most appropriate investigation?
A. Barium swallow
B. Endoscopy
C. Serum gastrin
D. Oesophageal manometry
E. Urea breath test

97. A 25-year-old man has sudden, sharp left-sided chest pain and shortness of breath. He came back from holiday 3 days ago where he went scuba diving. His respiratory rate is 23 breaths per minute and oxygen saturation of 98% on air. He has decreased breath sounds on left chest auscultation.

Investigations:
CXR: 2.4 cm rim of air.

Which is the most appropriate management?
A. Chest tube insertion
B. Immediate needle decompression
C. IV fluids
D. Needle aspiration
E. Observation

98. A 38-year-old man has 1 week of worsening left hip pain and difficulty weight bearing. He is an intravenous drug user. His temperature is 38.3°C and pulse 106 bpm. He has a tenderness, warm left hip, with erythema and boggy swelling over the left greater trochanter, with movement limited by pain.

Which test is most likely to confirm the diagnosis?
A. Arthrocentesis with synovial fluid MC&S
B. Deep tissue biopsy
C. Pelvic MRI
D. Pelvic X-ray
E. Ultrasound hip

99. A 46-year-old woman has had severe agitation and confusion after having a right-sided lobectomy for lung cancer 2 hours ago. She has Graves disease, managed with carbimazole. Her temperature is 38.8°C, pulse 114 bpm and BP 178/105 mmHg. She has a diffusely enlarged thyroid gland and bilateral protrusion of the eyes.

Investigations:
Serum TSH: 0.2 mU/L (0.4–5.0).
Serum-free T4: 26.4 pmol/L (10.0–22.0).

Which is the most appropriate management?
A. IV fluids
B. IV propranolol and propylthiouracil
C. Levothyroxine
D. Prednisolone
E. Radioactive iodine

100. A 29-year-old man has had recurrent genital and oral ulcers for a year, which often resolve spontaneously. He also had pain and redness of the eyes bilaterally. He has aphthous ulcers and tenderness and swelling of multiple joints.

Investigations:
Erythrocyte sedimentation rate (ESR): 25 mm/h (<20).
C-reactive protein (CRP): 14 mg/L (<10).

Which of the following HLA antigens is associated with the likely diagnosis?

A. HLA-B27
B. HLA-B51
C. HLA-Cw6
D. HLA-DR2
E. HLA-DR4

Section 6

UKMLA DIAGNOSTIC AND FULL MOCKS - ANSWERS

UKMLA diagnostic mock – medicine 34

CARDIOVASCULAR

Question 1

D. (Lateral STEMI) **Sudden, severe chest pain** radiating to the left shoulder combined with tachycardia, pallor and **ST elevation in leads I, V5 and V6** (lateral ECG leads). **Differentials: Inferior leads** (leads II, III and aVF), **Anterior leads** (leads V1-V4).

Question 2

C. (Stable angina) Recurrent **exertional central chest tightness**, relieved by **rest** on the background of hypercholesterolaemia combined with **ST depression** in the inferior leads and a normal troponin. **Differentials: Unstable angina** (pain at rest); **Prinzmetal angina** (not associated with ST changes)

Question 3

A. (Acute pericarditis) **Pleuritic chest pain** on the background of SLE combined with a scratchy sound accentuated by leaning forward **(friction rub)** and widespread **concave ST elevation**. **Differentials: Constrictive pericarditis** (elevated JVP, pericardial knock), **Pulmonary embolism** (sinus tachycardia, S1Q3T3 on ECG)

Question 4

D. (Pulmonary embolism) **Sudden dyspnoea** and **pleuritic chest pain** after **recent surgery** combined with tachycardia, tachypnoea with **dilated, swollen, tender lower leg veins** bilaterally. **Differentials: Congestive heart failure** (S3 heart sound, pitting oedema), **STEMI** (chest pain not usually pleuritic)

Question 5

B. (Cardiac arrest) **Sudden loss of consciousness** leading to **syncope** combined with pulseless, **unresponsive** and **ventricular fibrillation** on ECG. **Differentials: AF** (less chaotic rhythm and QRS narrow rather than absent), **HOCM** (FH of sudden cardiac death, younger patient),

Question 6

B. (Heart failure) **Increasing fatigue** and dyspnoea, on the background of hypertension and type 2 diabetes mellitus combined with **bilateral pitting oedema, S3 heart sound** and **bibasal crepitations** on examination. **Differentials: Aortic stenosis** (ejection systolic murmur), **pulmonary embolism** (pleuritic chest pain)

Question 7

A. (Cardiac tamponade) **Hypotension, elevated JVP with absent y descent, muffled heart sounds** (Beck's triad) and **electrical alternans** on ECG. **Differentials: constrictive pericarditis** (both x and y JVP descent present), **tension pneumothorax** (tracheal deviation).

Question 8

C. (Infective endocarditis) Chest pain and dyspnoea, on the background of **IV drug use** combined with a high-grade fever, **Janeway lesions** (painless) and a **tricuspid regurgitation murmur** (consistent with IV drug use). **Differentials: atrial myxoma** (waxing-waning presentation rather than subacute), **rheumatic fever** (polyarthritis, chorea)

Question 9

A. (Atrial fibrillation) **Intermittent palpitations** and dyspnoea, on the background of hypertension combined with tachycardia and **irregularly irregular R-R intervals** and absent p waves. **Differentials: TdP** (long QT interval), **WPW syndrome** (short PR interval and wide QRS complexes)

Question 10

B. (Aortic stenosis) Exertional dyspnoea and chest pain, on the background of hypertension and an **ejection systolic murmur radiating to the carotids** with an otherwise clear chest. **Differentials: Aortic regurgitation** (early diastolic murmur), **Atrial septal defect** (fixed splitting of S2), **HOCM** (syncope history, younger patient)

GASTROENTEROLOGY

Question 1

E. (Ulcerative colitis) **Bloody diarrhoea** associated with abdominal cramping and tenesmus combined with left lower quadrant pain, **anterior uveitis** and **pseudopolyps (regenerating mucosa)** on colonoscopy. Differentials: Coeliac disease (autoimmune history, recurrent fatigue), Crohn (Nonbloody diarrhoea, anterior uveitis unlikely)

Question 2

C. (Crohn disease) **Right lower quadrant pain**, **nonbloody diarrhoea** combined with **perianal skin tags, mouth ulcers** and arthralgia with **skip lesions** on colonoscopy. **Differentials: IBS** (abdominal bloating, alternating bowel habit), **UC** (Bloody diarrhoea, pseudopolyps)

Question 3

A. (Coeliac disease) Stomach cramps and pale diarrhoea, on the background of type 1 diabetes mellitus combined with abdominal bloating and dermatitis herpetiformis on examination and raised IgA tissue transglutaminase and villous atrophy and crypt hyperplasia on biopsy (usual villous:crypt ratio is >3:1). **Differentials: Duodenal ulcer** (pain relieved by eating), **SBBOS** (jejunum aspirate Ix not duodenal biopsy)

Question 4

E. (Liver cirrhosis) Fatigue and appetite loss for 4 months on the background of **chronic alcohol abuse** combined with **jaundice, caput medusae and RUQ tenderness**. **Differentials: Hepatitis B** (infected blood history and fever), **liver abscess** (hepatomegaly, right lobe mass)

Question 5

A. (Hepatitis A) **Fever and right upper quadrant pain** after recent foreign travel where meals were from **street food vendors** combined with **scleral icterus, hepatomegaly and RUQ tenderness**. **Differentials: Hepatitis B** (Infected blood/bodily fluids), **Hepatitis C** (IV drug users)

Question 6

D. (Irritable bowel syndrome) **Crampy abdominal pain** and a **change in bowel habits** for 8 months, worsened by stress and meals. **Differentials: Coeliac disease** (just diarrhoea, autoimmune history), **diverticulitis** (more severe pain and acute history)

Question 7

E. (Liver failure) Right upper quadrant pain and **confusion (encephalopathy)**, on the background of chronic alcohol misuse, with RUQ tenderness, **jaundice** and **prolonged prothrombin time (coagulopathy). Differentials: acute cholecystitis** (no coagulopathy), **Hepatitis B** (no confusion)

Question 8

E. (Wilson disease) **Declining academic performance** and increased irritability combined with a **resting tremor** (neurological symptoms), jaundice (liver symptoms) and **Kayser-Fleischer rings**. **Differentials: Haemochromatosis** (hyperpigmentation), **Parkinson disease** (no liver symptoms)

Question 9

A. (Achalasia) **Progressively worsening dysphagia to solids and liquids,** causing central chest pain and unintentional weight loss combined with a **bird's beak appearance** (oesophageal dilation and tapering). **Differentials: GORD** (not progressively worsening), **hiatus hernia** (regurgitation symptoms)

Question 10

B. (Haemochromatosis) Bilateral **arthralgia in the hands** and RUQ pain combined with **hepatomegaly** and **skin hyperpigmentation** and **raised serum iron. Differentials: Hepatocellular carcinoma** (systemic signs of malignancy), **Wilson** (raised copper not iron)

RESPIRATORY

Question 1

A. (Asthma) **Dyspnoea** and **cough worse at night**, on the background of **atopy (eczema)**, combined with **bilateral expiratory wheeze** and an **obstructive spirometry** pattern. **Differentials: COPD** (smoking history), **pneumonia** (productive cough)

Question 2

D. (COPD) **Progressive dyspnoea** and a chronic cough producing more sputum recently, on the background of a **30-pack-year smoking history**, combined with decreased breath sounds, **scattered bilateral expiratory wheezes** and an **obstructive spirometry** pattern. **Differentials: A1AT** (young patient, with no smoking history), **asthma** (atopic history), **bronchiectasis** (coarse crackles).

Question 3

A. (Bronchiectasis) Chronic cough producing **copious amounts of sputum** associated with occasional haemoptysis, on the background of **recurrent respiratory infections** combined with **coarse crepitations. Differentials: Chronic sinuisitis** (clear chest), **pulmonary fibrosis** (dry not productive cough)

Question 4

B. (Pneumonia) **Productive cough** and **progressive dyspnoea** for 5 days, on the background of hypertension combined with **crepitations and bronchial breath sounds** in the left lower lobe on examination. **Differentials: pulmonary embolism** (no productive cough), **sarcoidosis** (dry cough), **tuberculosis** (more chronic history)

Question 5

E. (Tuberculosis) **Productive cough** for 3 weeks after recently being exposed to a **patient with a chronic cough** combined with **decreased breath sounds** and **fine upper lobe crepitations**. **Differentials: Lung cancer** (systemic signs of malignancy), **sarcoidosis** (dry cough)

Question 6

D. (Simple pneumothorax) Sudden dyspnoea and left-sided **pleuritic chest pain**, on the background of **Marfan syndrome** combined with left-sided decreased breath sounds and **hyperresonant** percussion and **absent left-sided lung markings** on CXR. **Differentials: Pulmonary embolism** (CXR normal), **tension pneumothorax** (tracheal deviation away from pneumothorax)

Question 7

B. (Lung cancer) **Persistent cough with haemoptysis** and **unintentional weight loss,** on the background of a **35-pack-year** smoking history combined with decreased left upper lobe breath sounds. **Differentials: amyloidosis** (paraesthesia and fatigue), **tuberculosis** (infection history not smoking history)

RENAL

Question 1

B. (Acute interstitial nephritis) **Right flank pain** and decreased urine output, on the background of antibiotic treatment of a UTI combined with a diffuse **maculopapular rash**, right costovertebral angle tenderness with raised urea and creatinine and **eosinophilia. Differentials: glomerulonephritis** (haematuria), **eosinophilic granulomatois with polyangiitis** (asthma, pANCA)

Question 2

B. (Chronic kidney disease) Fatigue and nocturia, on the **background of hypertension and type 2 diabetes mellitus** combined with bilateral oedema to the knees with **elevated urea and creatinine** and **decreased eGFR (stage 3a is between 45 and 59). Differentials: nephrotic syndrome** (proteinuria, hypoalbuminuria), **urinary tract infection** (fever, no oedema)

Question 3

D. (Minimal change disease) **Periorbital oedema** and **pitting oedema to the knees** with frothy urine and appetite loss combined with mild pallor, **proteinuria and hypoalbuminaemia** on urinalysis. **Differentials: Alport syndrome** (hearing loss), **IgA nephropathy and poststreptoccoal glomerulonephritis** (preceding sore throat, infection)

Question 4

C. (IgA nephropathy) **Painless haematuria** and intermittent flank pain after a **URTI 2 days ago** combined with pitting leg oedema, proteinuria and haematuria on urinalysis with **mesangial hypercellularity**. **Differentials: Henoch-Schonlein purpura** (rash), **poststreptococcal glomerulonephritis** (2 weeks after URTI)

Question 5

C.. (Polycystic kidney disease) Recurrent abdominal pain and **intermittent haematuria**, on the background of a **family history of renal failure** combined with **bilateral flank masses**. Differentials: **tuberous sclerosis** (no haematuria), **urinary tract calculi** (unlikely to have masses or family history of renal failure)

NEUROLOGY

Question 1

D. (Subarachnoid haemorrhage) **Sudden severe, occipital headache** on the background of **polycystic kidney disease** combined with **photophobia, neck stiffness** and **basal cistern hyperdensities** on CT head. **Differentials: Extradural** (lucid interval, lemon-shaped hyperdense collection), **subdural haematoma** (banana-shaped collection)

Question 2

E. (Total anterior circulation infarct) **Sudden right-sided hemiparesis** and **Broca aphasia** combined with hypertension, right facial droop and **right homonymous hemianopia** with a left MCA hypodensity. **Differentials: lateral medullary syndrome** (Horner's syndrome), **partial** (only 2/3 of hemiparesis, aphasia and homonymous hemianopia).

Question 3

A. (Bacterial meningitis) **Severe headache and low-grade fever**, with signs of **meningism** (neck stiffness and photophobia) and Kernig sign and LP showing **low glucose, high protein and neutrophil predominance**. **Differentials: fungal** and **viral meningitis** (lymphocyte predominance).

Question 4

B. (Migraine) **Severe unilateral headaches** lasting several hours preceded by a **visual aura**, exacerbated by **menstruation** and improved by going into a **dark, quiet room**. **Differentials: Cluster** (no aura, stabbing pain around eye), **temporal arteritis** (palpable temporal artery, scalp tenderness)

Question 5

B. (Encephalitis) **Severe headache,** acute **confusion/altered mental status**, a high-grade fever **and increased signal intensity in the mediotemporal lobes** bilaterally. **Differentials: Brain tumour** (commonly mets so other system signs like lung cancer), **meningitis** (Signs of photophobia)

Question 6

A. (Alzheimer's disease) **Memory decline, difficulty performing routine tasks**, forgetting important events and misplacing her belongings on the background of her **mother having similar symptoms** combined with **disorientation to time and place and moderate cognitive impairment**. **Differentials: FTD** (behaviour changes), **Lewy body** (Parkinsonism, Visual Hallucinations)

Question 7

D. (Generalized tonic–clonic seizure) **Sudden loss of consciousness** causing syncope, followed by **body stiffness (tonic)** and **rhythmic jerking of arms and legs (clonic),** with no memory of the event. **Differentials: Absence** (blank episodes), **myoclonic** (just jerking movements, no stiffness)

Question 8

E. (Parkinson disease) **Resting tremor,** increased bilateral muscle tone **(rigidity)** and a shuffling gait **(bradykinesia)** without cognitive impairment or autonomic failure. **Differentials: essential** (worse tremor if outstretched), **multiple sclerosis** (double vision caused by optic neuritis)

Question 9

A. (Cluster headache) Severe **unilateral stabbing pain around the eye** lasting for **45 minutes**, on the background of a 10-pack-year smoking history combined with **nasal stuffiness** and unilateral **ptosis. Differentials: Migraine** (aura signs), **subarachnoid haemorrhage** (thunderclap headache)

Question 10

D. (Multiple sclerosis) **Double vision** with **numbness and tingling bilaterally** in her legs and **weakness** in her left leg, on the background of similar episodes 18 months ago that **eventually self-resolved** combined with **Lhermitte sign** (paraesthesia on neck flexion). **Differentials: GBS** (ascending paralysis), **motor neuron disease** (upper and lower motor neuron signs)

RHEUMATOLOGY

Question 1

D. (Rheumatoid arthritis) **Bilateral pain and stiffness** in the wrists and hands, with stiffness **worse in the morning** combined with bilateral swelling and tenderness in the wrists and **positive metacarpal squeeze. Differentials: Osteoarthritis** (stiffness and pain worsens with activity), **septic arthritis** (fever and red, warm joint)

Question 2

B. (Osteoarthritis) **Gradually worsening pain** and stiffness in her right hand after **periods of immobility** for **2 years**, on the background of hypertension combined with **Heberden nodes**. **Differentials: Ankylosing spondylitis** (lower back pain, reduced lateral flexion), **rheumatoid arthritis** (positive squeeze test, swan-neck deformity)

Question 3

A. (Gout) **Sudden pain and swelling** of the **left big toe**, on the background of spironolactone, combined with erythema and tenderness of the left first metatarsophalangeal joint and **negatively birefringent needle-shaped crystals**. **Differentials: Pseudogout** (positively birefringent, chondrocalcinosis), **septic arthritis** (leucocytosis with neutrophil predominance)

Question 4

E. (Systemic lupus erythematosus) **Hand and wrist joint pain** and fatigue combined with a **butterfly-shaped rash** over her cheeks and nose and **metacarpophalangeal joint tenderness** with **positive ANA**. **Differentials: Psoriatic arthritis** (scaly rash on extesnors), **Sjogren's** (dry eyes, mouth)

Question 5

D. (Polymyalgia rheumatica) **Shoulder + hip pain and stiffness** with appetite loss and fatigue combined with **limited ROM and tenderness in shoulders + hips** on examination with a **raised ESR and CRP. Differentials: Fibromyalgia** (ESR and CRP are normal), **Polymyositis** (elevated CK levels and positive EMG)

Question 6

D. (Sjögren syndrome) **Oral and ocular dryness** for 3 months, on the background of **rheumatoid arthritis**, combined with **swollen, tender hand joints** bilaterally with **anti-Ro and anti-La antibody positive**. **Differentials: Limited cutaenous systemic sclerosis** (CREST syndrome, anticentromere antibody), **SLE** (butterfly rash, positive ANA)

ENDOCRINOLOGY

Question 1

C. (Cushing's syndrome) **Rapid unintentional weight gain** for 4 months with **muscle weakness** and **easy bruising** combined with **hypertension, purple striae** and muscular atrophy. **Differentials: Addison** (hyperpigmentation, hyponatraemia), **PCOS** (amenorrhoea, polycystic ovaries)

Question 2

A. (Addison disease) Proximal muscle weakness and **unintentional weight loss**, on the background of **recent tuberculosis** combined with **hyperpigmentation of the palmar creases, hyponatraemia and hyperkalaemia**. **Differentials: Cushing** (hypernatraemia, hypokalaemia), **primary hyperaldosteronism** (hypertension, hypokalemia)

Question 3

B. (Graves' disease) Unintentional weight loss and **palpitations** for 3 months, on the background of a **family history of autoimmune disease** combined with **exophthalmos, pretibial myxoedema and thyroid acropachy**. **Differentials: de Quervain** (hypothyroid then hyperthyroid), **thyroid adenoma** (primary hyperparathyroidism).

Question 4

D. (Primary hyperparathyroidism) **Fatigue and polydipsia** for 4 months, on the background of **familial renal stones** combined with hypertension, **loss of sensation** in the hands and feet and **generalized bone pain** on examination with **hypercalcaemia and hypophosphataemia**. **Differentials: hyperthyroidism** (weight loss, palpitations), **secondary hyperparathyroidism** (hyperphosphataemia, hypocalcaemia)

Question 5

E. (Type 2 diabetes mellitus) **Polydipsia** and **blurry vision**, on the background of **hypertension and obesity** combined with an **HbA1c >48 mmol/mol**. **Differentials: Nephrogenic diabetes insipidus** (water deprivation test result), **type 1 diabetes mellitus** (younger patient, family history of diabetes)

Question 6

A. (Acromegaly) **Enlarged hands and feet** and **knee pain** over 3 years, on the background of **hypertension** combined with **coarse facial features** and **elevated IGF-1. Differentials: Cushing syndrome** (moon face not coarse facial features), **gigantism** (elevated IGF-1 before growth plates fuse)

Question 7

E. (Polycystic ovarian syndrome) **Oligomenorrhoea**, with heavy bleeding and severe cramping combined with an **obese BMI and hirsutism** with **elevated LH, FSH and testosterone. Differentials: Hypogonadotropic hypogonadism** (low LTH and FSH), **Premature ovarian failure** (unlikely to have hirsutism)

HAEMATOLOGY

Question 1

D. (Sickle cell disease) **Sudden severe joint pain** in his limbs, dyspnoea, fatigue, **pale conjunctivae, bilateral finger swelling**, anaemia and **reticulocytosis**. **Differentials: G6PD deficiency** (jaundice), **haemophilia** (haemarthroses, bleeding rather than joint pain)

Question 2

C. (Hodgkin lymphoma) **Painless swelling of her cervical lymph nodes** and unintentional weight loss combined with enlarged, firm lymph nodes in the axilla with normocytic anaemia, **eosinophilia** and **Reed-Sternberg cells** on lymph node biopsy. **Differentials: AML** (Auer rods), **Non-Hodgkin lymphoma** (presence of more B symptoms)

Question 3

C. (Chronic lymphocytic leukaemia) **Night sweats and unintentional weight loss**, on the background of hypercholesterolaemia combined with enlarged neck and axillae lymph nodes with **anaemia, thrombocytopenia** and **smear cells** on blood film. **Differentials: AML** (Auer rods), **CML** (splenomegaly and thrombocytosis)

Question 4

E. (Multiple myeloma) **Bone pain worse in the lower back** and ribs and **unintentional weight loss** combined with pallor and lower back tenderness on examination and **anaemia, hypercalcaemia** and **Rouleaux formation** on blood film. **Differentials: CLL** (often asymptomatic, smear/smudge cells), **Hodgkin** (Reed-Sternberg cells)

Question 5

A. (Haemophilia) **Persistent bleeding** after a **fall,** with knee pain and swelling combined with a **warm left knee with a limited ROM** and an isolated aPTT. Differentials: ITP (isolated thrombocytopenia), von Willebrand disease (prolonged PT)

UKMLA diagnostic mock – surgery 35

GENERAL SURGERY

Question 1

C. (Gastroesophageal reflux disease) **Central chest discomfort associated with meals, nausea and regurgitation**, with risk factors of obesity and smoking suggests GORD. **Differentials: Duodenal ulcer** (epigastric pain, relieved by meals), **hiatus hernia** (barium swallow would be provided),

Question 2

C. (Duodenal ulcer) **Chronic, severe epigastric pain, worse at night and relieved by meals, with weight gain**, suggests duodenal ulcer. NSAIDs and alcohol use are risk factors. **Differentials: Chronic pancreatitis** (pancreatic calcification, steatorrhoea), **gastric ulcer** (pain worse with eating causing weight loss)

Question 3

C. (Cholecystitis) **Fevers and RUQ pain, with positive Murphy's sign** (RUQ pain on inspiration during palpation), suggest cholecystitis. **Differentials: Biliary colic** (postprandial upper abdominal pain), **Cholangitis** (additional jaundice secondary to biliary flow obstruction).

Question 4

C. (Cholangitis) **Right upper quadrant pain, fever and jaundice**,ares Charcot's triad of acute cholangitis, obstruction and infection of a gallstone in the common bile duct. Haemodynamic instability is common. Hepatitis is associated with viral infection or autoimmune inflammation. Differentials: cholecystitis (Murphy's sign), Hepatitis (viral infection, history of F-O transmission)

Question 5

B. (Acute pancreatitis) **Severe epigastric pain radiating to the back, vomiting and fever** following **alcohol excess** suggest pancreatitis. Pancreatic inflammation can lead to ascites and ileus, resulting in abdominal distention and reduced bowel sounds. **Differentials: chronic pancreatitis** (steatorrhoea, pain after meals), **perforated peptic ulcer** (pneumoperitoneum, history of peptic ulcer).

Question 6

E. (Pancreatic cancer) Anorexia, **weight loss**, nausea and steatorrhoea with **jaundice and a painless abdominal mass** represent **Courvoisier sign,** suggesting cancer of the pancreatic head (cancer of the tail typically doesn't present with jaundice). **Differentials: Cholangiocarcinoma** (painless obstructive jaundice but no pancreatic mass), **chronic pancreatitis** (pancreatic calcifications)

Question 7

B. (Colorectal carcinoma) **Abdominal pain, unintentional weight loss and changes in bowel habits** are red flags for colorectal carcinoma. Fatigue suggests anaemia, relating to occult bowel blood loss. **Differentials: Diverticular disease** (no weight loss or anaemia), **Ulcerative colitis** (bloody diarrhoea)

Question 8

A. (Appendicitis) **Migratory abdominal pain, nausea and anorexia,** with low-grade fever suggest appendicitis. Pain at **McBurney point and Rovsing sign** (pain in the RLQ on palpation of the LLQ) are key features. **Differentials: Ectopic pregnancy** (positive pregnancy test), **ovarian torsion** (whirlpool sign on imaging)

Question 9

A. (Acute mesenteric ischaemia) AMI presents with sudden severe **abdominal pain and bloody diarrhoea**, commonly with a past medical history of **AF**, risking acute embolic occlusion of the mesenteric arteries. **Differentials: angiodysplasia** (aortic stenosis, melaena if upper GI), **colonic ischaemia** (bleeding secondary to concurrent systemic illness and transient colonic hypoperfusion)

Question 10

A. (Direct inguinal hernia) A **reducible groin lump superomedial to the pubic tubercle** suggests inguinal hernia. Heavy lifting risks direct protrusion of the bowel contents through the posterior wall of the inguinal canal. **Differentials: Femoral hernias** (inferolateral to pubic tubercle), **indirect inguinal hernia** (positive cough impulse)

Question 11

B. (Biliary colic) Biliary colic presents with **postprandial abdominal pain, nausea and indigestion**. Risk factors include diabetes and high cholesterol. **Differentials: cholecystitis** (fever, Murphy's sign positive), **pancreatitis** (alcohol or gallstone history)

TRAUMA

Question 1

E. (Splenic rupture) Splenic rupture presents with **diffuse abdominal pain radiating to the shoulder, abdominal guarding and rigidity** and dullness to percussion. Trauma is the most common aetiology. **Differentials: Pneumothorax** (absent lung markings, hyperresonant percussion)

Question 2

B. (Extradural haematoma) An extradural haematoma presents with **transient loss of consciousness followed by a lucid interval** with subsequent **deterioration in consciousness** following a head injury. Dilation of the ipsilateral pupil can develop secondary to oculomotor nerve palsy. **Differentials: Basal skull fracture** (periorbital bruising and Battle sign), **Subdural** (fluctuating consciousness, biconcave collection)

Question 3

E. (Tension pneumothorax) Chest pain, respiratory distress, reduced breath sounds, **hyperresonant percussion and tracheal deviation** suggest tension pneumothorax. **Differentials: Flail chest** (multiple rib fractures, paradoxical movement of the chest wall), **pulmonary embolism** (pleuritic chest pain, bibasilar crackles)

CARDIOTHORACIC AND VASCULAR SURGERY

Question 1

D. (Intermittent claudication) **Intermittent calf pain worse on exertion, relieved by rest,** suggests intermittent claudication. Hypertension and high cholesterol are risk factors for PAD. **Differentials: Acute Limb Ischaemia** (severe pain and pulselessness), **Critical Limb Ischaemia** (rest pain, gangrene and ulcers)

Question 2

A. (Acute limb ischaemia) Sudden severe **pain, paralysis, pallor, pulselessness paraesthesia and poikilothermia (coldness)** are the 6 Ps of ALI. **Differentials: Compartment syndrome** (tight swelling and a history of trauma or limb compression), **deep vein thrombosis** (no pulselessness, calf swelling)

Question 3

A. (Abdominal aortic aneurysm) **Dull lower back pain and an expansile mass with audible bruit,** with associated vascular risk factors, suggest AAA, which are common in older males. **Differentials: Aortic dissection** (tearing chest pain), **Mesenteric Ischaemia** (GI bleed, AF)

Question 4

B. (Aortic dissection) **Sudden tearing chest pain,** nausea and dizziness, **with tachycardia and a pulse difference between arms**, suggest aortic dissection. Hypertension and IHD increase the risk. **Differentials: Oesophageal perforation** (haematemesis), **thoracic aortic aneurysm** (back pain that spreads downwards)

Question 5

C. (Deep vein thrombosis) **Left calf swelling, pain and erythema**, with risk factors for VTE including flights, the oral contraceptive pill, smoking and diabetes suggest DVT. **Differentials: cellulitis** (shin swelling rather than calf), **superficial thrombophlebitis** (less serious presentation as superficial veins affected not deep).

Question 6

E. (Venous ulcer) Venous ulcers present as **painless itchy, shallow irregular ulcers, commonly on the medial malleoli**. Vascular risk factors and previous DVTs increase the risk of lower limb venous insufficiency and ulcer formation. **Differentials: arterial ulcer** (punched out, on toes and heels), **Marjorlin** (lipodermatosclerosis, eczema)

ORTHOPAEDICS

Question 1

A. (Neck of femur fracture) **Groin pain and a shortened and externally rotated right leg** following a fall suggest NOF fracture. Levothyroxine use and smoking increase the risk of osteoporosis and fractures.

Differentials: Posterior hip dislocation (hip pain radiating to the knee and shortened internally rotated leg), **pubic rami fracture** (no limited ROM)

Question 2

D. (Necrotizing fasciitis) Necrotizing fasciitis presents with diffuse **erythema, skin necrosis, crepitus and bullae formation, with severe pain**, fevers and confusion. **Differentials: Cellulitis** (systemic illness but no skin necrosis)

Question 3

D. (Septic arthritis) **Joint pain, warmth and swelling, reduced range of motion and fever** suggest septic arthritis. Joint injections can risk direct joint contamination and septic arthritis. Type 2 diabetes increases the risk. **Differentials: Osteomyelitis** (haematogenous or local spread of infection), **trochanteric bursitis** (lateral thigh pain)

Question 4

B. (Compartment syndrome) Compartment syndrome presents with severe limb **pain and swelling following trauma, with paralysis, sensory loss and impaired circulation**. Crush injuries risk bleeding into fixed lower limb compartments, elevated compartment pressures and muscle ischaemia. **Differentials: ALI** (6 P's), **DVT** (calf erythema)

Question 5

B. (Osteoarthritis) Osteoarthritis presents with joint **pain worse on exertion relieved by rest, with morning stiffness, reduced range of motion and palpable joint crepitu**s. **Differentials: Gout** (acute severe pain and erythema of distal joints) and **rheumatoid arthritis** (small joints in the hands)

Question 6

C. (Lateral malleolar fracture) **Lateral ankle pain following forced foot eversion, with pain, swelling, bruising and inability to weight bear**, suggest lateral malleolar fracture. **Differentials: Fibular fractures** (pain in the lateral distal third of leg), lateral ligament sprain (forced inversion but weight bearing preserved)

Question 7

B. (Anterior shoulder dislocation) **Shoulder pain and inability to weight bear** following a fall on an outstretched hand, with a **humeral head palpable below the coracoid process** suggest shoulder dislocation. Anterior dislocations are much more common, and typically the arm is held in external rotation and slight abduction. **Differentials: adhesive capsulitis** (active and passive movement affected, young females), **posterior shoulder dislocation** (adducted and internally rotated).

Question 8

A. (Anterior cruciate ligament injury) A **loud popping sound followed by pain, swelling and inability to weight bear** after trauma suggests ACL rupture. A positive Lachman test is the most sensitive test. **Differentials: PCL injury** (hyperextension injury), **MCL injury** (unstable when in valgus position)

UROLOGY

Question 1

D. (Renal stones) Renal colic presents with severe, **paroxysmal loin to groin pain with nausea, haematuria and agitation**. **Differentials: epididymo-orchitis** (+ve sexual history, testicular pain/ swelling), **pyelonephritis** (high-grade fever, rigors)

Question 2

A. (Benign prostatic hyperplasia) Six **months of LUTS** with DRE findings of **symmetrical prostate enlargement** suggests BPH, which is common in older males. **Differentials: UTIs and prostatitis** (acute presentation, signs of infection)

Question 3

C. (Prostate cancer) **LUTS** and constitutional features including **fatigue, poor appetite and unintentional weight loss** suggest prostate cancer. The DRE findings are highly suggestive of malignancy. **Differentials: BPH** (LUTS and a symmetrically enlarged, smooth prostate), **prostatic abscess** (fluctuant mass and fever)

Question 4

C. (Pyelonephritis) **Flank pain, fevers and rigors** suggest pyelonephritis. **Differentials: pelvic inflammatory disease** (deep dyspareunia), **renal colic** (no fevers/rigors)

Question 5

A. (Bladder cancer) **Painless gross haematuria** is a red flag for bladder cancer. Smoking increases the risk. **Differentials: interstitial cystitis** (irritative LUTS), **renal stones** (significant flank pain)

Question 6

C. (Testicular torsion) **Sudden testicular pain, hemiscrotal elevation and a transverse lie** suggest testicular torsion. An absent cremasteric reflex and negative Prehn's sign (no reduction of pain on elevation of the affected hemiscrotum). **Differentials: epididymo-orchitis** (positive Prehn sign), **varicocele** (bag of worms appearance)

Question 7

A. (Epididymo-orchitis) **Scrotal pain, LUTS and fevers**, with a **positive Prehn sign and preserved cremasteric reflex** suggest epididymo-orchitis. **Differentials: Hydrocele** (transilluminates), **testicular torsion** (absent cremasteric reflex)

Question 8

A. (Bladder outlet obstruction) **A sudden painful inability to pass urine** suggests acute urinary retention. The most likely aetiology is bladder outlet obstruction relating to BPH. **Differentials: detrusor-sphincter dyssynergia** (LUTS in spinal cord injuries), **urethral stricture** (multiple traumatic catheterizations)

BREAST SURGERY

Question 1

E. (Mastitis) A **warm, erythematous, tender breast and difficulty in breastfeeding** suggest mastitis. **Differentials: breast abscess** (localized, fluctuant mass and purulent nipple discharge), **duct ectasia** (yellow-green discharge)

Question 2

A. (Breast abscess) **Breast pain, erythema and oedema** with a fluctuant breast mass and purulent nipple discharge, with fever and tachycardia suggest breast abscess. **Differentials: galactocele** (women not breastfeeding), **mastitis** (no fluctuant mass)

Question 3

B. (Breast cancer) Breast cancer presents with a **painless breast lump with skin and nipple changes** and **axillary lymphadenopathy**. Hormonal contraception, smoking and alcohol use increase the risk of cancer. **Differentials: fat necrosis** (trauma to the breast in obese patient), **fibroadenoma** (firm, mobile mass with no nipple changes)

POSTOPERATIVE SURGERY

Question 1

B. (Atelectasis) Atelectasis is a common cause of early postoperative fever. Postoperative pain leads to diaphragmatic splinting and lung collapse, presenting with **respiratory distress, reduced lung sounds and fever**. **Differentials: Pneumonia** (lung field crepitations and a productive cough), **pneumothorax** (no fever)

UKMLA mixed topics mock – medicine and surgery 100 Qs 36

Question 1

B. (NSAID + colchicine) Pleuritic chest pain, on the background of Hashimoto's thyroiditis, combined with a fever and pericardial friction rub on examination and widespread concave ST elevation and PR depression on ECG suggests pericarditis (inflammation of the pericardium). An NSAID such as naproxen is given to reduce the inflammation, with colchicine given to reduce recurrent pericarditis.

Question 2

E. (Supportive care and avoiding triggers) Sudden abdominal pain and dark urine after having broad beans combined with mild pallor, jaundice and generalized abdominal tenderness with anaemia and Heinz bodies (small, cytoplasmic inclusions) suggest an inherited haemolytic disorder. The most common is glucose-6-phosphate dehydrogenase deficiency, which increases red cell susceptibility to oxidative stress causing the constellation of symptoms seen. Supportive care and avoiding triggers such as broad beans is the management for an acute attack without severe anaemia (<70 g/L)

Question 3

B. (CT abdomen) Painless jaundice and a palpable mass in the right upper quadrant is known as Courvoisier sign, suggesting cancer of the pancreas. Constitutional features of malignancy such as fatigue, weakness and weight loss are also common, with smoking and diabetes being important risk factors. CT abdomen is the diagnostic investigation for pancreatic malignancy, with a common sign observed being the "double duct sign", which is the simultaneous dilatation of the common bile duct and pancreatic duct.

Question 4

D. (Serum IgA tissue transglutaminase [tTG] antibodies) Chronic diarrhoea and abdominal bloating, worsening after consuming gluten, on the family background of autoimmune disease combined with dermatitis herpetiformis on examination suggest coeliac disease. The first-line investigation for coeliac disease is serum IgA tissue transglutaminase (tTG) antibodies, which is the most sensitive test for coeliac, with antigliadin antibodies not recommended despite coeliac disease being caused by a gliadin deficiency.

Question 5

B. (Medication overuse headache) Daily, dull headaches for a month, increasing in intensity throughout the day, on the background of postoperative pain, suggests a medication overuse headache. A tension-type headache would typically present with a tight band headache, with the other headaches presenting with more severe pain.

Question 6

B. (Disseminated intravascular coagulation) DIC can occur after significant blood loss, which in this case is likely secondary to haemothorax caused by trauma and overaction of the clotting cascade, resulting in consumptive coagulopathy with elevated APTT, PT and low platelet count. Fibrinogen can be high in DIC if caused by sepsis, but in this case the blood loss results in a low fibrinogen. Management involves blood transfusions and treatment of the underlying cause.

Question 7

D. (Propylthiouracil) A diffuse goitre and pretibial myxoedema on examination with elevated T4 and decreased TSH suggests autoimmune hyperthyroidism, specifically Graves disease. As the woman is in the first trimester of her pregnancy (9 weeks), propylthiouracil is preferred over carbimazole to reduce foetal malformation risks.

Question 8

A. (Arterial brachial pressure index) Cramping leg pain on exertion suggests intermittent claudication relating to PAD. The ulcer on the leg represents an arterial ulcer, which is typically painful, small and punched out with well-defined borders. An ABPI <0.9 will confirm the diagnosis.

Question 9

D. (Endoscopy) Oesophageal cancer presents with progressive swallowing difficulties and retrosternal pain, anaemia and lymphadenopathy. Barrett oesophagus risks malignant transformation of the oesophagus into adenocarcinoma. Smoking is a key risk factor.

Question 10

D. (Lateral STEMI) Sudden left-sided chest pain radiating to the left arm, on the background of hypertension combined with tachycardia, raised troponin and ST elevation in leads I, V5 and V6.

Question 11

A. (Crypt abscesses) Bloody diarrhoea and tenesmus for 4 months, on the background of rheumatoid arthritis combined with left lower quadrant pain and erythema nodosum, suggest ulcerative colitis. Crypt abscesses are one of the changes seen on a patient's biopsy with ulcerative colitis, which is the collection of neutrophils and apoptotic cells in the intestinal crypts.

Question 12

D. (Physiotherapy) Adhesive capsulitis results from inflammation, fibrosis and contracture of the shoulder joint, presenting with pain and stiffness. Diabetes and hypothyroidism are common associations. Management is with early physiotherapy. NSAIDs should be avoided in those with CKD.

Question 13

D. (Secondary hyperparathyroidism) Symptomatic hypocalcaemia (Chovstek's sign) and hyperphosphatemia with an increased PTH, suggest secondary hyperparathyroidism. This is caused by chronic kidney disease which causes a vitamin D deficiency, resulting in reduced absorption of calcium and consequently increased release of PTH.

Question 14

D. (Pelvic floor exercises) Stress incontinence typically presents with leakage of small volumes of urine upon sneezing or coughing. Initial management involves pelvic floor exercises to strengthen the muscles, holding the external urethral sphincter closed. If this fails following a 6–8 week trial, options include duloxetine, vaginal pessaries, urethral slings or colposuspension.

Question 15

E. (Widening of the mediastinum) Sudden, severe chest pain radiating to the back, on the background of hypertension combined with a difference in BP between the arms and early diastolic murmur over the left sternal border suggests aortic dissection. Widening of the mediastinum due to the aortic dilatation is a classic X-ray finding associated with aortic dissection.

Question 16

B. (Montelukast) Symptoms consistent with poorly controlled asthma despite being on salbutamol and beclomethasone inhalers suggests escalation of her asthma management. The next step in the asthma management ladder in both the NICE and BTS guidelines is leukotriene receptor antagonists, i.e., Montelukast indicated due to the night-time waking.

Question 17

D. (Surgical excision) Thrombosed external haemorrhoids result from thrombus formation in the inferior haemorrhoidal plexus and present with perineal pain and bleeding and a tender, purple mass at the anal canal. Management of acute presentations (within 72 hours) is with surgical excision, with patients otherwise being managed with stool softeners, ice packs and analgesia.

Question 18

E. (Verapamil) Severe unilateral orbital pain lasting 45 minutes to an hour associated with nasal congestion and signs of sympathetic hypoactivity like ptosis of the right eye suggests a cluster headache. Verapamil is the prophylaxis of choice for a cluster headache, and it is thought that blocking the L-type calcium channel which may modulate neurotransmitter release implicated in the pathogenesis of cluster headaches.

Question 19

C. (Manual reduction) Posterior hip dislocation is suggested by a shortened and internally rotated left leg, with superolateral dislocation of the femoral head. There is no cortical disruption to suggest fracture. Management is with manual reduction first and open reduction if this fails.

Question 20

B. (Bisoprolol) Worsening weakness and vision problems (bilateral ptosis and diplopia) suggest exacerbation of myasthenia gravis by medication. Beta-blockers are the class of antihypertensive known to exacerbate myasthenia gravis because they are known to reduce acetylcholine release, which is the pathophysiology behind myasthenia gravis.

Question 21

D. (Lupus nephritis) Lupus nephritis is a type of glomerulonephritis caused by systemic lupus erythematosus and presents with features of nephritic syndrome (oedema, proteinuria, haematuria) and a photosensitive malar rash (not seen with the other given differentials). Severe lupus nephritis is marked by >90% of sclerosis and is classed as ISN class VI

Question 22

D. (Percutaneous drainage) Breast abscesses present with a fluctuant mass in the breast with localized pain, oedema and erythema and is more common in lactating women. Management is with abscess drainage and then oral antibiotic therapy. Continuing breastfeeding is suggested in mastitis which is an inflammation of the breast tissue that can develop into a breast abscess if not treated.

Question 23

A. (Anti-CCP antibodies) Intermittent pain and stiffness of the hands bilaterally combined with PIP and wrist swelling bilaterally, and positive metacarpal squeeze suggest rheumatoid arthritis. Anti-CCP antibodies are the investigation of choice due to their high sensitivity, although rheumatoid factor is often performed first line. This is due to rheumatoid arthritis being characterised by the conversion of arginine to citrulline by immune responses to citrullinated self-antigens.

Question 24

A. (Cessation of transfusion) Acute haemolytic transfusion reaction presents with jaundice and haemodynamic instability during blood transfusion. The most important initial management step is a cessation of transfusion, following which the patient's identity needs to be confirmed, with blood sent for a direct Coombs test, repeat typing and cross-matching. After this fluid resuscitation may be initiated as part of supportive care.

Question 25

D. (Intravenous fluids) Variceal bleeding presents with sudden frank haematemesis in those with a history of chronic liver disease, evidenced by a history of alcohol excess, jaundice and portosystemic anastomoses on examination. The priority is resuscitation, initially with intravenous fluids before endoscopy. A blood transfusion is performed if haemoglobin is under >70 mg/dL once blood results are available. Sengstaken-Blakemore tube is indicated if uncontrolled haemorrhage after medical management.

Question 26

B. (Cardiac tamponade) An absent y descent in JVP, muffled heart sounds and hypotension suggest cardiac tamponade, which is caused by an accumulation of fluid in the pericardium. Therefore the management is an urgent pericardiocentesis.

Question 27

A. (Autosomal dominant) Irregular, jerky movements of the limbs for 4 months, on the family background of similar symptoms (albeit at an older age) combined with unsteady gait on tandem walking and slurred speech suggests Huntington disease, which is an autosomal dominant condition. Huntington disease is caused by a trinucleotide repeat (CAG) disorder causing degeneration of cholinergic and GABAergic neurons in the striatum of the basal ganglia, with genetic anticipation being a key feature (successive generations getting symptoms earlier).

Question 28

C. (Stage 3a) Fatigue and pitting lower limb oedema, on the background of hypertension combined with multiple excoriations on her shins, likely due to itching with raised urea and creatinine and an eGFR of 56, making it Stage 3a CKD (45-59 mL/min/1.73 m^2)

Question 29

D. (Intravenous antibiotics) Wet gangrene refers to infectious gangrene (dry gangrene is ischaemic gangrene), with the two most common types being necrotising fasciitis (commonly caused by Enterobacteriae) and gas gangrene (most commonly caused by clostridium perfringens). Wet gangrene presents with well-demarcated black discolouration of the foot, oedema, pain, skin blistering and discharge. Autoamputation of affected digits can occur. The most important initial treatment is intravenous antibiotics to control the rapid spread of sepsis before debridement of necrotic tissue and attempts at revascularization or amputation.

Question 30

B. (DEXA scan) An atraumatic vertebral fracture is evident on MRI, suggesting osteoporosis. DEXA scan will demonstrate reduced bone mineral density, with a T score (comparison of your BMD to average healthy adult) of less than -2.5 suggestive of osteoporosis

Question 31

D. (Septic arthritis) Swollen painful knee for 24 hours with a high-grade fever, erythema, tenderness and a limited range of motion in the knee with raised inflammatory markers suggests septic arthritis. Whilst transient synovitis is an important differential, the high-grade fever and the positive sexual history make this less likely.

Question 32

E. (Polycythaemia rubra vera) Weakness and dizziness with severe pruritus, especially after a hot bath combined with hypertension, splenomegaly and engorged veins with neutrophilia and thrombocytosis suggest polycythaemia vera. Polycythaemia rubra vera is caused by a clonal proliferation of marrow stem cells resulting in polycythaemia, as well as thrombocytosis and neutrophilia.

Question 33

C. (CT chest) Oesophageal rupture presents with retrosternal pain, haemodynamic instability and subcutaneous crepitus following multiple vomiting episodes. In this case given the history of alcoholic binge, it is likely to be Boerhaave syndrome; CT chest is diagnostic with features such as oesophageal wall oedema, subcutaneous emphysema and oesophageal wall thickening seen. A chest X-ray is the initial investigation which would show mediastinal free air, whilst a barium swallow is not usually indicated first-line it can cause an inflammatory response due to barium spillage into the mediastinum.

Question 34

E. (Mammogram) Breast cancer presents with a painless firm breast lump with skin changes. Hormonal therapies and smoking are risk factors. The triple assessment is indicated for all breast lumps, including clinical assessment, imaging and biopsy. In patients >35, mammography is preferred over ultrasound because as women age their breasts become less dense (due to processes such as involution where the breast lobules are replaced with fat tissue) hence ultrasound becomes less sensitive.

Question 35

C. (Penicillamine) Difficulty writing and slurred speech combined with irritability and a bilateral resting tremor with decreased serum caeruloplasmin and an increased 24-hour urinary copper suggest Wilson's disease. Penicillamine is the management of choice for Wilson's disease, as it is a copper chelating agent hence directly targeting the cause of Wilson's disease (excessive copper deposition in tissue).

Question 36

B. (Nucleic acid antigen testing) Epididymoorchitis presents with scrotal pain, erythema and swelling. With the history of UPSI with a new partner, STI organisms, including *Chlamydia trachomatis* or *Neisseria gonorrhoeae*, are the most likely cause. NAAT testing of the urine will confirm the diagnosis as the cause is an STI; in older patient where the most common cause is Escherichia coli, the most appropriate investigation would be urinalysis.

Question 37

B. (Bridging vein) Intermittent headaches and confusion after a slip in the bathroom 2 months ago, despite no immediate symptoms, on the background of atrial fibrillation combined with left-sided limb weakness and pronator drift with a right-sided crescentic hypodensity suggests a chronic subdural haemorrhage. Bridging veins are the vessels affected by subdural haemorrhages, with patients with cerebral atrophy like an elderly patient being more prone to the shearing forces that might cause a bridging vein tear.

Question 38

E. (Variable rate insulin infusion) Patients with insulin-controlled diabetes mellitus are at high risk of perioperative hypoglycaemia. VRII is the most appropriate regimen as it offers the best control of blood sugar throughout the perioperative period. Once daily, long-acting insulins should be given at 80% of the normal dose, and short-acting insulin doses omitted. VRII can be stopped when eating and drinking, and the normal insulin regimen continues.

Question 39

B. (IV antibiotics) Right upper quadrant pain and fever for 3 hours, on the background of COPD, combined with a high-grade fever, scleral icterus and RUQ tenderness with bile duct stones on the US, suggest ascending cholangitis. IV antibiotics are the initial management of choice for ascending cholangitis, followed by ERCP 24-48 hours later to relieve any obstruction.

Question 40

D. (Hypertrophic obstructive cardiomyopathy) Progressive steadiness and frequent stumbling affecting daily activities, on the background of similar issues in his older sister combined with absent ankle jerks, optic atrophy and kyphoscoliosis suggest Freidreich's ataxia. Hypertrophic obstructive cardiomyopathy is seen in 90% of patients with Friedreich's ataxia and is the most common cause of death in these patients.

Question 41

B. (Acute pancreatitis) Jaundice, RUQ pain and fever, with evidence of cholestasis (↑ALP) on blood results, suggest ascending cholangitis. Distal common bile duct stones which could have caused the cholangitis can also obstruct the pancreatic duct, causing acute pancreatitis. Further, the management of ascending cholangitis involves ERCP, which can also cause acute pancreatitis.

Question 42

C. (Lamotrigine) Sudden loss of consciousness causing syncope, followed by body stiffness (tonic phase) before her limbs rhythmically jerked (clonic phase), combined with post-ictal confusion and fatigue, suggests a generalized tonic-clonic seizure. Lamotrigine is the management for generalized tonic-clonic seizures in women due to sodium valproate being teratogenic.

Question 43

A. (Chest X-ray) Sudden, severe epigastric pain, on the background of recurrent peptic ulcers combined with hypotension, epigastric rebound tenderness and guarding, suggests a peptic ulcer perforation. A CXR is the investigation of choice to look for pneumoperitoneum caused by peptic ulcer perforation.

Question 44

D. (Warfarin for 6 months) Sudden pleuritic chest pain and dyspnoea, on the background of a 38-pack-year smoking history combined with decreased right base breath sounds with a positive CTPA suggests an unprovoked pulmonary embolism, as there is no preceding surgery or immobility that could have caused this. The history of a metallic valve and unprovoked PE means that DOACs are contraindicated; therefore, warfarin for 6 months is appropriate.

Question 45

C. (Lumbar puncture) Subarachnoid haemorrhages present with a sudden, severe headache and can occur secondary to traumatic brain injury or, in this case, more likely, a spontaneous intracranial aneurysmal rupture. Risk factors include smoking and hypertension. For acute presentations, CT head is the best initial test to confirm the diagnosis; after 12 hours, intracranial resorption of the blood makes lumbar puncture more likely to confirm the diagnosis, with xanthochromia of the CSF due to bilirubin from RBC breakdown.

Question 46

E. (Vascular dementia) Cognitive decline, which was initially forgetfulness and aphasia, before suddenly getting lost in familiar places and having difficulty following conversations (stepwise decline), on the background of hypertension and hypercholesterolaemia combined with MMSE showing moderate cognitive impairment, suggests vascular dementia.

Question 47

C. (Hiatus hernia) Recurrent central chest pain and regurgitation, particularly after meals, on the background of hypercholesterolaemia combined with a very obese BMI and the gastroesophageal junction being above the diaphragm suggests hiatus hernia, specifically a sliding hiatus hernia.

Question 48

B. (Bilateral reticular opacities) Dry cough and progressive exertional dyspnoea for a year combined with bilateral finger clubbing and bibasal end-inspiratory fine crepitations with a restrictive pattern on spirometry suggest idiopathic pulmonary fibrosis (IPF). Bilateral reticular opacities would be seen in the CXR of a patient with IPF, which presents with a "ground-glass" appearance before progressing to "honeycombing" of the lung in the later stages of IPF.

Question 49

B. (Heparinoid) Superficial thrombophlebitis results from inflammation and thrombosis of a superficial leg vein, presenting with leg pain, erythema and a palpable inflamed vein. This case likely relates to a superficial branch of the great saphenous vein. Management is with an NSAID such as ibuprofen or a topical heparin called heparinoid and compression stockings. If the diagnosis is in doubt, US to exclude DVT can be performed.

Question 50

E. (Wernicke's aphasia) Unilateral hemiparesis and speech problems, on the background of hypertension, with impaired comprehension but intact fluency, suggest Wernicke aphasia due to a stroke (easy way to remember between Broca and Wernicke is that **Bro**ca's speech is **Bro**ken)

Question 51

E. (Whipple disease) Whipple disease is a multisystem disorder caused by *Tropheryma whipleii* and presents with diarrhoea, hyperpigmentation and confusion due to vitamin B3 deficiency. The key pathological hallmark macrophage deposition containing periodic acid-Schiff granules on a jejunal biopsy.

Question 52

A. (Closed reduction) Distal radius fracture typically occurs after a fall on an outstretched hand. The distal fragment is dorsally displaced and dorsally angulated, suggesting Colles fracture. Management is with closed reduction and backslab immobilization for 6 weeks.

Question 53

E. (Weight loss) Severe headache, worse in the morning, on the background of COCP usage, combined with an obese BMI, enlarged blindspot, sixth nerve palsy and bilateral papilloedema on fundoscopy suggests idiopathic intracranial hypertension (IIH). Weight loss is the initially recommended management for IIH, before treatment with carbonic anhydrase inhibitors such as acetazolamide as they reduce the rate of CSF production

Question 54

B. (Postvoid residual bladder scan) Chronic urinary retention presents gradually progressive painless difficulty in passing urine with urinary retention. Nocturnal enuresis is common. A postvoid residual bladder scan demonstrating >300 mL in the bladder is diagnostic. Multiparametric MRI is the investigation of choice for prostate cancer, which can cause chronic urinary retention; however the lack of systemic signs of malignancy points away from this.

Question 55

E. (*Streptococcus pneumoniae*) Sudden high-grade fever and increased dyspnoea combined with tachycardia and tachypnoea combined with decreased breath sounds and crepitations at the right lower lung base suggest typical pneumonia. The most common causative organism for typical pneumonia is *Streptococcus pneumoniae*.

Question 56

D. (Omeprazole) Central chest pain and regurgitation for 4 months, with symptoms worse when lying down and improved by antacids combined with an obese BMI and barium swallow showing the gastroesophageal junction above the diaphragm suggest a sliding hiatus hernia. Omeprazole is the management for a sliding hiatus hernia.

Question 57

D. (Nasogastric tube insertion and intravenous fluids) Acute bowel obstruction presents with abdominal pain, vomiting and obstipation, abdominal distention, a tympanic abdomen and high-pitched bowel sounds. Initial management involves bowel decompression and resuscitation, with NG tube insertion, free drainage and IV fluids.

Question 58

E. (Sacroiliitis) Lower back pain and stiffness, progressively worsening for 6 months, with pain worse in the morning and improved by exercise, on the background of anterior uveitis combined with limited lumbar spinal mobility and spinal tenderness, suggest ankylosing spondylitis. Sacroiliitis, on imaging, is most commonly associated with ankylosing spondylitis, with other common features being squaring of the lumbar vertebrae and syndesmophytes.

Question 59

A. (Chest physiotherapy and postural drainage) Chronic cough and exertional dyspnoea, on the background of recurrent sinus infections and steatorrhoea combined with bilateral finger clubbing, coarse crepitations and a sweat chloride level >60 mmol/L, is diagnostic for cystic fibrosis. The initial management for cystic fibrosis is chest physiotherapy and postural drainage, with options such as Lumacaftor/Ivacaftor used to treat CF if patients have a homozygous delta F508 mutation (however this is not currently recommended by NICE)

Question 60

C. (Smoking cessation) Risk factors for an AAA include hypertension, PAD, smoking and alcohol use. Smoking is the most important risk factor to address as it has the most significant association with disease progression, complications and treatment failure.

Question 61

E. (Progressive supranuclear palsy) Parkinsonian symptoms (bradykinesia, pill-rolling right-sided tremor and cogwheel rigidity) combined with impairment of vertical gaze, despite her pupils being equal and reactive to light, suggest progressive supranuclear palsy. The visual signs in PSP are thought to be caused by tau protein accumulation in the tectum, which is where the gaze centres are located.

Question 62

D. (Scrotal exploration and bilateral orchidopexy) Testicular torsion presents with sudden testicular pain and swelling and presents with acute scrotal pain and swelling. Urgent surgical exploration is required within a 6-hour window to save the testis. Bilateral orchiopexy should be performed to reduce the risk of future torsion.

Question 63

A. (*Haemophilus influenzae*)

Chronic cough and decreased exercise tolerance, on the background of recurrent childhood ear infections combined with bilateral finger clubbing and coarse crepitations with thick-walled dilated bronchi on CXR, suggest bronchiectasis. *Haemophilus influenzae* is the most likely causative organism for bronchiectasis.

Question 64

C. (Rouleaux formation) CRAB features (Hypercalcaemia, Renal failure, Anaemia and Bone pain) suggest multiple myeloma. Rouleaux formation, RBCs linked into chains resembling a "stack of coins", would be seen on the blood film of a patient with multiple myeloma, and is thought to occur due to the excess of immunoglobulins seen in MM causing hyperviscosity and RBC's to adhere to themselves.

Question 65

C. (CT angiogram) The classic triad of Acute Mesenteric Ischaemia (AMI) is severe abdominal pain, bloody diarrhoea and AF. Diagnosis will be confirmed with contrast CT angiography, which would often show a central lucency in the mesenteric veins. However, if there are signs of peritonitis or sepsis, an urgent laparotomy should be performed.

Question 66

A. (Liver abscess) Right upper quadrant pain and jaundice for a week, on the background of a recent *E. coli* infection (most likely cause of epididymo-orchitis in the elderly) combined with RUQ tenderness and hepatomegaly and a liver US showing a fluid-filled cavity in the right lobe of the liver, suggests a liver abscess.

Question 67

A. (Ann Arbor staging) Painless lymph node swelling, night sweats and unintentional weight loss, on the background of Epstein-Barr virus combined with a palpable, rubbery and nontender right cervical area with normocytic anaemia, eosinophilia and Reed-Sternberg cells on biopsy suggest Hodgkin lymphoma. Ann Arbor staging is the staging criteria for Hodgkin lymphoma, with stage I being a single lymph node affected and stage IV being spread beyond the lymph nodes. FAB staging is used for leukaemias, not lymphomas.

Question 68

A. (Increase weight-bearing exercise) Osteoarthritis is suggested by bilateral asymmetrical knee pain and stiffness with reduced range of motion and palpable crepitus. Management is with regular analgesia and lifestyle measures. Weight loss can be recommended if overweight, but increased weight-bearing exercise should be recommended as a first line in all patients.

Question 69

B. (Implantable cardioverter-defibrillator) Syncope without associated palpitations or dyspnoea, on the background of sudden cardiac death combined with convex ST elevation in leads V1–V3 followed by a negative T wave (a type I Brugada pattern, suggests Brugada syndrome. A dual-chamber implantable cardioverter-defibrillator is the management for Brugada syndrome, if there is a spontaneous type I Brugada pattern to reduce the potential for sudden cardiac death occurring. Sodium channel blockers like ajmaline are used to make type I Brugada pattern more apparent.

Question 70

B. (CT angiography) Aortic dissection presents with sudden central chest pain radiating to the back, nausea and presyncope. Relevant risk factors include hypertension, diabetes and smoking. CT angiography will demonstrate a double lumen resulting from an intimal tear of the aorta.

Question 71

C. (Pseudogout) Sudden, severe right knee pain and swelling, on the background of Wilson disease, combined with a warm right knee that she is unable to bear weight on and has a limited ROM with rhomboid-shaped, weakly positively birefringent crystals on synovial fluid analysis suggests pseudogout (**P**seudogout = Calcium **P**yrophosphate = **P**ositively birefringent). Gout is negatively birefringent and presents classically with pain in the 1st metatarsophalangeal joint rather than the knee.

Question 72

D. (IV saline) Confusion and polydipsia for 4 days, on the background of type 2 diabetes mellitus, combined with hypertension, tachycardia and dry mucous membranes with severe hyperglycaemia, minor ketonaemia and elevated serum osmolality suggest hyperosmolar hyperglycaemic state (HHS). IV fluids with saline is the management of choice for HHS, to replace the fluid losses with insulin not indicated unless the blood glucose stops dropping with the IV fluids.

Question 73

D. (Prostate adenocarcinoma) There is extensive bony metastatic disease, with multiple sclerotic lesions in the vertebra, pelvic bones and proximal femora, resulting in a pathological vertebral fracture. The most likely aetiology in this demographic for sclerotic metastasis is prostate cancer, which is commonly asymptomatic in the early stages, only picked up through screening, and may present late with metastatic disease.

Question 74

C. (Faecal elastase) Chronic pancreatitis presents with abdominal pain, bloating, nausea and steatorrhoea, relating to pancreatic exocrine insufficiency. Chronic alcohol abuse and smoking are key risk factors. Faecal elastase is a noninvasive measure of pancreatic exocrine function and has shown excellent correlation with duodenal juice amylase, lipase and trypsin values

Question 75

C. (HIV-associated nephropathy) Leg swelling and decreased urine output, on the background of IV drug use combined with hypertension, proteinuria and haematuria on urinalysis and a low CD4 cell count suggest HIV-associated nephropathy. HIV-associated nephropathy is associated with massive proteinuria and renal biopsy would show focal segmental glomerulosclerosis with focal capillary collapse.

Question 76

A. (Cranial diabetes insipidus) Polydipsia and nocturia, despite no changes in fluid intake on the background of haemochromatosis combined with normal blood glucose, low urine osmolality initially after water deprivation test with increased urine osmolality with desmopressin administration suggest cranial diabetes insipidus. Cranial diabetes insipidus is caused by an underproduction of ADH by the posterior pituitary, hence why it reacts to desmopressin administration.

Question 77

C. (Mitral regurgitation) Dyspnoea and an irregular heartbeat, on the background of hypertension combined with a pansystolic murmur best heard on expiration at the apex radiating to the axilla, suggest mitral regurgitation. A pansystolic murmur best heard on inspiration suggests tricuspid regurgitation.

Question 78

B. (Compartmental pressures) Compartment syndrome presents with severe pain, swelling and neurological deficits of a limb. Following revascularization, ischemia-reperfusion oedema can occur, resulting in swelling in the closed limb compartments and muscle ischaemia. Diagnosis is with compartmental pressure measurement, with >40 mmHg being a diagnostic intracompartmental pressure.

Question 79

D. (Collagen type IV) Haematuria for a week, on the background of similar shorter episodes combined with a soft, non-tender abdomen with bilateral sensorineural hearing loss and raised urea and creatinine suggests Alport syndrome. Alport syndrome is an X-linked dominant condition caused by mutations in the genes encoding collagen type IV, which causes a thinning and splitting of the basement membrane.

Question 80

D. (Turner syndrome) Mid-systolic murmur and bilateral radio-femoral delay suggest coarctation of the aorta. Coarctation of the aorta is associated strongly with Turner syndrome despite coarctation of the aorta being more common in males. Turner syndrome is caused by the presence of only one X chromosome (45, X0) which commonly presents with a short stature, webbed neck and widely spaced nipples along with raised gonadotropins levels which causes primary amenorrhoea.

Question 81

D. (Lumbosacral MRI) Lumbar spinal stenosis presents with back pain and calf claudication on walking and standing due to nerve root compression by a narrowed central spinal canal. Symptoms are worse with positions that narrow the spinal canal, typically walking downhill and standing, relieved by forward flexion (i.e., sitting down). MRI will confirm the diagnosis, which would demonstrate canal narrowing.

Question 82

C. (Small bowel obstruction) Sudden abdominal pain and bilious vomiting for 48 hours on the background of a caesarean section, combined with a distended abdomen, high-pitched bowel sounds, and a small bowel diameter >3 cm suggests small bowel obstruction. The most likely cause of the SBO is adhesions from a prior Caesarean section.

Question 83

E. (Vacuum-assisted erectile device) Erectile dysfunction can occur in cardiac disease due to atherosclerotic narrowing of the penile arteries, impairing blood flow and penile engorgement. For patients on nitrates and at high cardiac risk, PDE-5 inhibitors are contraindicated due to the risk of profound hypertension. In these cases, second-line management can include vacuum-assisted erection devices or intracavernous prostaglandin injections.

Question 84

B. (High cortisol and low ACTH) Weight gain, fatigue, easy bruising and skin thinning combined with hypertension, proximal muscle weakness and purple abdominal striae suggest Cushing syndrome. The right adrenal cortex mass suggests it is Cushing secondary to an adrenal adenoma; hence, cortisol would not be suppressed, and ACTH suppressed on a high-dose dexamethasone test because the tumour can produce cortisol autonomously despite pituitary ACTH suppression.

Question 85

C. (Intravenous flucloxacillin) Cellulitis presents with pain, swelling, warm and erythema of the lower leg and fevers. Diabetes increases the risk of skin infections due to elevated blood glucose levels, increasing susceptibility to infection. IV flucloxacillin is the management of this case over oral due to the presence of T2DM making this patient's Eron classification class II, for which IV antibiotics are suggested.

Question 86

E. (Sputum culture) Cough and night sweats for 3 weeks combined with decreased right upper lobe breath sounds and crepitations with a right upper lobe cavitary lesion on CXR suggest tuberculosis. Sputum culture is the gold-standard investigation for tuberculosis because it is the most sensitive and specific for mycobacterium tuberculosis.

Question 87

B. (Polyarteritis nodosa) Progressively worsening joint pain and fatigue combined with livedo reticularis and erythema nodosum with elevated pANCA, urea and creatinine suggest polyarteritis nodosa. Polyarteritis nodosa is a medium vessel vasculitis leading to aneurysm formation and is commonly associated with hepatitis B infection.

Question 88

B. (Intravenous antibiotics) Fever, abdominal guarding and rigidity suggest generalized peritonitis relating to diverticular perforation. Immediate management of sepsis with intravenous antibiotics is the most important first step before exploring surgical management options (part of the sepsis six).

Question 89

A. (Atrial septal defect) Dyspnoea and fatigue, on the background of multiple respiratory infections combined with a fixed, widely split S2 heart sound and ejection systolic murmur on examination and a left-to-right shunt suggest atrial septal defect. The most common ASD is an ostium secundum which would present with right axis deviation

Question 90

B. (Cystoscopy and biopsy) Painless haematuria is a red flag feature of bladder cancer. Smoking is a key risk factor. The diagnosis is confirmed with cystoscopy and biopsy to stage the cancer with TNM staging.

Question 91

A. (IM glucagon) Loss of consciousness preceded by weakness and shakiness, on the background of type 2 diabetes mellitus combined with mild pallor, diaphoresis and unresponsiveness with a significantly reduced blood glucose suggests hypoglycaemia causing loss of consciousness. IM glucagon is the management for an unconscious patient with hypoglycaemia.

Question 92

A. (Extracorporeal shock wave lithotripsy) There is a 12 mm stone in the ureter, resulting in renal colic as the ureter attempts to pass the stone with peristalsis. ESWL is the preferred management for urethral stones >10 mm. Medical expulsive therapy (with tamsulosin) can be attempted for smaller stones which fail to pass spontaneously.

Question 93

E. (Reassurance) Simple breast cysts are common in women aged 35–50 relating to physiological tissue involution. Asymptomatic simple cysts can be managed conservatively. Aspiration can be performed if symptomatic. Complicated cysts (if blood is filled or constantly refilled) should be biopsied.

Question 94

C. (Fanconi anaemia) Microcephaly and short stature combined with a family background of acute lymphoblastic leukaemia combined with cafe-au-lait spots and aplastic anaemia (pancytopenia and hypocellular marrow with fatty infiltrates) suggest an inherited haematological disorder. Fanconi anaemia is an autosomal recessive haematological disorder characterised by a defect in DNA repair genes, specifically homologous recombination which predisposes patients to a variety of haematological issues.

Question 95

A. (Brown granular casts) Nausea and decreased urine output, on the background of aminoglycoside use combined with hypertension and mild pallor with raised urea and creatinine, suggest acute tubular necrosis. Acute tubular necrosis is associated with brown granular casts, due to dead epithelial cells sloughing into the urine

Question 96

E. (Urea breath test) Duodenal ulcers present with gnawing epigastric pain, worse at night and relieved by eating. NSAID use and alcohol are risk factors. An *H. pylori* test and treatment strategy with a urea breath test is the most appropriate first step.

Question 97

D. (Needle aspiration) Sudden, sharp left-sided chest pain and dyspnoea, on the background of scuba diving while on holiday combined with tachypnoea and reduced left breath sounds and a >2 cm rim of air on CXR suggest a simple primary pneumothorax. A primary pneumothorax is when there is no underlying lung disease (often occurs in young tall, thin men), whilst in secondary, there is underlying lung disease such as COPD. The management for a simple primary pneumothorax >2 cm or with dyspnoea is needle aspiration.

Question 98

C. (Pelvic MRI) Osteomyelitis presents with fever, joint pain, swelling, warmth and redness. Intravenous drug use, particularly with local administration (i.e., the groin), is a significant risk factor. Diagnosis is confirmed with MRI, which will show cortical destruction, bone marrow inflammation and soft tissue oedema.

Question 99

B. (IV propranolol and propylthiouracil) Severe agitation and confusion combined with a high-grade fever, hypertension, tachycardia, a diffusely enlarged goitre and exophthalmos on examination with elevated T4 and reduced TSH suggest severe thyrotoxicosis. The history of Graves disease and preceding surgery suggests a thyroid storm. IV propranolol and propylthiouracil are the management for thyroid storm, to stabilise blood pressure and reduce levels of circulating T4 levels quickly

Question 100

B. (HLA-B51) The triad of oral ulcers, genital ulcers and anterior uveitis in a young man suggests Behcet disease. Behcet disease is associated with HLA-B51, with homozygotes for this gene being at particular risk which suggests a potential gene-dose relationship.

Images 37

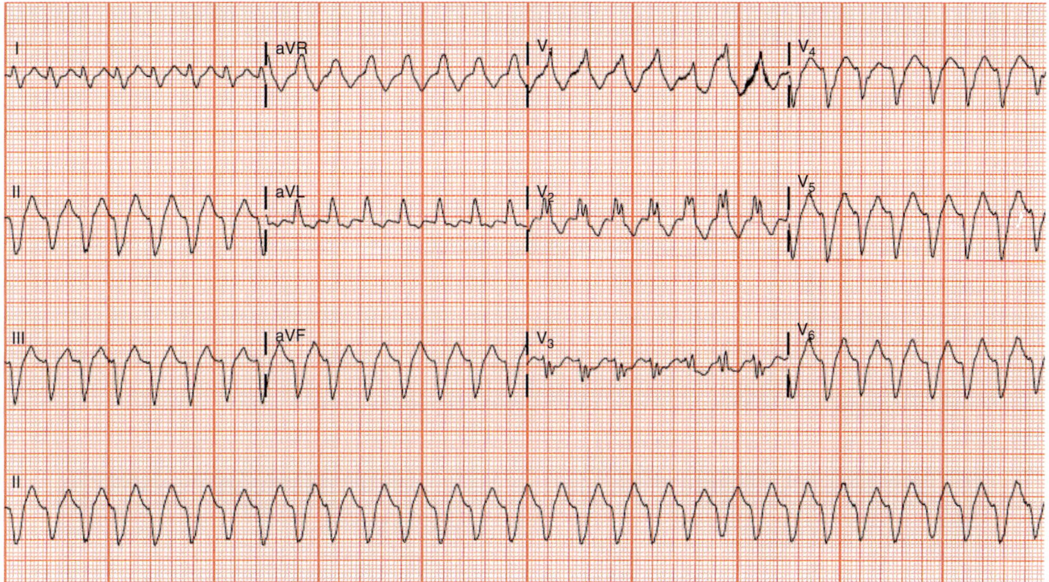

Fig. 1.1 ECG. (From Ziad Issa, John M. Miller et al. *Clinical Arrhythmology and Electrophysiology: A Companion to Braunwald's Heart Disease*. 4th ed. Copyright © 2024 by Elsevier Inc. All rights reserved.)

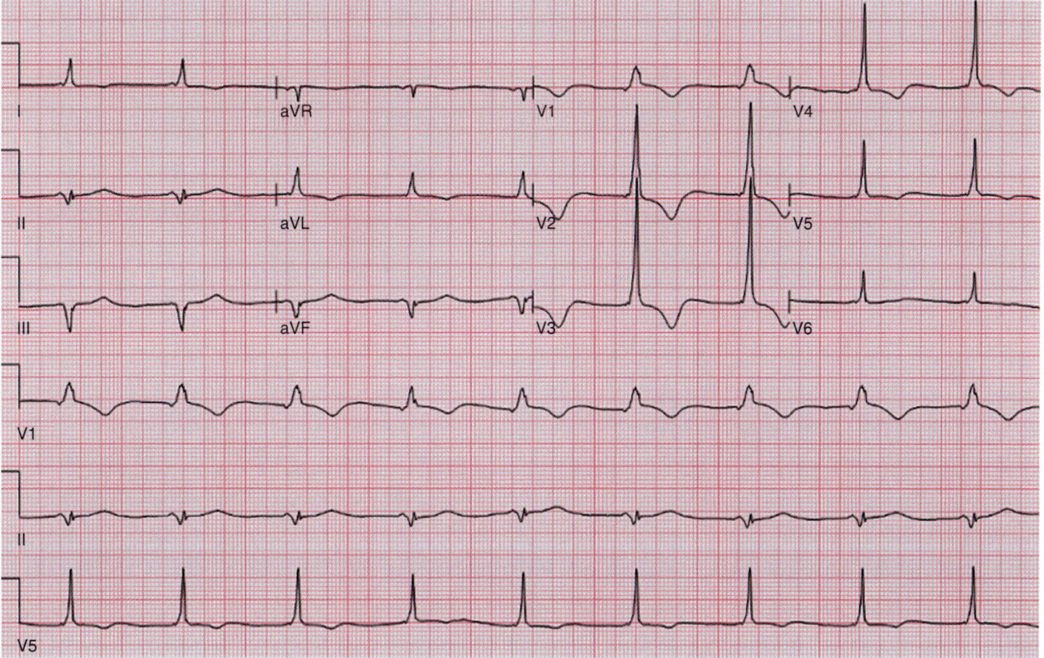

Fig. 1.2 ECG. (From Bonnie Halpern-Felsher. *Encyclopedia of Child and Adolescent Health*. 1st ed. Copyright © 2023 by Elsevier Inc. All rights reserved.)

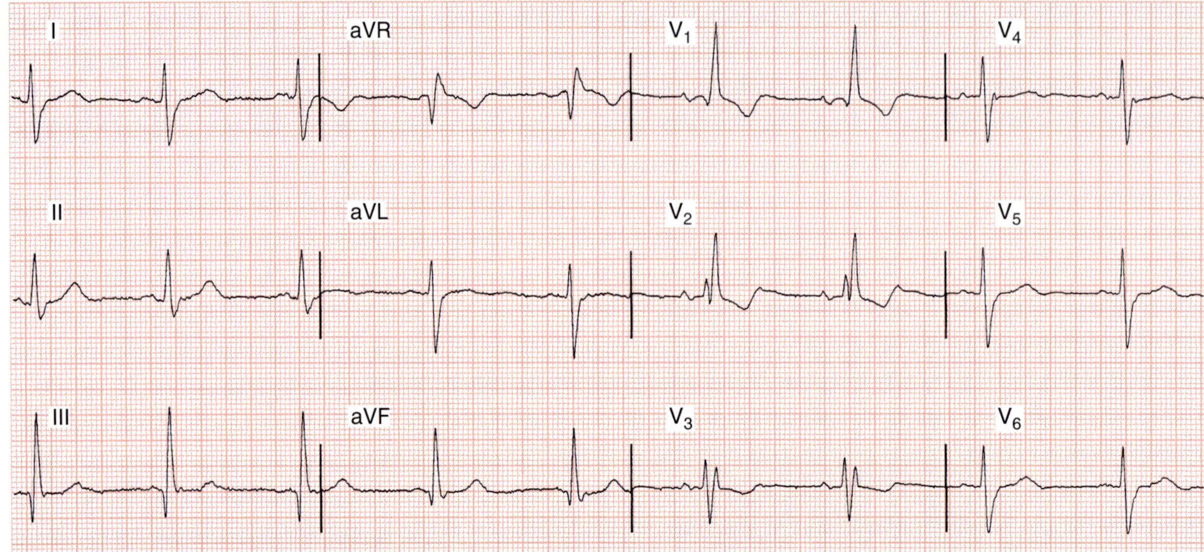

Fig. 1.3 ECG. (From Goldberger A L, Goldberger ZD et al. *Goldberger's Clinical Electrocardiography: A Simplified Approach*. 9th ed. Philadelphia: Elsevier; 2018.)

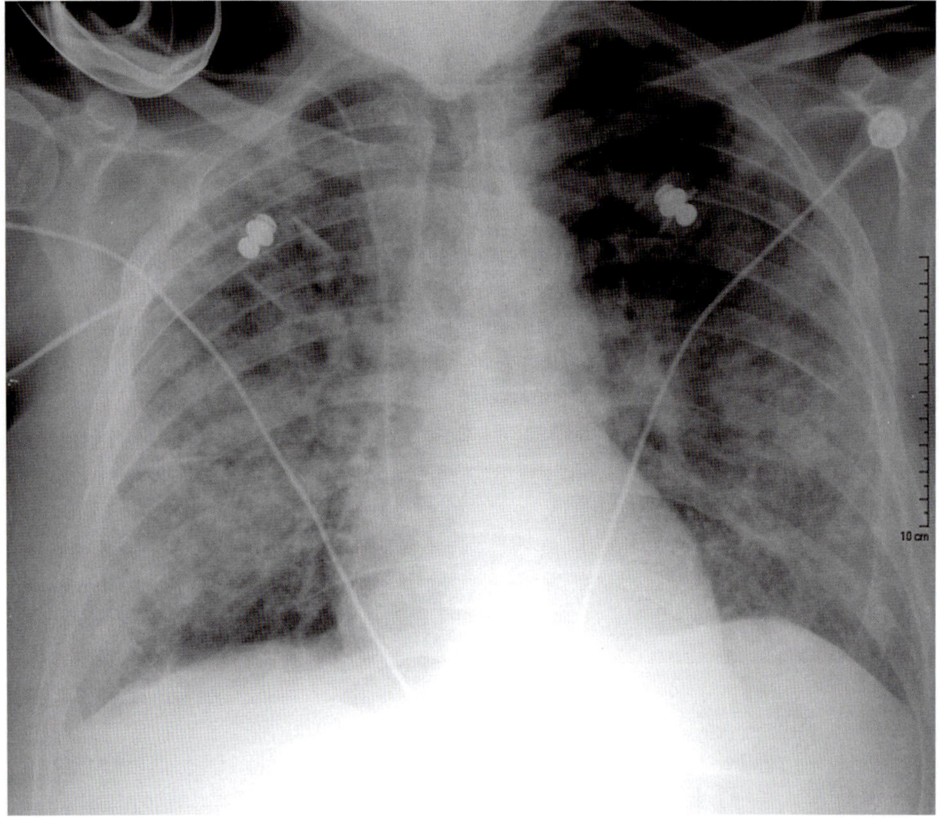

Fig. 4.1 CXR. (From Andy Adam et al. *Grainger & Allison's Diagnostic Radiology*. 7th ed. Copyright © 2021 by Elsevier Limited. All rights reserved.)

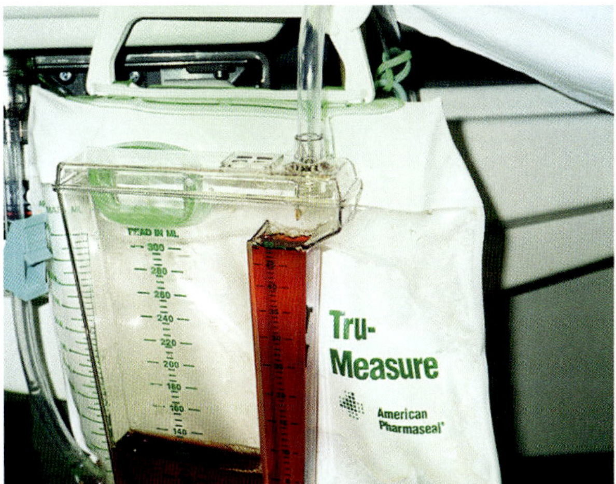

Fig. 9.1 Catheter output. (From Matthew S. Slater, Richard J Mullins. *Journal of the American College of Surgeons*, 1998 June 186(6):693–716, DOI: 10.1016/S1072-7515(28)00089-1.)

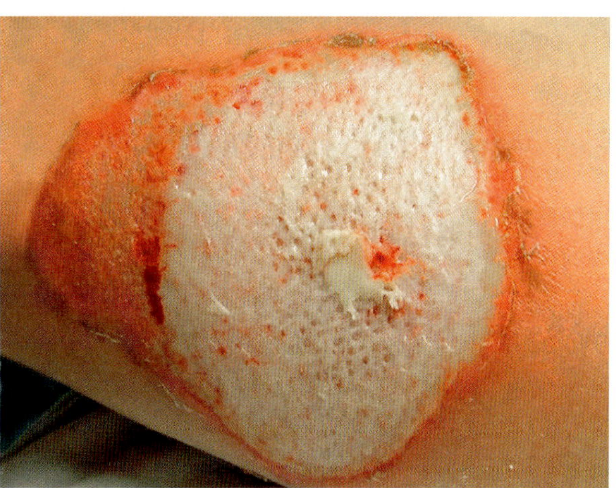

Fig 9.2 Burn injury. (From Linda D, Urden et al. *Priorities in Critical Care Nursing*. 9th ed. Elsevier; 2024.)

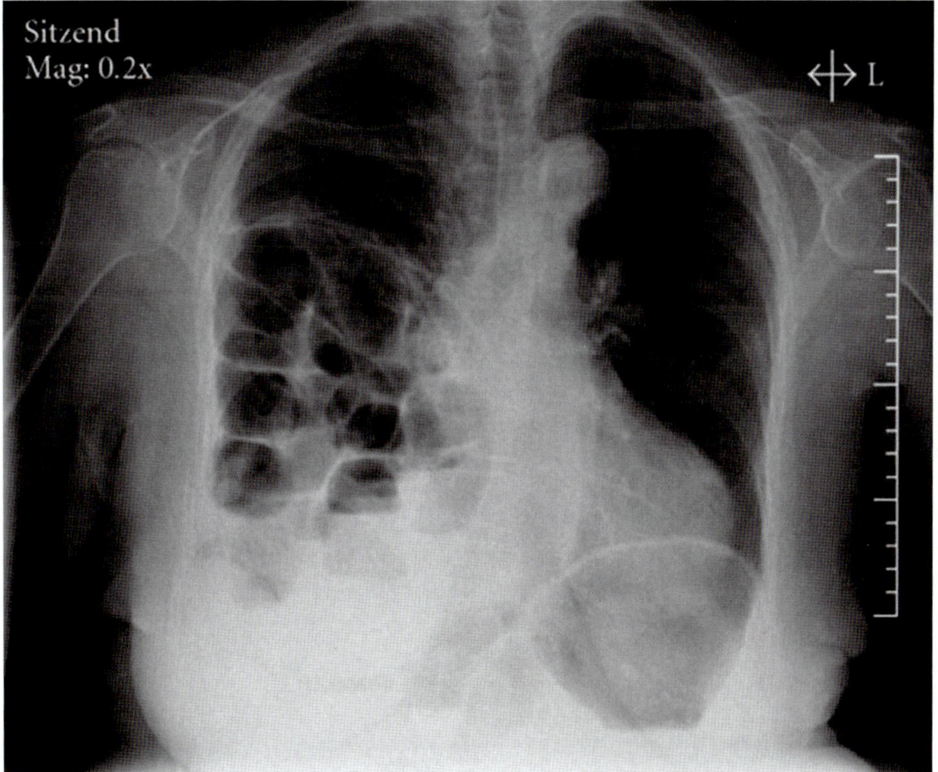

Fig 9.3 Chest X-ray. (From Edmond Cohen: *Cohen's Comprehensive Thoracic Anesthesia*. 1st ed. Copyright © 2022 by Elsevier Inc. All rights reserved.)

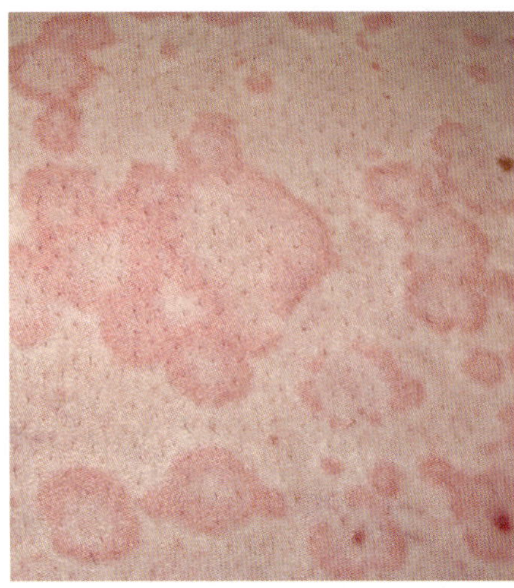

Fig 10.1 Cannula site. (From Habif TP. *Clinical Dermatology: A Color Guide to Diagnosis and Therapy*. 6th ed. St Louis: Elsevier; 2015.)

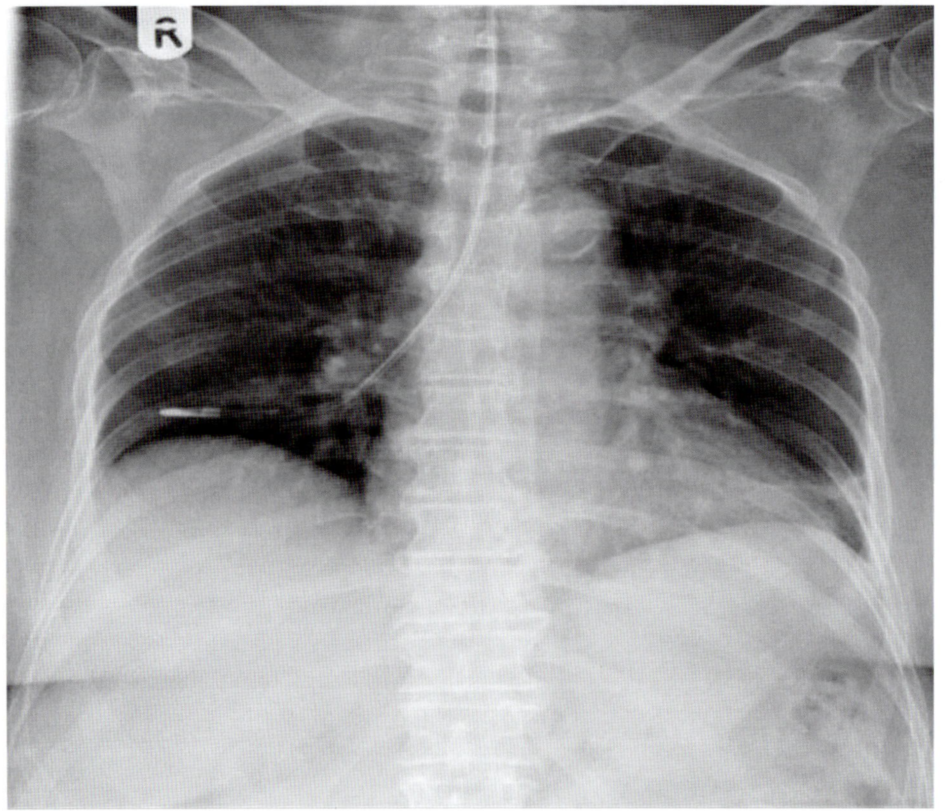

Fig 10.2 Chest X-ray. (From Berenice Aguirrezabala Armbruster, Hannah Punter, Gregory Oxenham et al. *Medicine in a Day*. 1st ed. Elsevier; 2023.)

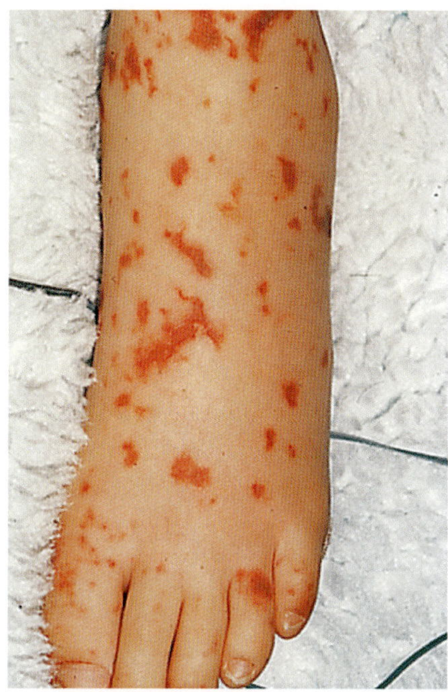

Fig 10.3 Right lower leg. (From Alyce Hayes, Andrei Pobischan et al. *Crash Course Paediatrics*, 6th ed. Elsevier; 2005.)

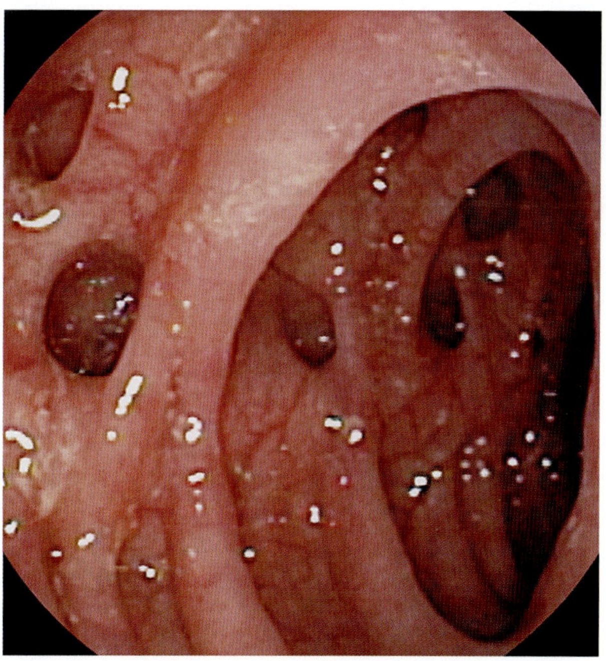

Fig 11.1 Colonoscopy. (From M. Feldman et al. *Sleisenger and Fordtran's Gastrointestinal and Liver Disease*. 11th ed. Copyright © 2021 by Elsevier, Inc. All rights reserved.)

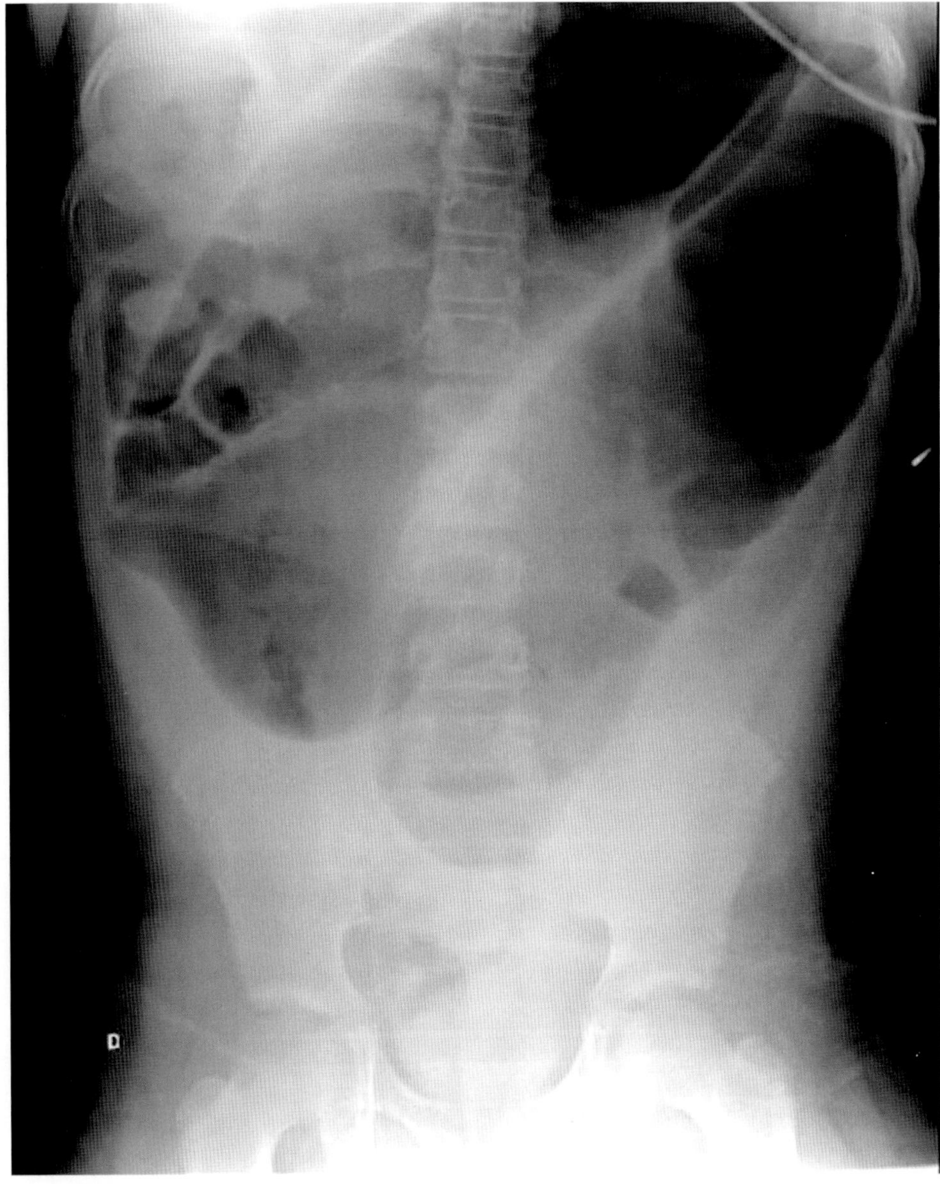

Fig 11.2 Abdominal X-ray. (From Abdillahi Omar. *USMLE Step 2 CK Plus*. 1st ed. Copyright © 2023 by Elsevier, Inc. All rights reserved.)

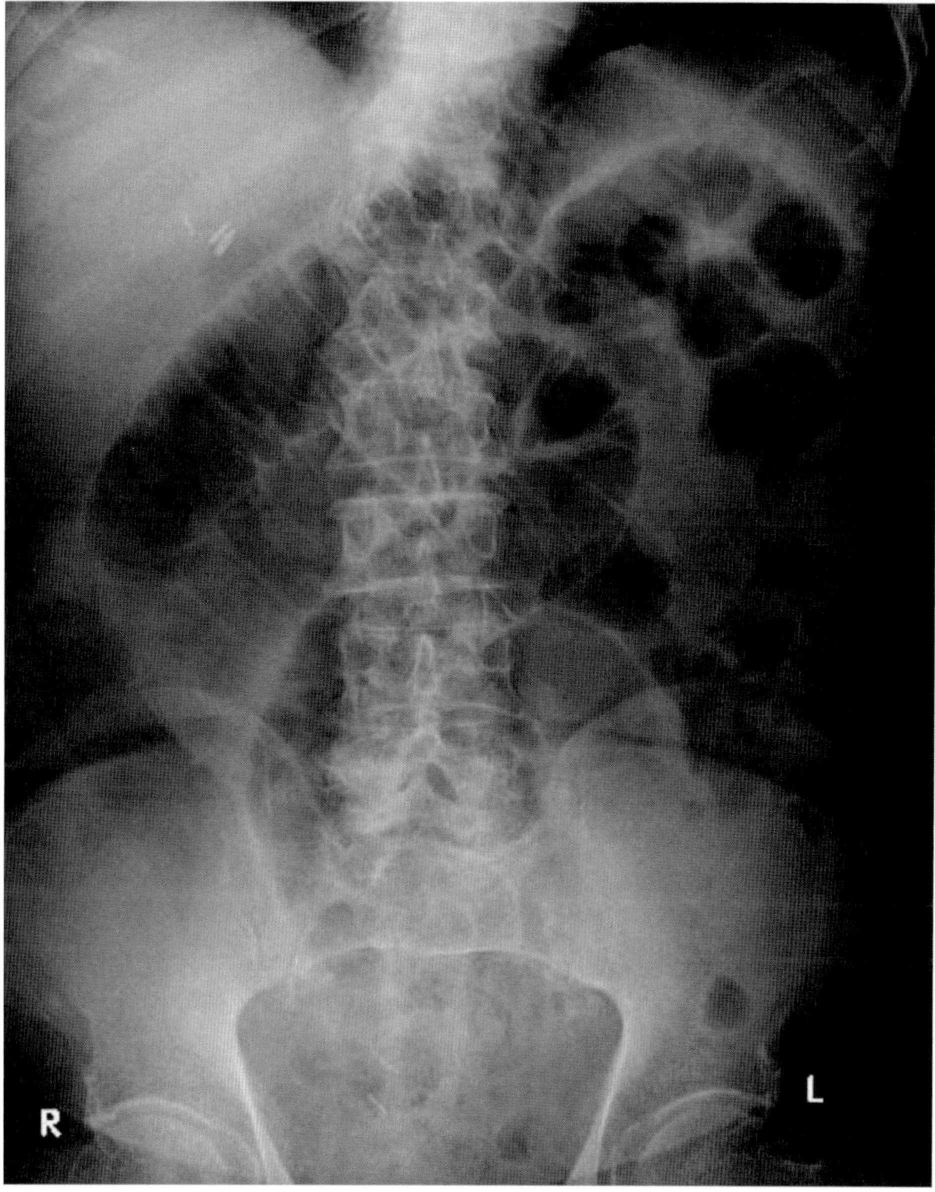

Fig 11.3 Abdominal X-ray. (From O. James Garden et al. *Principles and Practice of Surgery*. 8th ed.

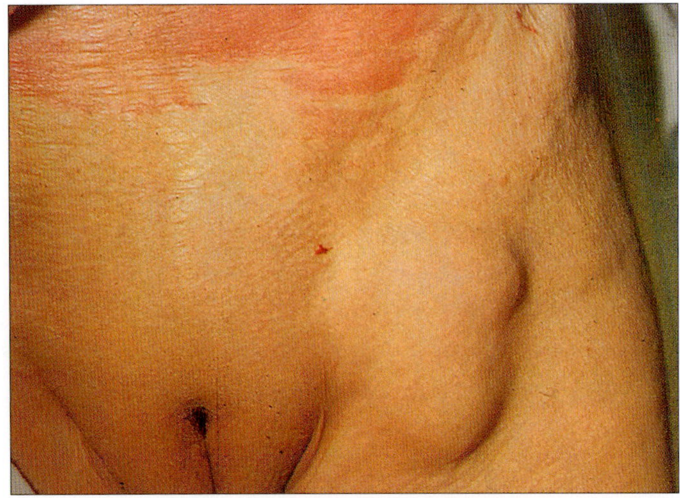

Fig 11.4 Left groin examination. (From Hagen-Ansert SL. *Textbook of Diagnostic Ultrasonography*. 7th ed. St Louis: Mosby; 2012.)

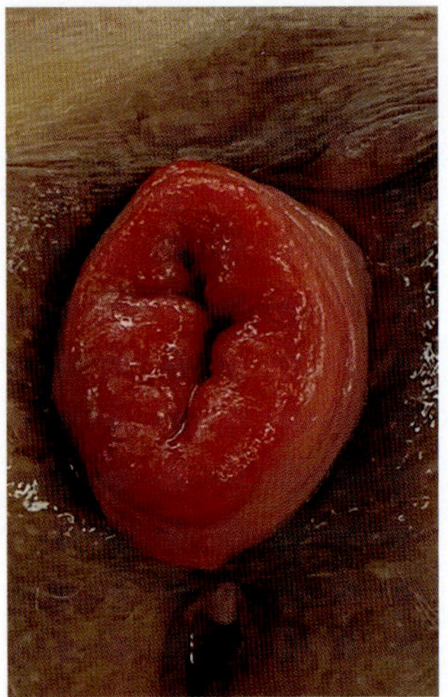

Fig 11.5 Digital rectal examination. (From Matthew D. Barber et al. *Walters & Karram Urogynecology and Reconstructive Pelvic Surgery*. 5th ed. Copyright © 2022 by Elsevier, Inc. All rights reserved.)

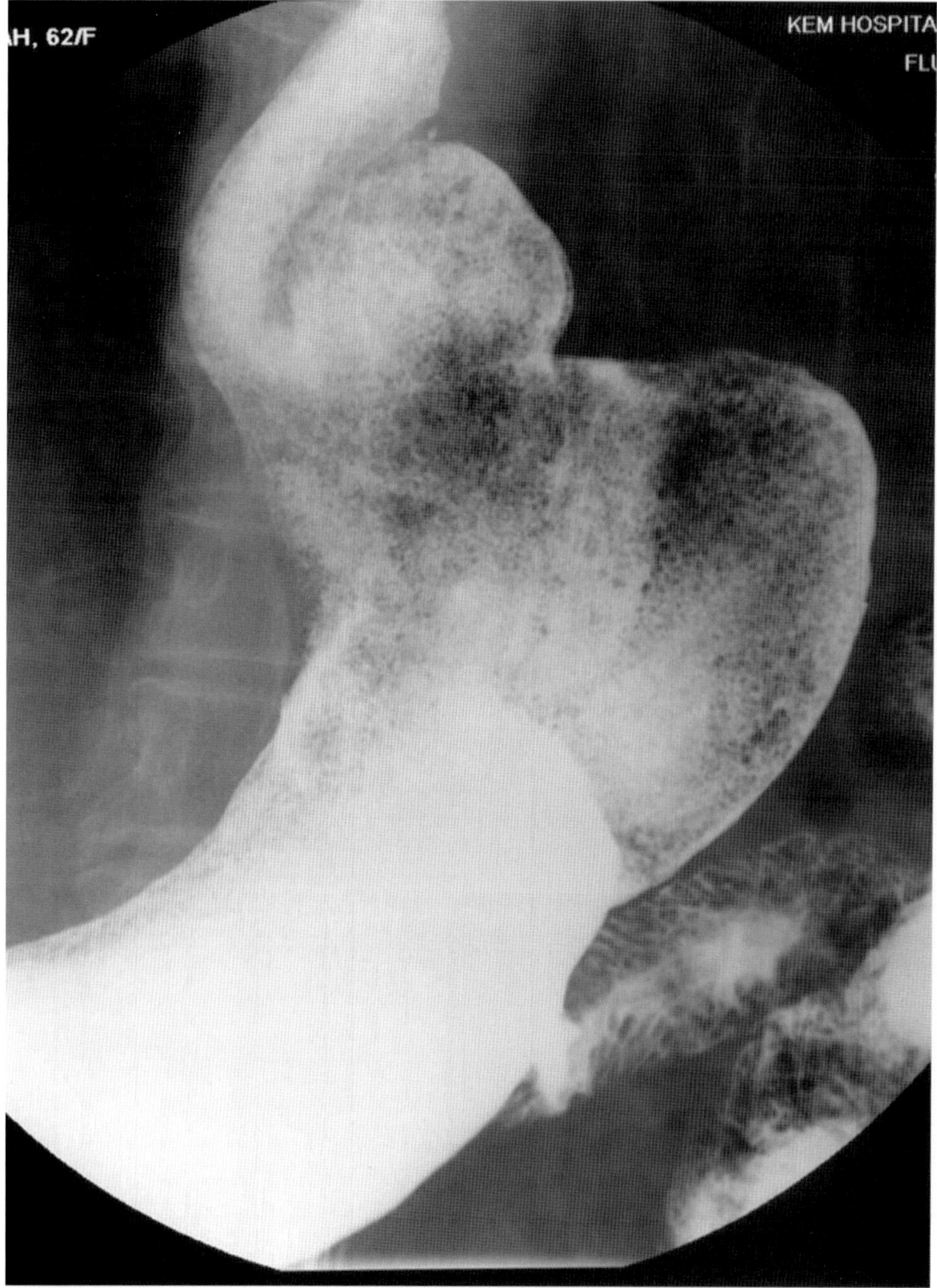

Fig 11.6 Barium swallow. (From Shrinivas Desai et al. *Comprehensive Textbook of Clinical Radiology Volume IV: Abdomen*. 1st ed.)

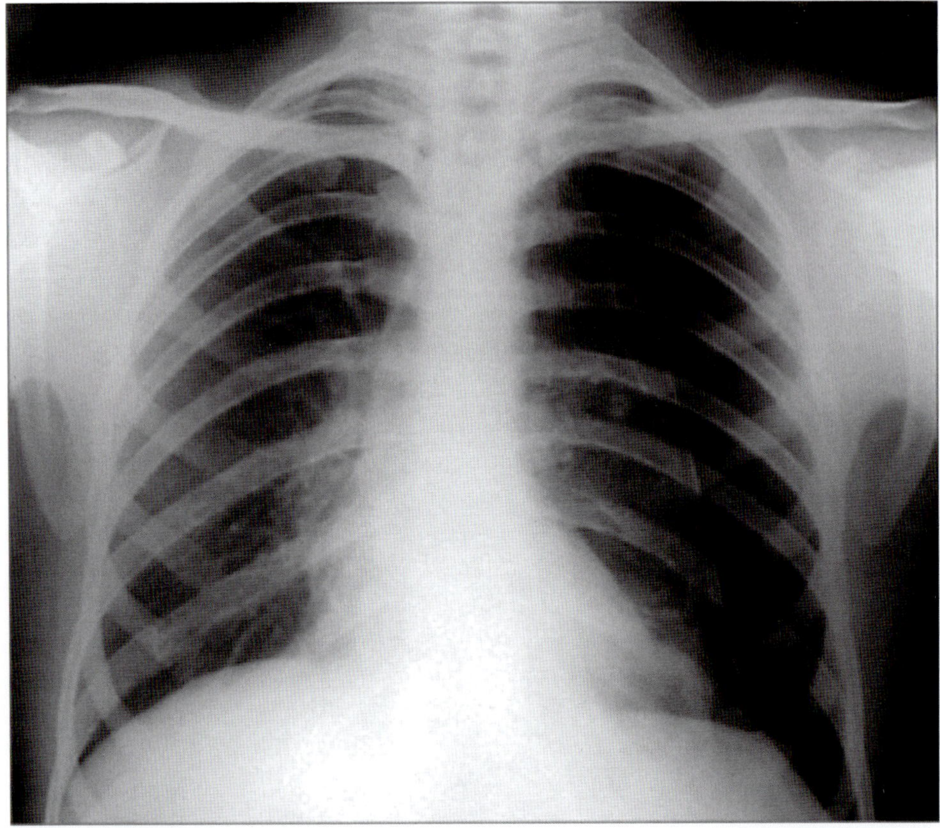

Fig 12.1 Chest X-ray. (From Lee P. *Lancet*, 2013 Apr 13;381(9874):1252–1254.)

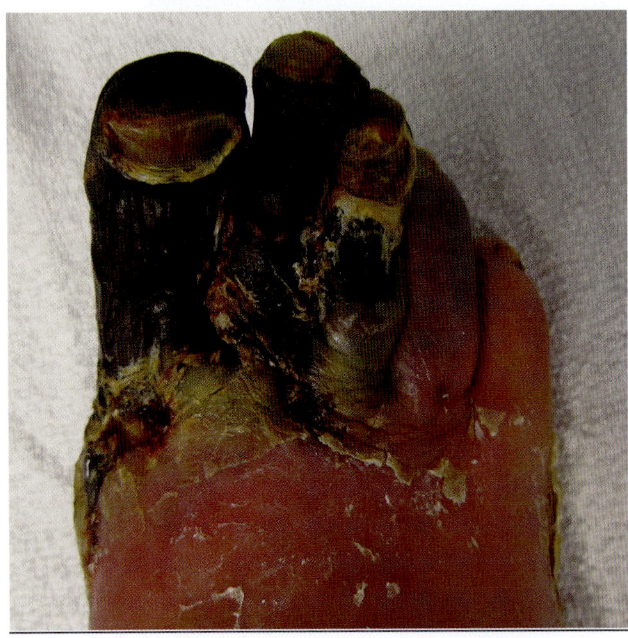

Fig 12.2 Right foot. (From Ken Zafren, MD, FAAEM, FACEP, FAWM International Commission for Mountain Emergency Medicine (ICAR MedCom) and Mountain Rescue Association Medical Committee Clinical Professor – Department of Emergency Medicine Stanford University Medical Center – Stanford, CA USA Staff Emergency Physician – Alaska Native Medical Center – Anchorage, AK USA.)

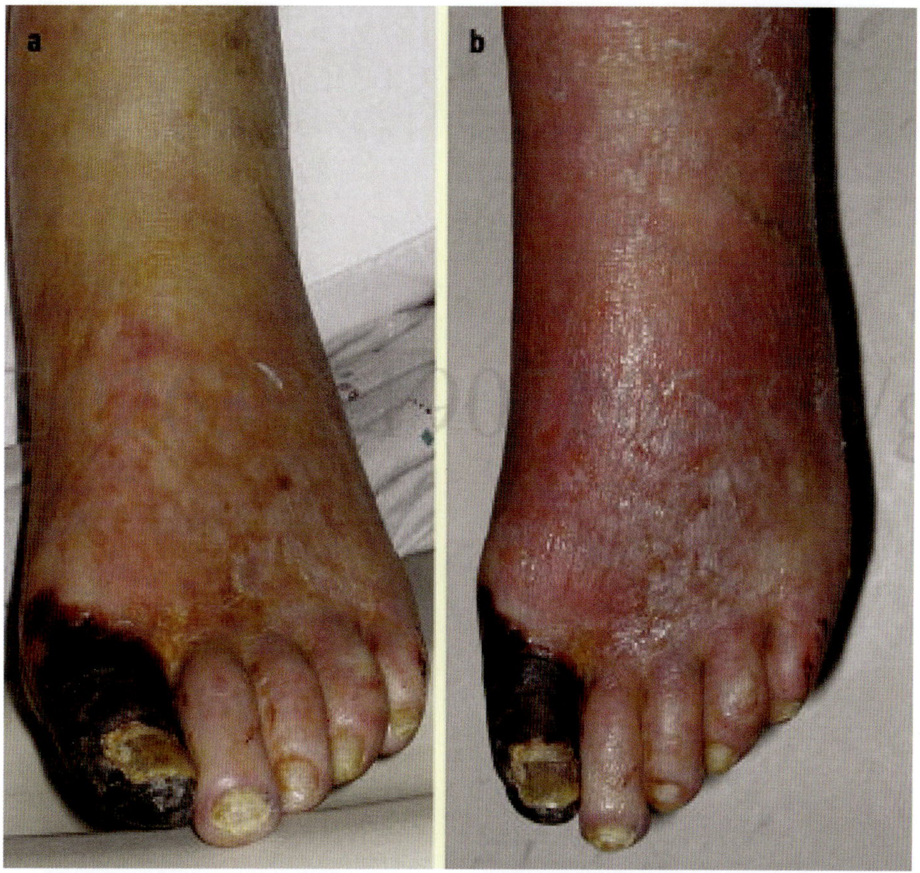

Fig 12.3 Left foot. (From Marcus Brooks, Michael P Jenkins. *Surgery (Oxford).* 2004 December 1; 22(12):331–334.)

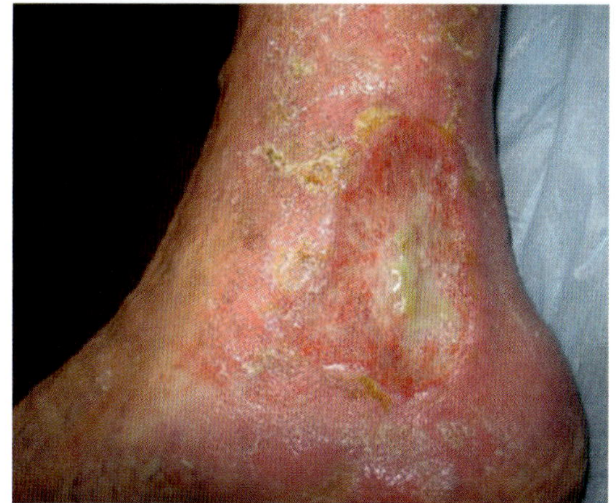

Fig 12.4 Lower limb ulcer. (From Jasmine Shen, Thomas Foster et al. *Crash Course Cardiology*, 6th ed. Elsevier; 2025.)

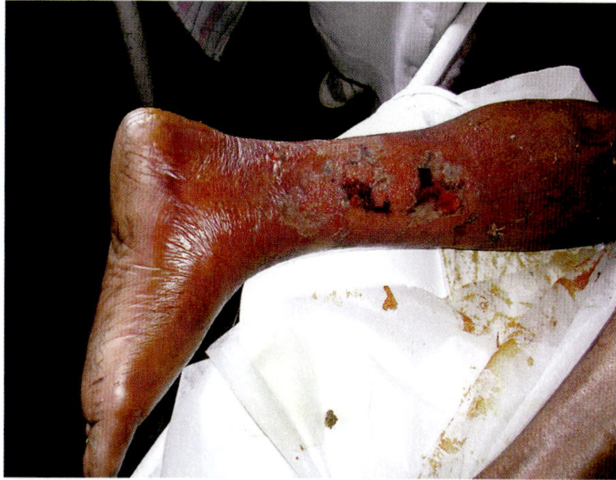

Fig. 13.1 Left leg. (From S. Devaji Rao, Kirthana Devaji Rao. *Essentials of Surgery for Dental Students*. 1st ed. Elsevier; 2016.)

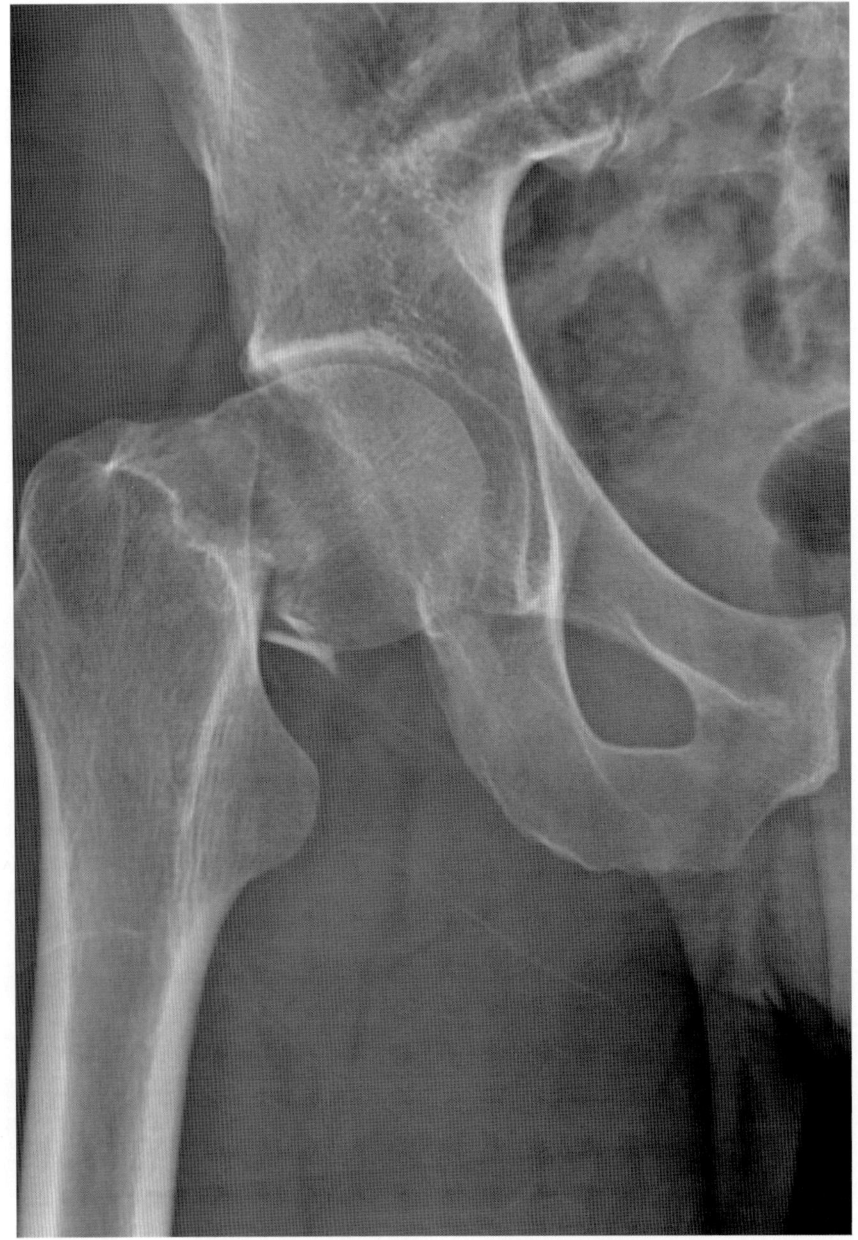

Fig. 13.2 X-ray pelvis. (From A. Waqar et al. *Advances in Medical and Surgical Engineering*. 1st ed. Copyright © 2020 by Elsevier, Inc. All rights reserved.)

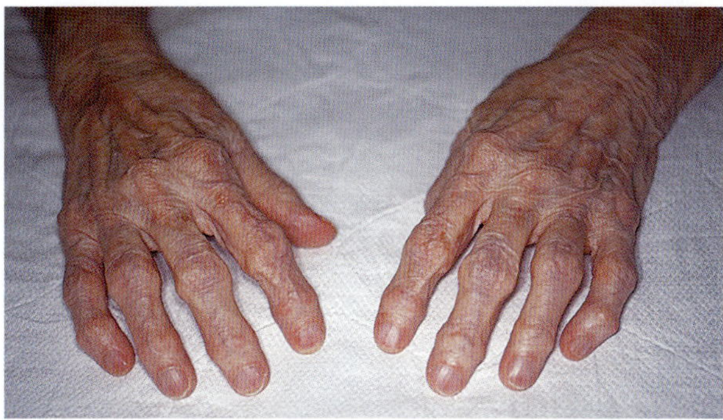

Fig. 13.3 Hand examination. (From Swartz MH. *Textbook of Physical Diagnosis: History and Examination*. 8th ed. Copyright © 2021 by Elsevier, Inc. All rights reserved.)

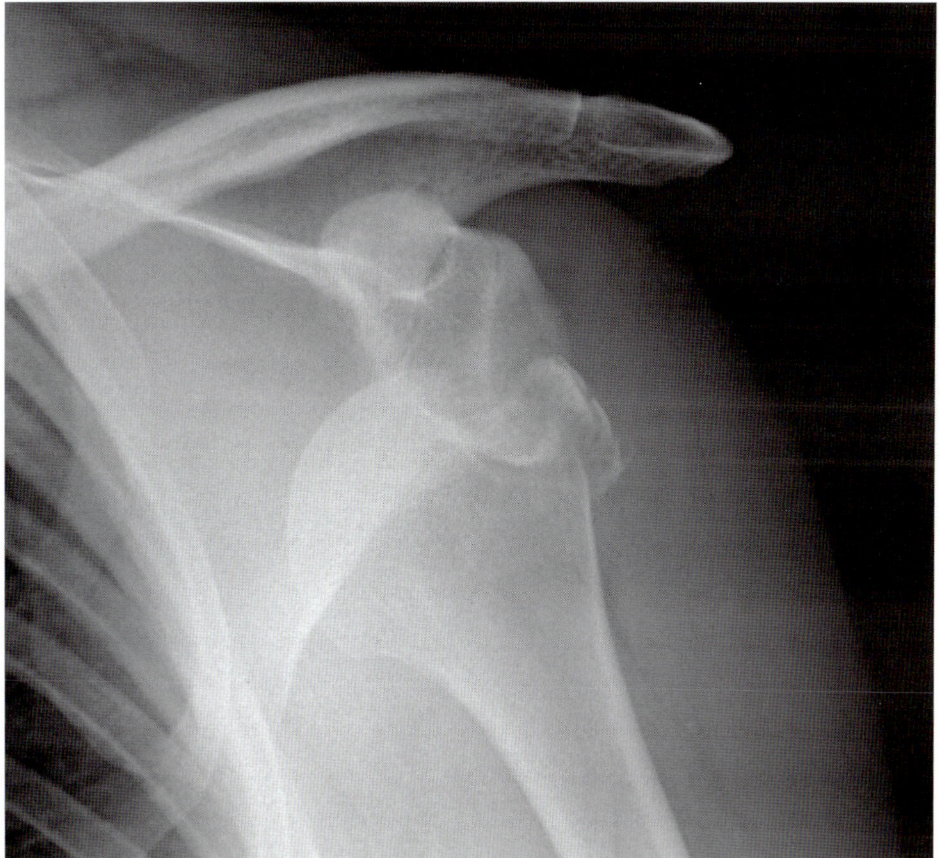

Fig. 13.4 X-ray shoulder. (From Richard L. Drake et al. *Gray's Anatomy for Students*. 5th ed. Copyright © 2024 by Elsevier Inc. All rights reserved.)

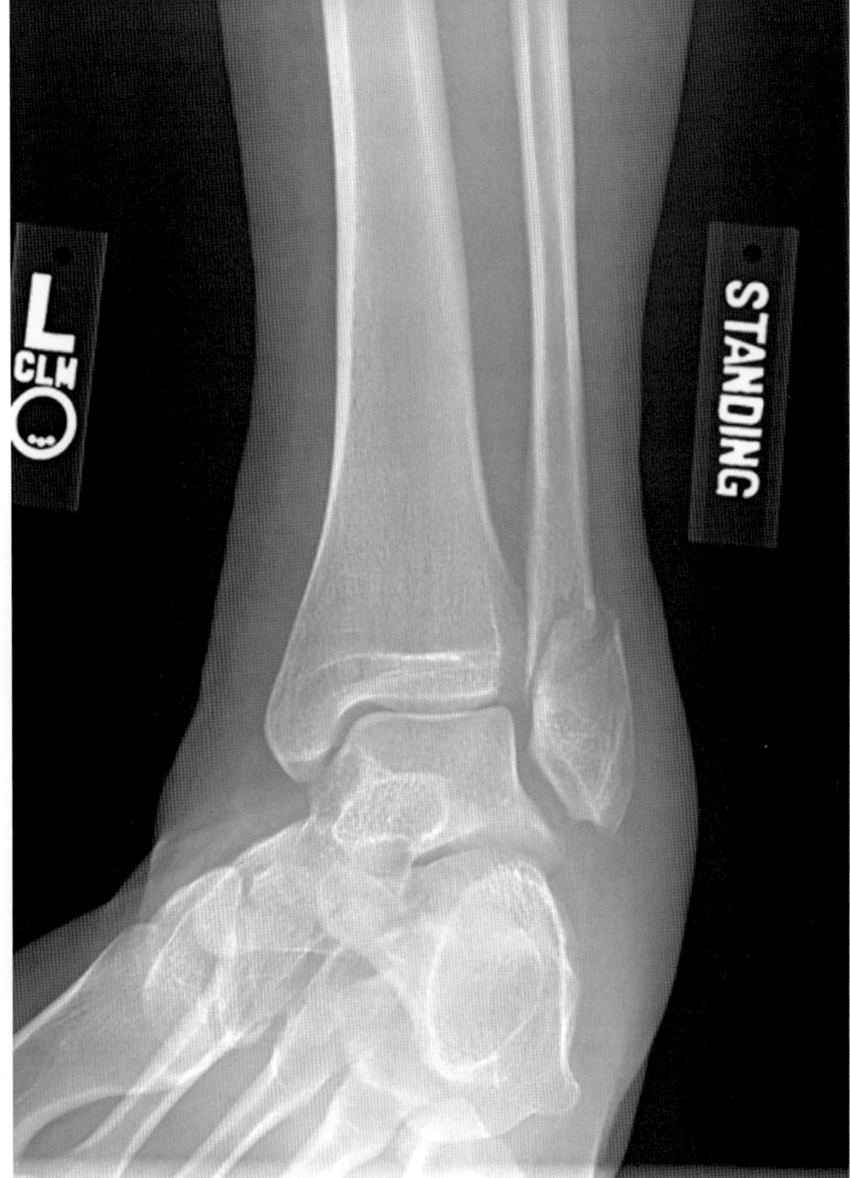

Fig. 13.5 X-ray ankle. (From Sara D. Rynders *Orthopaedics for Physician Assistants*. 2nd ed. Copyright © 2022 by Elsevier, Inc. All rights reserved.)

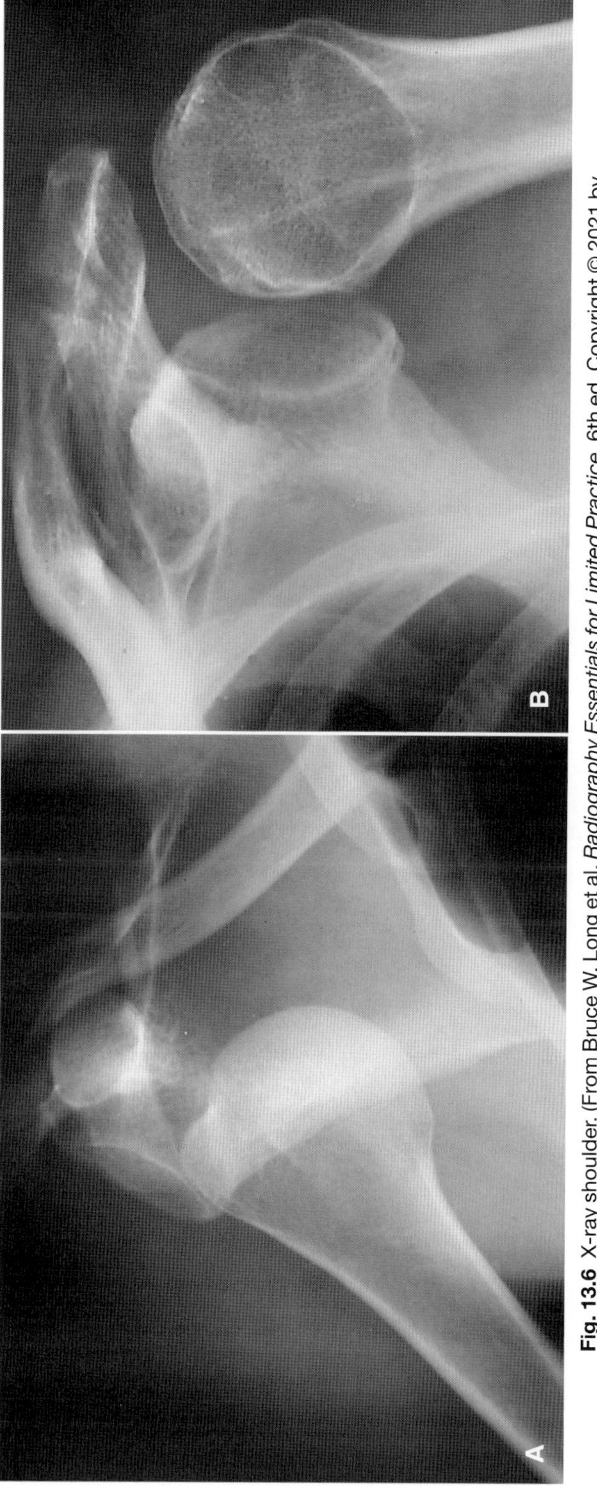

Fig. 13.6 X-ray shoulder. (From Bruce W. Long et al. *Radiography Essentials for Limited Practice*. 6th ed. Copyright © 2021 by Elsevier, Inc. All rights reserved.)

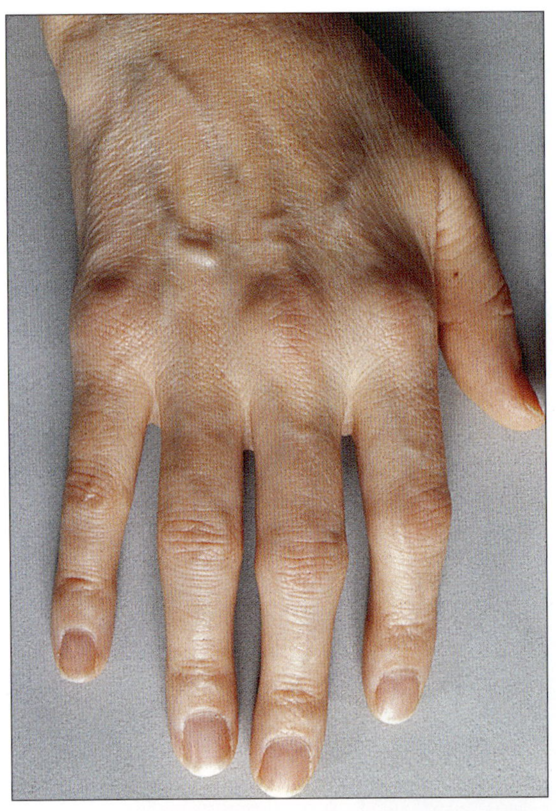

Fig. 13.7 Hand examination. (Reproduced with permission from P. Dieppe, P. A. Bacon, A. N. Bamji, I. Watt. *Slide atlas of clinical rheumatology*. London: Gower Medical; 1982.)

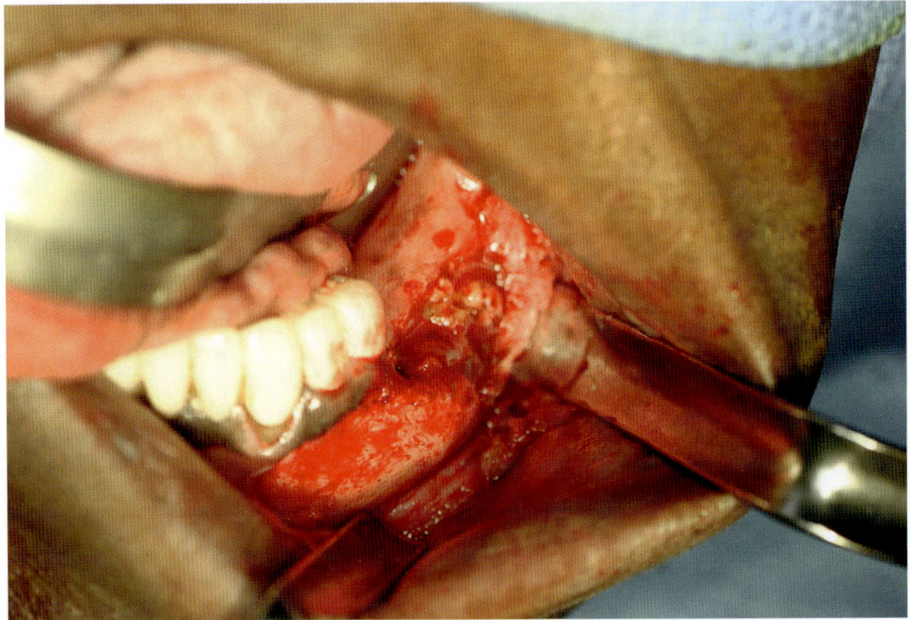

Fig. 13.8 Examination of the oral cavity. (From Constance G. Visovsky et al. *Introduction to Clinical Pharmacology*. 10th ed. Elsevier; 2020.)

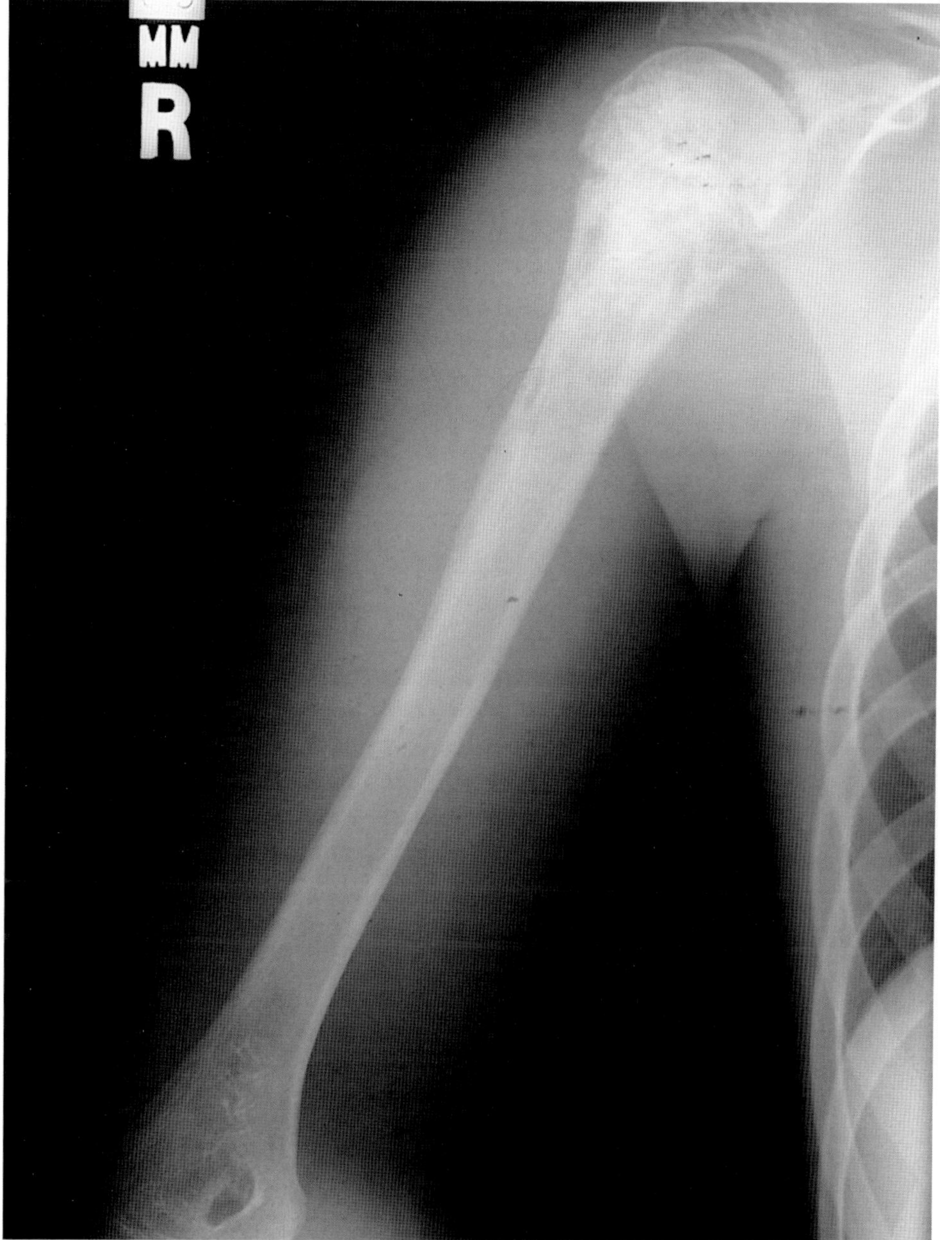

Fig. 13.9 X-ray shoulder. (From Charles M. Washington et al. *Washington and Leaver's Principles and Practice of Radiation Therapy*. 5th ed. Elsevier; 2021.)

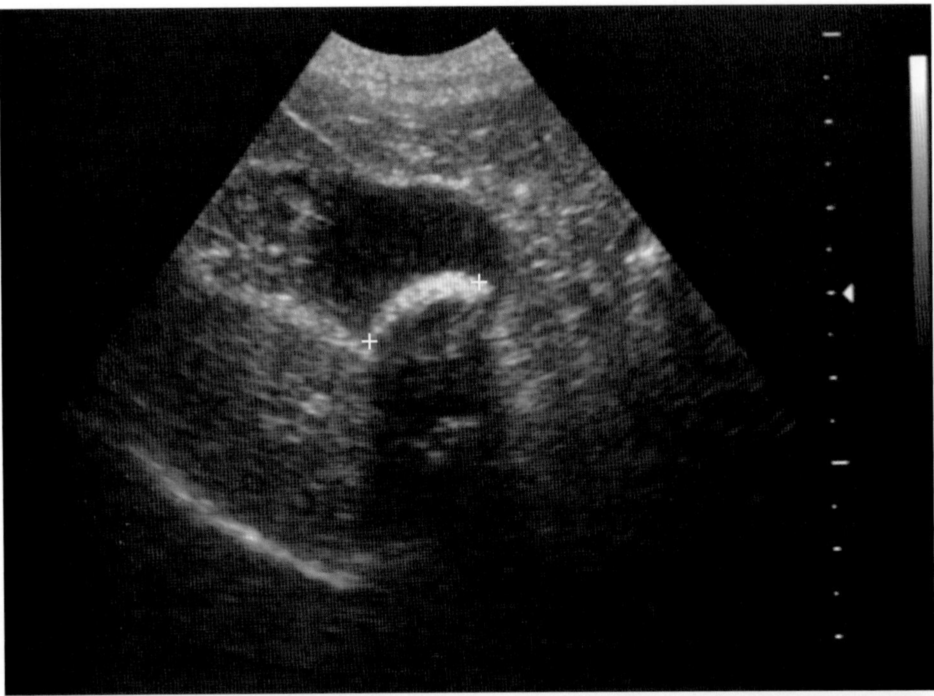

Fig 14.1 Ultrasound of bladder. (From Richard W. Nelson, C. Guillermo Couto. *Small Animal Internal Medicine*. 5th ed. Elsevier; 2014.)

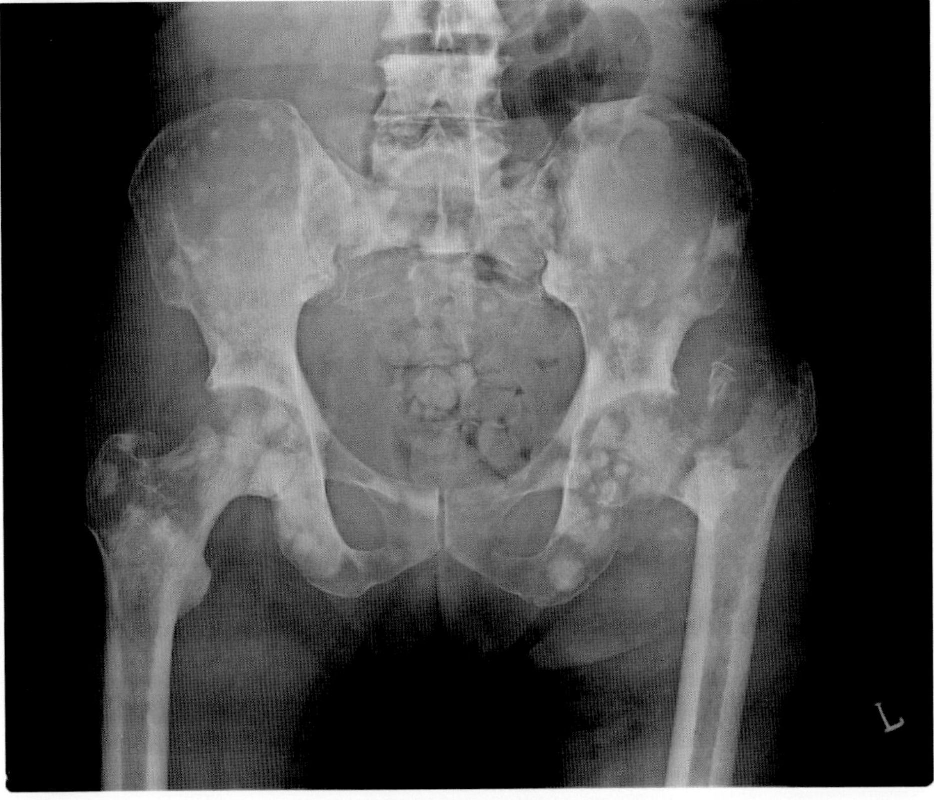

Fig. 14.2 X-ray of pelvis. (From Rajeswari Kathiah. *Textbook of Pathology*. 1st ed. Elsevier; 2022.)

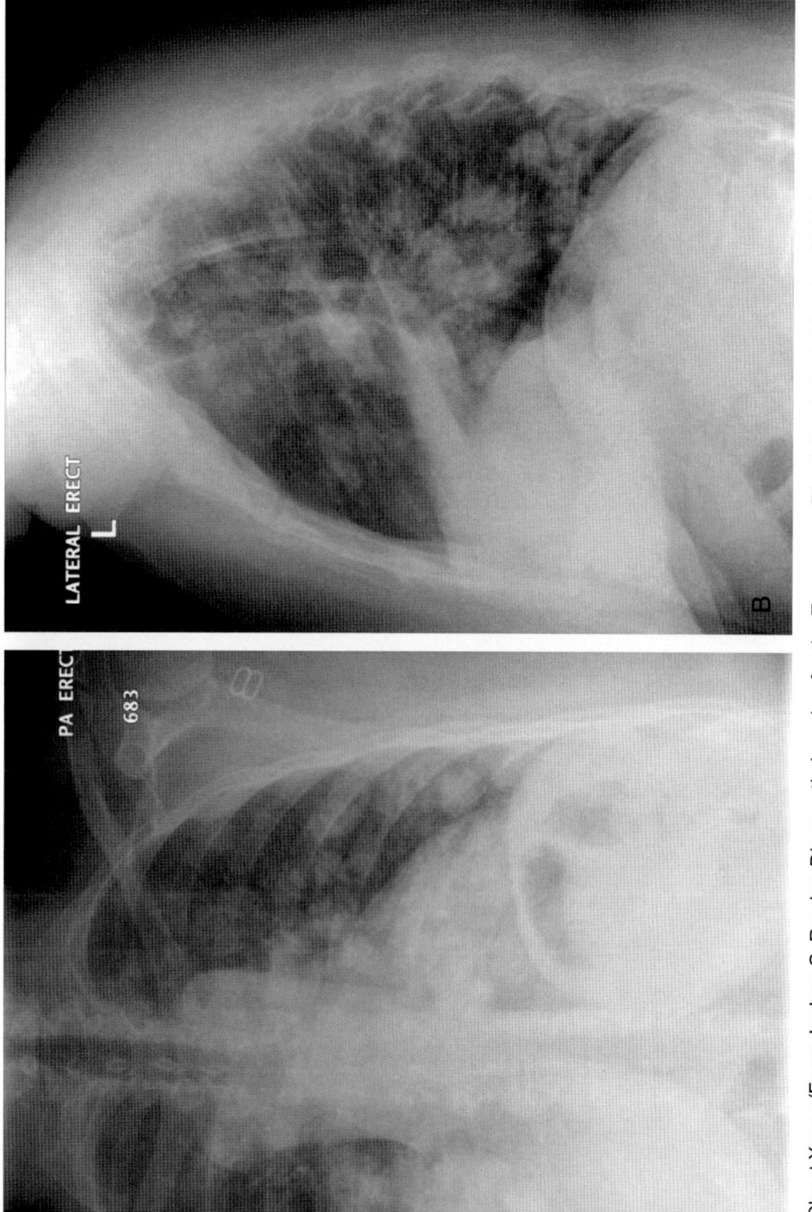

Fig 14.3 Chest X-ray. (From Joshua S. Broder. *Diagnostic Imaging for the Emergency Physician*. 1st ed. Elsevier; 2011.)

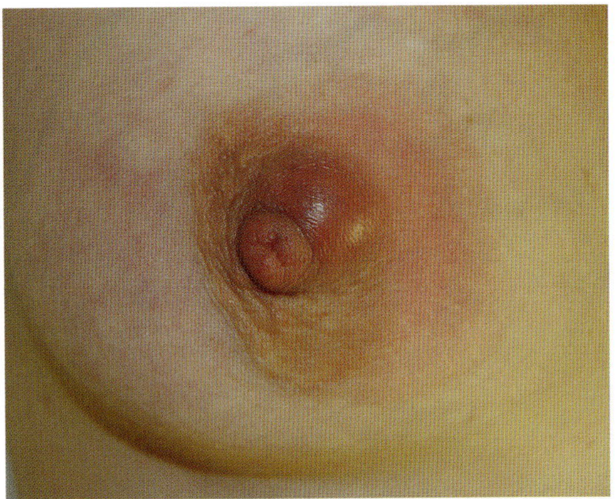

Fig. 15.1 Left breast. (From O. James Garden, Rowan W Parks. *Principles and Practice of Surgery*. 7th ed. © 2018 Elsevier Ltd. All rights reserved.)

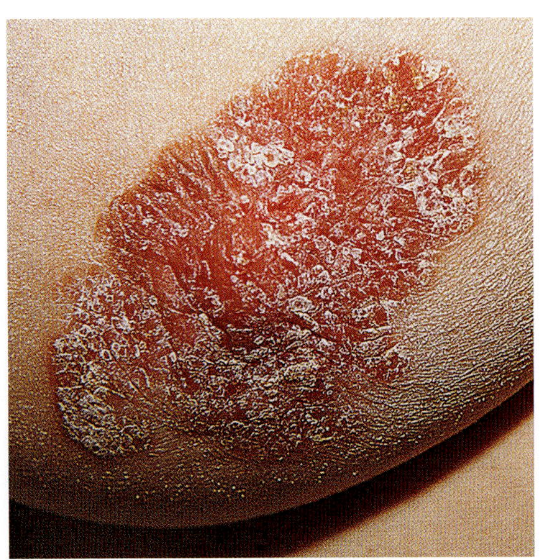

Fig. 15.3 Left breast. (From T. P. Habif. *Skin Disease: Diagnosis and Treatment*, First south Asia edition, 2018.)

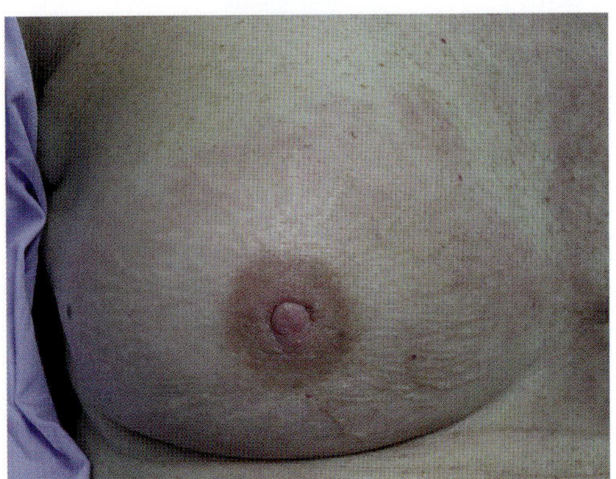

Fig. 15.2 Right breast. (From Anna R Dover et al. *Macleod's Clinical Examination*. 15th ed. Copyright © 2024 Elsevier Ltd. All rights reserved.)

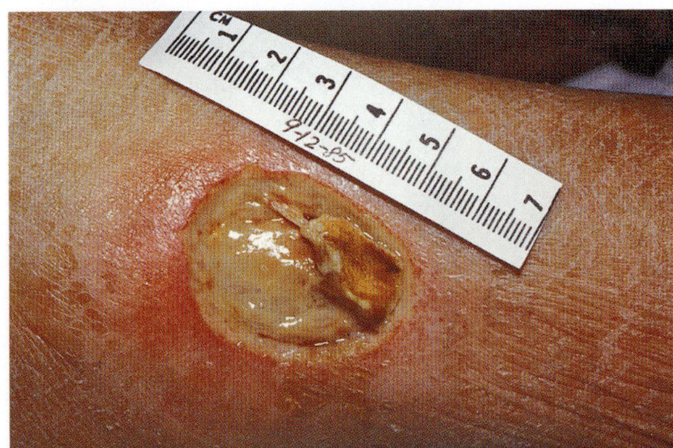

Fig 33.1 Ulcer. (From Ruth Bryant, Denise Nix. *Acute and Chronic Wounds*. 6th ed. Elsevier; 2024.)

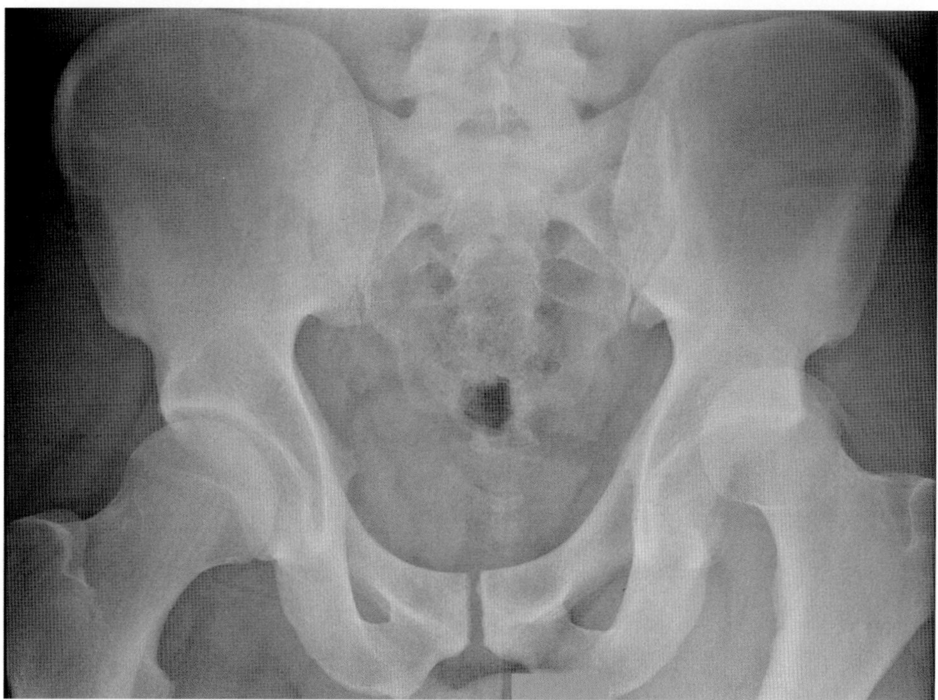

Fig 33.2 Pelvic X-ray. (From Timothy O White. *McRae's Orthopaedic Trauma and Emergency Fracture Management*. 4th ed. Elsevier; 2024.)

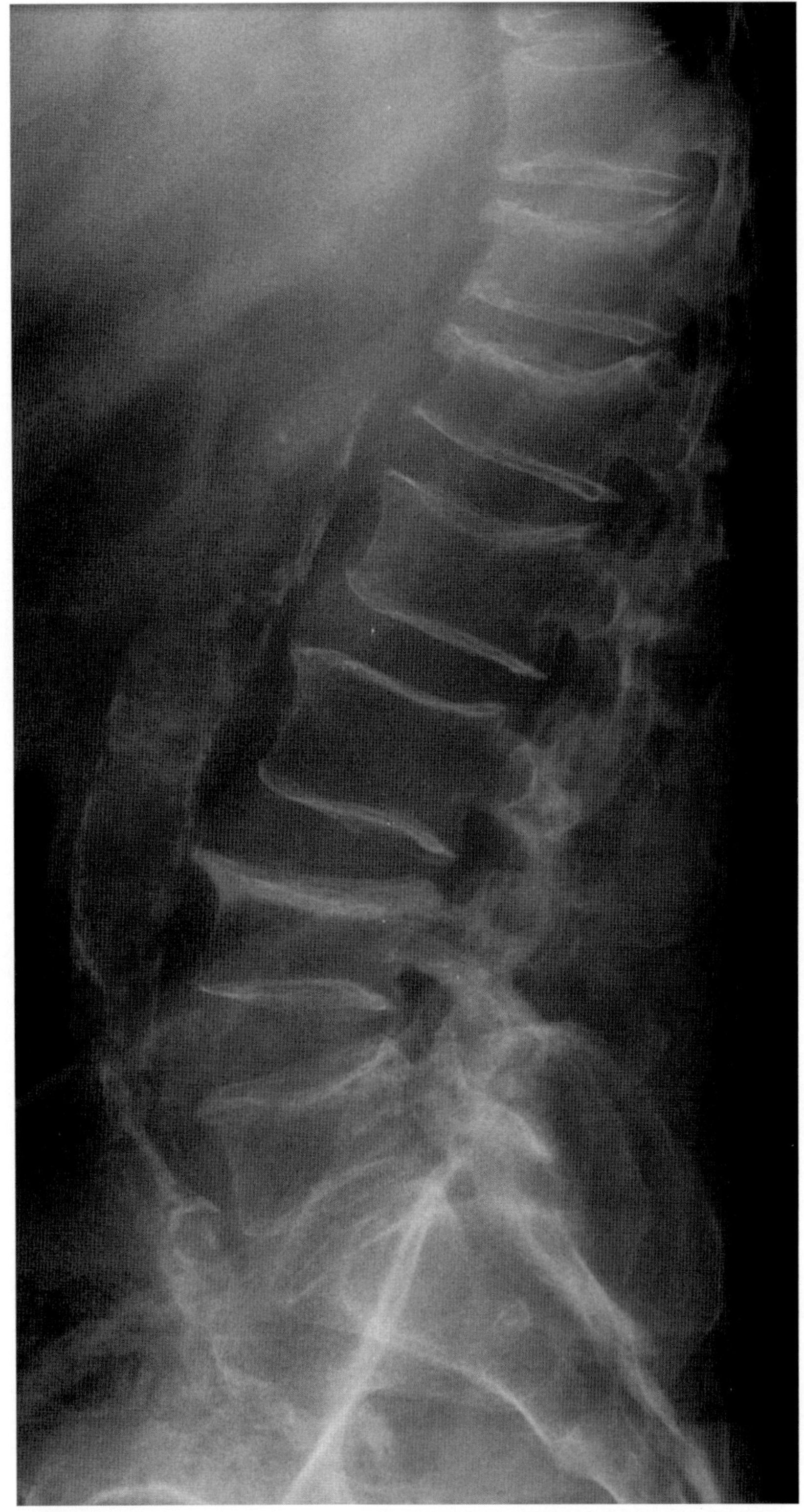

Fig 33.3 Lumbosacral MRI. (From Donald L. Resnick, Jon A. *Jacobson: Resnick's Bone and Joint Imaging*. 4th ed. Elsevier; 2024.)

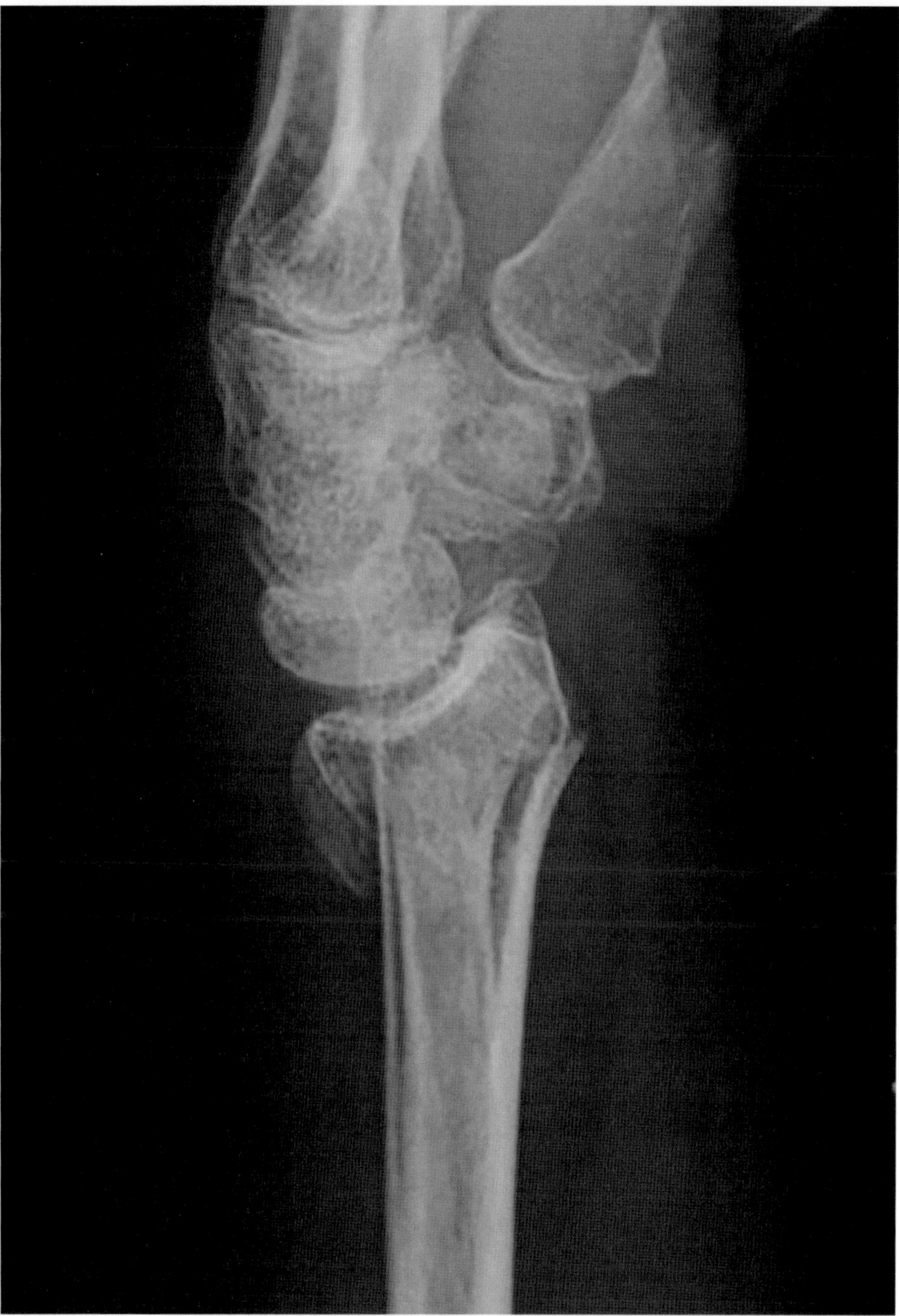

Fig 33.4 Lateral wrist X-ray. (From P. M. Hughes, A. Davies. Appendicular and pelvic trauma. In: Adam A, Dixon AK, Gillard JH, Schaefer-Prokop CM, eds. *Grainger & Allison's Diagnostic Radiology*. 7th ed. Elsevier; 2020:1142–1183.)

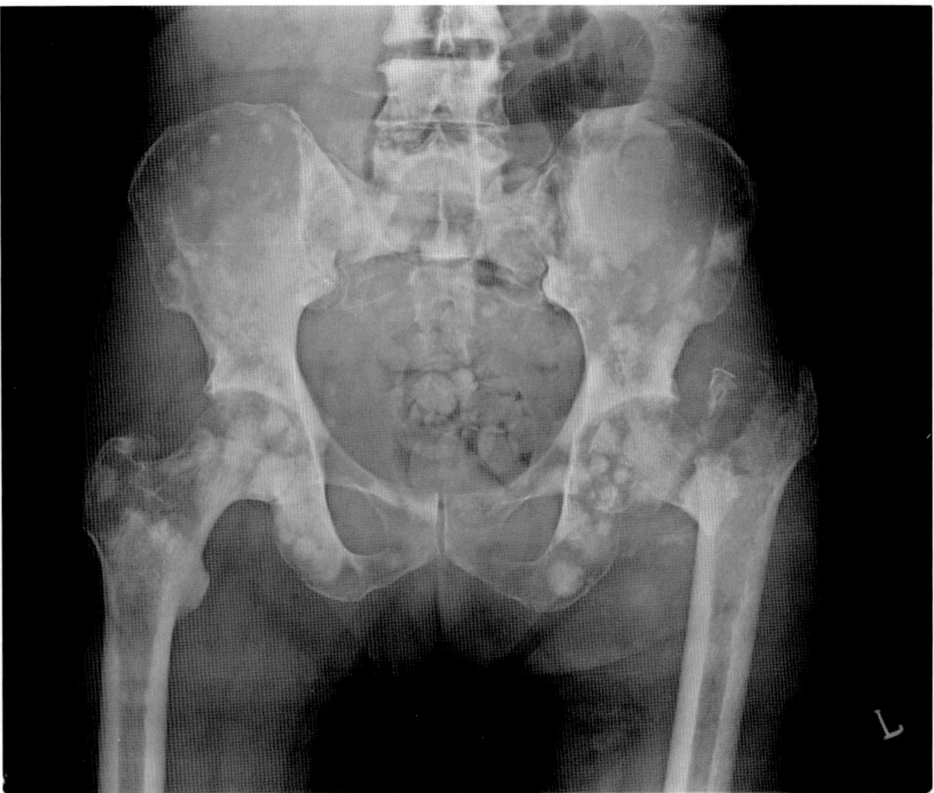

Fig 33.5 Pelvic X-ray. (From Rajeswari Kathiah. *Textbook of Pathology*. 1st ed. Elsevier; 2022.)

Index

Note: Page numbers followed by *f* indicate figures, *t* indicate tables.

A

B

C

D

E

J

K

L

M

N

R

S

T

U

V

W

X

Y

Z